ASSISTED LIVING ADMINISTRATION AND MANAGEMENT

Effective Practices and Model Programs in Elder Care

Darlene Yee-Melichar, EdD, CHES, is Professor and Coordinator of Gerontology at San Francisco State University (SF State). She received her BA in Biology from Barnard College, MS in Gerontology from the College of New Rochelle, and MS and EdD in Health Education from Columbia University. Dr. Yee-Melichar's research interests in healthy aging, long-term care administration, and minority women's health are reflected in 3 books; 90 journal articles, book chapters, book reviews, and technical reports; and numerous community and professional presentations. She is Vice President of the Board of Directors for the California Advocates for Nursing Home Reform; President of SF State's Chapter of Sigma Xi, the national research society; and Past Chair of the DHHS-OWH Minority Women's Health Panel of Experts. Dr. Yee-Melichar is a Fellow of the Gerontological Society of America, Association for Gerontology in Higher Education (AGHE), and AAHPERD's Research Consortium. She received the 1995 Distinguished Educator Award from the California Chapter of the American College of Health Care Administrators; 1998 Distinguished Service Award from the American Association of Homes and Services for the Aging; 2001 Distinguished Alumna Award from Teachers College, Columbia University; 2007 SF State Distinguished Faculty Award for Excellence in Service; and 2007 AGHE Distinguished Teaching Award.

Andrea Renwanz Boyle, DNSc, RN, BC, is a graduate of the University of California, San Francisco, where she received her DNSc in Nursing Science. Dr. Boyle received her MS in Nursing from Boston University and Nurse Practitioner certification from Peter Bent Brigham Hospital. Currently, Dr. Boyle is an Associate Professor and Director of the Family Nurse Practitioner Program at San Francisco State University (SF State). Dr. Boyle is the co-editor of the textbook *Aging in Contemporary Society: Translating Research into Practice,* has published on health-related issues in aging, and conducts research on evidence-based practice for nurses and problem-based learning strategies for undergraduate and graduate students. Additionally, Dr. Boyle has been certified as a Residential Care Facility for the Elderly (RCFE) administrator; and currently serves as a manuscript reviewer for a gerontology nursing journal. Dr. Boyle received the 2009 SF State Distinguished Faculty Award for Excellence in Service.

Cristina Flores, PhD, RN, is the Director of Health Services Research at the Institute on Aging in San Francisco; an Assistant Adjunct Professor in the Department of Social and Behavioral Sciences at the University of California, San Francisco; and a Lecturer in the Gerontology Program at San Francisco State University (SF State). She received her BS in Nursing from the California State University, Dominguez Hills; MA in Gerontology with an academic emphasis in Long-Term Care Administration from SF State, and PhD in Nursing Health Policy from University of California, San Francisco. Dr. Flores is a registered nurse specializing in elder care for 21 years, and an assisted living owner/operator for 14 years. She has completed several studies relative to long-term care for the elderly. Dr. Flores' current research projects include Developing a Consumer Information Website for Residential Care for the Elderly (California Health Care Foundation), A Community Approach to Improve Palliative Care Access (Sutter Health Institute for Research and Education), and Linking Affordable Senior Housing and Services (Institute on Aging). Her published work includes several journal articles and two book chapters on assisted living and quality of care.

ASSISTED LIVING ADMINISTRATION AND MANAGEMENT

Effective Practices and Model Programs in Elder Care

Darlene Yee-Melichar, EdD, CHES
Andrea Renwanz Boyle, DNSc, RN, BC
Cristina Flores, PhD, RN

SPRINGER PUBLISHING COMPANY

NEW YORK

Springer Publishing Company, LLC
11 West 42nd Street
New York, NY 10036
www.springerpub.com

Acquisitions Editor: Sheri W. Sussman
Senior Editor: Rose Mary Piscitelli
Cover design: David Levy
Project Manager: Amor Nanas
Composition: The Manila Typesetting Company
ISBN: 978-0-8261-0466-3
E-book ISBN: 978-0-8261-0467-0

10 11 12 13/ 5 4 3 2 1

The author and the publisher of this Work have made every effort to use sources believed to be reliable to provide information that is accurate and compatible with the standards generally accepted at the time of publication. The author and publisher shall not be liable for any special, consequential, or exemplary damages resulting, in whole or in part, from the readers' use of, or reliance on, the information contained in this book. The publisher has no responsibility for the persistence or accuracy of URLs for external or third-party Internet Web sites referred to in this publication and does not guarantee that any content on such Web sites is, or will remain, accurate or appropriate.

Library of Congress Cataloging-in-Publication Data

Yee-Melichar, Darlene.
  Assisted living administration and management : effective practices and model programs in elder care / Darlene Yee-Melichar, Andrea Renwanz Boyle, Cristina Flores.
    p. ; cm.
  Includes bibliographical references and index.
  ISBN 978-0-8261-0466-3
  1. Congregate housing–Management. I. Boyle, Andrea Renwanz. II. Flores, Cristina, Ph. D. III. Title.
  [DNLM: 1. Assisted Living Facilities–organization & administration. 2. Aged. 3. Homes for the Aged. 4. Nursing Homes. WT 27.1]
  HV1454.Y44 2010
  362.61068–dc22

                                                                                          2010028606

Printed in the United States of America by Hamilton Printing

In dedication to students and practitioners in health and human services who are committed to enhancing the quality of care and quality of life of older adults residing in assisted living facilities and other long-term care communities.

With love and gratitude to our families and friends for their continuing patience and moral support.

Darlene Yee-Melichar, EdD, CHES
Andrea Renwanz Boyle, DNSc, RN, BC
Cristina Flores, PhD, RN

Contents

PART I: ORGANIZATIONAL MANAGEMENT

1. **The Assisted Living Industry:**
   Context, History, and Overview   1

2. **Policy, Licensing, and Regulations**   21

3. **Organizational Overview (With Sarah Dillon, MA)**   53

PART II: HUMAN RESOURCES MANAGEMENT

PART III: BUSINESS AND FINANCIAL MANAGEMENT

CONTRIBUTORS

Clara Allen, MA
Program Director
Golden Gate Healthcare Center
San Francisco, CA

Anthony M. Chicotel, JD, MPP
Staff Attorney
California Advocates for Nursing Home Reform
San Francisco, CA

Sarah Dillon, MA
Administrator
Eden Villa
Castro Valley, CA

Sandi Flores, RN, ADN
President
Sandi Flores Consulting Group, Inc.
Temecula, CA

Joseph F. Melichar, PhD
President
Adaptive Systems Corporation
San Mateo, CA

Raymond Yee, MBA, MPH
Director of Finance and Administration
Healthdata EZ Consulting Corporation
Fair Lawn, NJ

FOREWORD

Supportive housing, whether known as assisted living, residential care, adult foster care, or numerous other labels, has long served a population approximately equal in size to that residing in nursing homes. Advocates and others involved in long-term care now recognize supportive housing (a.k.a. assisted living) as a vital component in the continuum of care. This recognition is partly attributable to assisted living advocates (and more recently public policy) who herald assisted living as an alternative to nursing home care. Such an assertion brings with it enormous responsibility. To be a reality, a facility must do more than serve the shelter and hotel service needs of individuals with moderate physical and/or cognitive limitations. They must provide appropriate assistance for such important daily tasks as getting out of bed, dressing, grooming, toileting, managing medications, or even getting to dining rooms. Meeting these needs requires a sufficient number of trained facility staffing; administrators capable and willing to collaborate with families; health care providers in planning and coordinating care; and business management that ensure adequate pricing and operational efficiency.

Much of the academic literature on assisted living has focused on describing residents and facility features. It has also looked at architecture and design, with the vision that assisted living could be more home-like than nursing homes. This notion is achieved with private rooms, softer lighting, carpeted hallways, attractive common spaces and furniture, and greater resident autonomy. There is less writing on assisted living operations, and what makes one facility successful while another fails. A polemic within the field between a "social" model of care and what was termed an institutional model, or even a medical model of care (said to be represented by nursing homes), has had to be negotiated before the field could move to effective solutions.

Those advocating the social model emphasized the home-like features, privacy, and autonomy, but they failed to notice that residents with limited mobility or confusion, or whose behavior or appearance was objectionable to other residents, were often segregated with assisted living facilities. They also did not effectively account for the diminishing capacity of some residents to take their own medications, dress, or ambulate without substantial assistance and the consequences such changes have for staffing levels, and even resident autonomy. The medical model perspective was often most evident in state regulations and fire and safety codes. These standards define the levels of care that can be served in a particular setting, and who is allowed to provide assistance. Such policies, among other things, affect building materials, internal design, and staffing. They also determine who can remain or has to be relocated.

It is now acknowledged that a continuum of capability exists within a population, and for those who are "aging in place" within a setting. Progression along this continuum necessarily obscures the distinction between the social and medical model. The use of medications illustrates this point. Initially residents may require assistance only in the storage of medications. However, an increase in the number of medications and the times of day these are taken frequently call for the facility to take on the role of supervising the use of medications or even their administration. Transitions like this are to be expected in a population whose members may have multiple chronic health conditions, and who require careful monitoring of medications, diet, and physical activity. These transitions inherently move the care management from social to more medical. Without the authority of facility staff to administer medications, many residents would have to be relocated—often to nursing homes.

Another reality is that assisted living operations have found that it is important for them and their residents that they communicate with the resident's health provider about appointments, changes in status, care plans, and care progression. All of these changes have left an assisted living provider with a choice. Do they broaden their services and abilities to accommodate the wide range of needs (some of which are medical) or do they require residents to relocate because of the problems of medication management, personal care assistance needs, or cognitive and/or behavioral problems? Such decisions are sometimes fundamental to a facility's design and operating philosophy. Sometimes they are individualized for particular residents.

This book is much needed. It offers a practical approach to key issues in the management of an assisted living facility. Among these are human resources issues like staff recruitment and training; business operations, like marketing; and legal and ethical issues. Moreover, the book transgresses the false social vs. medical model dichotomy and recognizes that assisted living must span the continuum of social and health needs. The authors are highly qualified advisors. They have practical experience in the day-to-day operations of facilities, and they bring a combination of background and skills to this subject. It is especially pleasing to see the long-needed collaboration between nursing, social services, and education that is reflected by the training of the authors. This book is an important milestone for the field of aging and assisted living administration.

Robert Newcomer, PhD
Professor of Medical Sociology
Department of Social and Behavioral Sciences
University of California
San Francisco, CA

PREFACE

Gerontology recognizes the country's growing elderly population, and the implications of this demographic trend for the field of long-term care. Long-term care is the fastest growing segment of the health care industry; there is a critical need to educate and train a core of professional personnel with the knowledge and skills to address the complex issues in aging, health, and human services. Long-term care administration is in a period of diversification and expansion. Professional requirements vary widely depending on state and federal regulations for the specific area of administration. Long-term care administrators manage and direct the daily operations of a variety of facilities.

This book was designed to provide a useful reference of content information, effective practices, and model programs in elder care related to the administration of assisted living facilities. It will be based on the core competencies required to operate assisted living facilities. This book contains five parts; each part will focus on a core competency in assisted living administration such as organizational management, human resources management, business and financial management, environmental management, and resident care management. This book will include learning objectives, case studies, effective practices, and model programs in elder care that apply to assisted living facilities.

Part I focuses on Organizational Management, and includes three chapters. Chapter 1 will introduce the reader to the assisted living concept. A historical background, nomenclature, definitions, and an overview description of the industry will be included. The evolution and emergence of assisted living will be discussed. Individual states are responsible for the licensing, monitoring, and oversight of assisted living. Chapter 2 will summarize basic laws and regulations regarding assisted living and will discuss some of the similarities and differences seen across states. A description of various regulatory models will be included. Chapter 3 is intended to provide an overview of the organizational models used in assisted living facilities. States' staffing requirements and staff educational requirements for assisted living facilities will be described.

Part II focuses on Human Resources Management, and includes four chapters. The success of an assisted living facility depends greatly on the hiring of appropriate staff that is based upon the specific needs of the facility. Chapter 4 will describe the recruitment and hiring of suitable staff persons, including the administrator and direct care workers. Factors influencing recruitment, recruitment sources, and hiring process will be included. Chapter 5 will describe the training processes of staff in assisted living. Concepts such as orientation, on-the-job training, and the evaluation of training processes will be included. A summary of the various state requirements regarding staff training will be incorporated. In Chapter 6, strategies for the retention of key and high quality personnel will be discussed. The needs of employees, such as economic security and job satisfaction, will be included. Strategies for empowering staff to participate in the vision of the assisted living facility will be described. Staff development concepts, including continuing education requirements, for personnel will be discussed in Chapter 7. An overview of the various state requirements for ongoing training and continuing education for the administrator and direct care staff will be included. Examples of important continuing education topics will be integrated into the chapter.

Part III focuses on Business and Financial Management, and includes three chapters. Chapter 8 is intended to present an introduction to business, management, and marketing in assisted living facilities with attention to management theories, management method and style, management and organizational structure, the business plan, operational plan and planning system, information and technology support services, and marketing approaches for assisted living facilities. Chapter 9 is intended to present information on accounting systems, organization, financial reporting, account procedures, accounts records, budget preparation, ratio analysis, risk management, and accounting terms used in assisted living facilities. Chapter 10 is intended to present information on tort law and negligence, *respondeat superior,* corporate negligence, governing body, contracts, evictions, wills, trusts, conservatorships, guardianships, advance directives, living wills, and durable power of attorney.

Part IV focuses on Environmental Management, and includes three chapters. Chapter 11 is intended to present effective practices and model programs that address accessibility, fire, and workplace safety as well as disaster preparedness in assisted living facilities. Chapter 12 will present the medical and social models of care in assisted living facilities. Effective practices and model programs (i.e., Eden Alternative) for each of these models will be described and discussed. Chapter 13 will examine the use of architecture and space management within assisted living facilities to improve quality of life for residents. Concepts of building and retrofitting facilities for aging in place will be explored, as will the use of design elements to create healing environments to benefit residents.

Part V focuses on Resident Care Management, and includes four chapters. Issues related to diversity, including cultural and sexual orientation as related to both caregivers and residents in assisted living facilities, will be examined in Chapter 14. Special attention will be given to issues that are connected to both caregiver and resident diversity. The physical aspects of aging of importance to residents in assisted living facilities will be identified and discussed in Chapter 15. Special attention will be paid to issues related to chronic pain assessment, nutritional assessment, and sleep assessment, as well as the assessment and prevention of falls. Many important issues related to the psychological aspects of aging will be examined in Chapter 16. Issues such as the evaluation, diagnosis, and treatment of delirium, depression, and dementia will be presented. Memory loss and memory enhancement training will be discussed. The issues related to alcohol and substance abuse in assisted living facilities will be explored. Chapter 17 will explore the significant challenges related to the rights of residents in assisted living facilities. Areas including ethical, legal, and social rights of residents will be examined and discussed.

Assisted Living Administration and Management: Effective Practices and Model Programs in Elder Care will be a helpful reference for professionals who are associated with the American Association of Homes and Services for the Aging, American College of Healthcare Administrators, American Society of Aging, Association for Gerontology in Higher Education, Gerontological Society of America, and other aging and long-term care administration organizations. It will also be a useful textbook for undergraduate and graduate students in gerontology, health administration, and long-term care administration, as well as for practitioners in counseling, dietetics, health education, kinesiology, nursing, physical therapy, recreation, social work, and other health and human service providers.

Darlene Yee-Melichar, EdD, CHES
Andrea Renwanz Boyle, DNSc, RN, BC
Cristina Flores, PhD, RN

ACKNOWLEDGMENTS

We are grateful to the many people who have contributed meaningfully to the successful completion of this book.

In particular, we thank Sheri Wynne Sussman, Senior Vice President, Editorial, at Springer Publishing Company, who helped to conceive the idea of this book and invited us to develop it. We appreciated very much the encouragement and support that our colleagues at Springer have provided during the past year in finalizing the manuscript.

We especially want to thank all the contributing authors who have shared their respective areas of expertise within this publication. Clara Allen, Tony Chicotel, Sarah Dillon, Sandi Flores, Joseph F. Melichar, and Raymond Yee have provided insightful contributions.

For their assistance with literature and Web site searches and updating references, we are grateful for the helpful work of San Francisco State University graduate assistants Jaclyn Smith and Kimberly Weber.

Our families and friends have been a mainstay of encouragement and support throughout the preparation of this book, and we take this opportunity to express our gratitude to all of them.

One of us is especially grateful to her husband and brother who, as contributing authors, helped to make this book the best it could be; you're the best—many thanks.

Darlene Yee-Melichar, EdD, CHES
Andrea Renwanz Boyle, DNSc, RN, BC
Cristina Flores, PhD, RN

List of Figures

List of Tables

CHAPTER **1**

The Assisted Living Industry: Context, History, and Overview

Learning Objectives

Upon the completion of Chapter 1, the reader will be able to:

- *Describe assisted living in the context of the continuum of long-term care services.*
- *Discuss the historical evolution of assisted living.*
- *Cite a variety of common definitions of assisted living.*
- *Describe the characteristics of assisted living residents, such as resident profiles and sources of payment.*
- *Discuss the challenges faced by the assisted living industry, such as quality of care and safety concerns.*
- *Describe quality improvement strategies of the assisted living industry.*

INTRODUCTION

The purpose of this first chapter is to introduce the reader to the assisted living industry. First, the context of long-term care services, needs, and associated costs is described. Next, the historical evolution of assisted living is included to help the reader understand the background and development of today's assisted living facilities. Because there is no single nationally accepted definition of assisted living, multiple definitions, along with their sources are provided. A description of common resident characteristics is incorporated, including resident profiles, length of stay averages, reasons residents leave assisted living facilities, and common payment sources. This chapter closes with an overview of some of the challenges related to quality of care in assisted living, highlighting the important need for knowledgeable administrators in the industry.

Context

Assisted living is a prominent and significant component of long-term care for older persons in the United States. Concerns regarding nursing home quality, states' interests in containing long-term care costs, as well as consumer demand have produced a dramatic growth in the industry. The number of assisted living beds doubled between 1990 and 2002 (Harrington, Chapman, Miller, Miller, & Newcomer, 2005) and the assisted living industry is often referred to as the fastest growing segment of long-term care. In 2007, states reported 38,373 licensed residential care facilities with 974,585 units/beds, compared to 36,218 facilities with 935,364 units/beds in 2004 (Mollica, Sims-Kastelein, & O'Keeffe, 2007). Compared to 2004, the supply of licensed facilities rose 6% and the number of units rose 4%.

Long-Term Care

Long-term care (LTC) has been defined "as an array of health care, personal care and social services generally provided over a sustained period, 90 days or more, to persons with chronic conditions and with functional limitations" (Wunderlich & Kohler, 2001).

Functional limitations include limitations with activities of daily living (ADLs) and/or instrumental activities of daily living (IADLs). *Activities of daily living (ADLs)* typically refer to basic functions that include bathing, dressing, eating, transferring in and out of bed (mobility), and toileting. *Instrumental activities of daily living (IADLs)* are considered additional activities that are necessary to live independently such as light housework, shopping, managing money, using the telephone, communicating verbally or in writing, preparing meals, and taking medications.

Long-term care is distinct from acute care in duration and emphasis concerning personal and social services. Services may be regular or intermittent and occur over months, years, or a lifetime. Services include personal care, rehabilitation, social services, medical care coordination, transportation, skilled and custodial care, and more. Services are delivered in a variety of settings, from individual homes to institutional environments. *Formal long-term care* refers to a variety of supportive and health care services provided by organizations and persons paid to provide services. *Informal long-term* care remains a more common form of long-term care, where care is provided by family members and friends on an unpaid basis.

Traditionally, much of formal long-term care was provided in institutional settings such as large state hospitals and skilled nursing facilities. Today, the focus of long-term care has shifted to consumer-centered care. *Consumer-centered care* (also referred to as patient-centered care) is care that is aligned with the needs, wants, and preferences of the person requiring care. Developments in legislation, such as the Americans with Disabilities Act (ADA) of 1990, have supported the growth and acceptance of consumer-centered care. The Patient Self-Determination Act of 1990 requires all health care facilities that participate in Medicare or Medicaid to inform adult patients about advanced directives. Furthermore, the U.S. Supreme Court's 1999 landmark *Olmstead* decision concluded that confining persons with disabilities in institutions without adequate medical reasons is a form of discrimination that violates the Americans with Disabilities Act. In the *Olmstead* decision, the Supreme Court held that states cannot make institutionalization a condition for publicly funded health coverage unless it is clinically mandated. Instead, states must direct their health programs to persons with disabilities towards providing community-based care. Therefore, the growth of community-based long-term care, including assisted living facilities, has been rapid.

Need for Long-Term Care

The steady increase of an aging population and an increase in life expectancy present many challenges to the formation of public policy in the United States. The population is aging and the elderly population is growing older and living longer. The fastest growing age group in the country is 85 years and older. As the "baby boom" generation begins to age, the demand for long-term care services is expected to increase. The number of elderly persons needing long-term care is estimated to double, reaching over 14 million people over the next 20 years (U.S. GAO, 1999).

Although people of many ages may need long-term care, older persons are the primary recipients of long-term care services because functional disability increases with advancing age. According to a public policy analysis from American Association of Retired Persons (AARP) in 2005, about 10 million people age 18 or older needed assistance from others to perform everyday activities (see Figure 1.1) and more than 30 million had some type of activity limitation (Houser, 2007). The majority (about 60%) were adults needing help with everyday activities and about 40% with any activity limitation were 65 or older. As the U.S. population

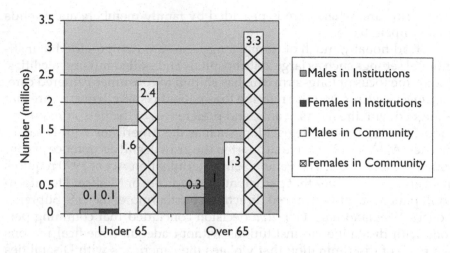

Source: Adapted from Houser, 2007 – Data from AARP Public Policy Institute Analysis

FIGURE 1.1   Adults in United States needing assistance with everyday activities by age, gender, and setting.

ages, the number of people needing long-term care will rise. About 69% of people age 65 today will need long-term care. The average duration of need over a lifetime is usually about 3 years (Kemper, Komisar, & Alecixh, 2005). Women live longer and have higher rates of disability than men, so older women are more likely to need care and on average need care for a longer period of time (Houser, 2007). While most people will need some long-term care, only 20% are expected to need it for 5 years or more.

Long-Term Care Providers

The majority of long-term care continues to be provided by unpaid family and friends often in the home setting. Others require care in long-term care facilities. Although the majority of public funding supports persons residing in skilled nursing facilities (commonly called nursing homes), long-term care is largely and increasingly provided outside of these institutions in community-based group residential settings, such as assisted living. In 2004, about 1,500,000 people received long-term care in certified nursing facilities and nearly 1,000,000 people lived in assisted living facilities (Spillman & Black, 2006). Table 1.1 illustrates many of the long-term care options available today.

TABLE 1.1	Long-Term Care Options
Home Care	Home care can include medical care (nursing, social work, rehabilitation therapies) and also help around the home. Skilled professionals come directly to the home to provide care. Home health aides or personal care service workers can visit daily or as needed to help with activities of daily living, such as bathing and grooming. They can also assist with housekeeping, meals, and shopping.
Adult Day Care (ADC) *Adult Day Health Care (ADHC)*	Adult care programs are a type of long-term care that offers social interaction and meals from one to five days a week, depending on the program. Some adult care programs provide transportation to and from the care center. Activities often include exercises, games, trips, art, and music. Some adult care programs include medical services, such as help taking medications or checking blood pressure.
Senior Housing	This type of housing is often rental apartments that have been adapted for seniors, including railings installed in the bathrooms and power outlets placed higher on the walls. Other services offered by senior housing communities include meals, transportation, housekeeping, and activities.
Assisted Living/Community Based Residential Care	Assisted living facilities offer room and board with provisions for assistance with activities of daily living (ADLs) such as bathing, dressing, eating, grooming, continence, and eating. In addition, assistance with transportation, housekeeping, laundry, obtaining medical and social services, and the supervision of medications and other medical needs is often offered.
Skilled Nursing Facility (SNF) *Nursing Home*	Skilled nursing facilities or nursing homes offer 24-hour nursing care. These services are for those who need more medical care than other long-term care options can offer, such as wound care, rehabilitative therapy, and help with respirators or ventilators.
Continuing Care Retirement Community (CCRC)	Continuing Care Retirement Communities offer several levels of care in one setting. They can enable persons to remain in one place for the rest of their life rather than moving each time a new level of care is needed. Typically, there are senior housing apartments, assisted living units, and skilled nursing facilities in a CCRC. A fee or endowment is often required to enter a CCRC.

TABLE 1.2	Long-Term Care Payment Sources
Medicare	A federal health insurance program for people 65 and older and younger people with disabilities. Medicare will pay part of the cost for skilled nursing and rehabilitative services in a skilled nursing home (up to 100 days) following a recent related stay in a hospital. Medicare will pay for some home health care such as skilled nursing services or therapy through a Medicare-certified home health agency if ordered by a physician. In addition, Medicare will also pay for medical and support services from a Medicare-approved hospice agency for the terminally ill. Many seniors believe that the federal Medicare program will pay for long-term care costs, such as costs for a nursing home or assisted living, but this is not true.
Medicaid	A federal and state funded program run by states that helps certain low-income individuals and families pay for some or all of their medical bills. People must meet eligibility criteria set by federal and state law. Medicaid may help pay for nursing home care and sometimes services at home. People whose income is higher, but who have high medical or long-term care bills, can also become eligible for Medicaid. Certain income and assets rules apply. Some states have home and community based waiver programs where Medicaid can help pay some costs associated with assisted living – their programs are limited and differ by state policy.
Veterans Affairs (VA)	Provides long-term care for service-related disabilities or for certain eligible veterans. Veterans who do not have service-related disabilities, but who are unable to afford to pay for long-term care are also eligible for assistance.
Long-term Care Insurance	Some, but few persons, purchase private long-term care insurance. It is specifically designed to cover the costs of long-term care services. Depending on the policy, long-term care insurance may pay for care in nursing homes, assisted living facilities, and/or at home. The cost of long-term care insurance depends on what type of coverage you buy and at what age you buy it. Coverage is variable and often quite expensive to purchase.
Personal Saving and Investments	Personal savings and investments is how most people who are not on Medicaid pay for long-term care services.

The Cost of Long-Term Care

Long-term care is very expensive. For example, a survey from the MetLife Mature Market Institute (2006) reported that (1) the average cost in the United States for a nursing home was about $67,000 for a shared room and $75,000 for a private room; (2) the average cost for a home health aide was $19.00 per hour; and (3) assisted living room rates averaged $35,600 per year. These costs are extremely variable throughout the country and vary considerably relative to the region, accommodations, amenities, services, and staffing availability.

There are a variety of payment sources for long-term care. Medicare generally doesn't pay for long-term care. Medicare also doesn't pay for help with activities of daily living or other care that most people can do themselves. Some examples of activities of daily living include eating, bathing, dressing, and using the bathroom. Medicare will help pay for skilled nursing or home health care when certain criteria are met (e.g., rehabilitation services after an acute event). If income and resources are limited, persons may qualify for Medicaid benefits. Private long-term care insurance, personal savings, and assets are other options people utilize to finance long-term care. Table 1.2 summarizes some of the public and private funding sources frequently utilized for the payment of long-term care services.

HISTORICAL EVOLUTION OF ASSISTED LIVING

Assisted living is not a new phenomenon in long-term care. Historically, some form of residential and community-based care arrangements or supportive housing has long been available. Residential settings for older people with health problems, ranging from ordinary boarding homes to philanthropically funded organizations often called *homes for the aged*, typically predate the 1965 enactment of Medicare and Medicaid (Cohen, 1974). After 1965, some homes for the aged converted into nursing facilities with encouragement from state governments. These facilities received matching federal money to help state and local governments finance long-term care services. Some residential care facilities did not convert into nursing facilities, either because they did not want to become medical facilities or because they could not meet the regulatory standards. These types of facilities are known by more than 30 different names across the country, including residential care, community care, personal care, domiciliary care, supervisory care, sheltered care, adult foster care, board and care, and family, group and boarding homes (Newcomer & Grant, 1990). Even as the demand for nursing facility beds grew, the residential care industry continued to develop and expand.

An overlapping type of residential care, termed assisted living, has become increasingly popular in the last decade (American Seniors Housing Association, 1998; Assisted Living Federation of America, 2000; Assisted Living Workgroup, 2003). Twenty-nine states and the District of Columbia report provisions regarding assisted living concepts (e.g., privacy, autonomy, and decision making) in their regulations, while many other states continue to utilize a variety of traditional names (Mollica et al., 2007).

It is difficult to identify the exact beginnings of assisted living. Recently, Keren Brown Wilson (2007) explored the historical evolution of assisted living. She wrote,

> To my knowledge, the first written use of the term (and my first such use of it) was in a 1985 proposal to the State of Oregon to fund a pilot study whereby the services for 20 nursing-home-level Medicaid recipients would be covered in a new residential setting. By 1988, assisted living was being used in presentations at professional meetings and in early trade publication articles. By 1991, when Hawes, Wildfire, & Lux (1991) published a national study of board and care homes, many residential care facilities that offered or arranged care were calling themselves assisted living, and the study included assisted living as an explicit subset of residential care.

In this book, the term assisted living is used to describe all types of group residential care settings for the elderly, because many states use the term assisted living generically to cover every type of group residential care on the continuum between home care and nursing homes (Mollica et al., 2007). We also acknowledge that for some stakeholders the term assisted living represents a unique model of residential care that differs significantly from traditional types of residential care. We include a discussion of the distinct assisted living philosophy that is included in some states' regulations in Chapter 2.

DEFINING ASSISTED LIVING

The setting for the delivery and receipt of long-term care is often discussed as a continuum, with one's own home at one end and the nursing home on the other. These end points also are used to symbolize the continuum from personal independence to institutionalization. Assisted living is typically considered as somewhere in between these extreme ends where personalized care and supervision can be provided outside of an institutionalized environment, with an emphasis of optimizing physical and psychological independence.

In general, assisted living facilities offer room and board with provisions for assistance with activities of daily living (ADLs) such as bathing, dressing, eating, grooming, continence, and eating. In addition, assistance with transportation, housekeeping, laundry, obtaining medical and social services, the supervision of medications, as well as other medical needs is often offered.

It is noted that the exact definition of assisted living remains a question, and that the ambiguity surrounding the various definitions and regulatory models used throughout the country make for great confusion for providers, consumers, and researchers. Some see this as a unique mix of services and privacy, while others view it as a new term for the type of care and assistance that has been available historically.

There has never been a single nationally accepted definition of an assisted living facility. Instead, states that have the responsibility for regulating the supportive housing industry have each developed their own definitions and guidelines. While there is much in common among the states, there are also differences in the terms used to label various housing types and levels of care, and variation in the standards and restrictions for which these operations are held accountable. Provider and trade associations, formal associations, and governmental agencies, as well as academic researchers have developed a vast variety of definitions designed to capture both the definition and essence of assisted living facilities and suit their own needs and purposes. In 1992, Lewin-VHI, Inc. (1996) conducted a literature review and policy synthesis for the Office of the Assistant Secretary for Planning and Evaluation, Administration on Aging, and the U.S. Department of Health and Human Services. They determined that overall, assisted living was used to refer to housing for the elderly with supportive services in a homelike environment; the term was used interchangeably throughout the states with other common labels, such as residential care and board and care. However, it was also determined that proponents of assisted living often assert that assisted living offers a special philosophy that includes maximizing functional capability and autonomy, and utilizing the environment as an aid for independence and socialization that makes assisted living distinguishable from other types of supportive housing for the elderly (Lewin-VHI, Inc., 1996). Over time, additional definitions have been suggested. Table 1.3 illustrates some selected definitions for assisted living and residential care.

TABLE 1.3 Selected Definitions of Assisted Living	
Association or Researcher	**Definition**
American Association of Homes and Services for the Aging (AAHSA)	"Assisted living is a program that provides and/or arranges for the provision of daily meals, personal and other supportive services, health care, and 24-hour oversight to persons residing in a group residential facility who need assistance with activities of daily living and instrumental activities of daily living. It is characterized by a philosophy of service provision that is consumer driven, flexible, individualized care and maximizes consumer independence, choice, privacy, and dignity."
Assisted Living Facilities Association of America (ALFAA)	"Assisted living is a special combination of housing supportive services, personalized assistance, and health care designed to respond to the individual needs of those who need help in activities of daily living. Supportive services are available 24 hours a day, to meet scheduled and unscheduled needs, in a way that promotes maximum independence and dignity for each resident and encourages the involvement of a resident's family, neighbors, and friends."
Assisted Living Quality Coalition (1998): Alzheimer's Association, the American Association of Retired Persons (AARP), the American Association for Homes and Services for the Aging (AAHSA), the American Health Care Association, the American Senior Housing Association, and the Assisted Living Federation of America (ALFA)	Their definition combined previous definitional characteristics into a concept including five categories: 1. A congregate residential setting that provides or coordinates personal services, 24-hour supervision and assistance, activities and health-related services; 2. Designed to minimize the need to move; 3. Designed to accommodate individual resident's changing needs and preferences; 4. Designed to maximize the residents' dignity, autonomy, privacy, independence, and safety; and 5. Designed to encourage family and community involvement.
Assisted Living Workgroup (ALW)	"Assisted living is a state regulated and monitored residential long-term care option. Assisted living provides or coordinates oversight and services to meet the residents' individualized scheduled needs, based on the residents' assessments and service plans and their unscheduled needs as they arise. Services that are required by state law and regulation to be provided or coordinated must include but are not limited to:

(Continued)

TABLE 1.3	Selected Definitions of Assisted Living (*Continued*)
Association or Researcher	**Definition**
	1. 24-hour awake staff to provide oversight and meet scheduled and unscheduled needs
	2. Provision and oversight of personal and supportive services (assistance with activities of daily living and instrumental activities of daily living)
	3. Health-related services (e.g. medication management services)
	4. Social services
	5. Recreational activities
	6. Meals
	7. Housekeeping and laundry
	8. Transportation
	"A resident has the right to make choices and receive services in a way that will promote the resident's dignity, autonomy, independence, and quality of life. These services are disclosed and agreed to in the contract between the provider and resident. Assisted living does not generally provide ongoing, 24-hour skilled nursing."
American Seniors Housing Association (ASHA)	"A coordinated array of personal care, health services, and other supportive services available 24 hours a day to residents who have been assessed to need those services. Assisted living promotes resident self direction and participation in decisions that emphasize independence, individuality, privacy, and dignity in residential surroundings."
Kane and Wilson (1993)	"Assisted living is any group residential program that is not licensed as a nursing home that provides personal care to persons with need for assistance in the activities of daily living and that can respond to unscheduled need for assistance that might arise."
National Association of Residential Care Facilities	"Residential care facility means a home or facility of any size, operated for profit, which undertakes through its owners or management to provide food, housing, and support with activities of daily living and/or protective care for two or more adult residents not related to the owner or administrator. Residential care homes are also known as assisted living facilities, foster homes, board and care homes, sheltered care homes, etc."

(Continued)

TABLE 1.3	Selected Definitions of Assisted Living (*Continued*)
Association or Researcher	**Definition**
National Center for Assisted Living	"Assisted living provides relatively independent seniors with assistance and limited health care services in a home-like atmosphere. Assisted living services include 24-hour protective oversight, food, shelter, and a range of services that promote the quality of life of the individual. The philosophy of assisted living emphasizes the right of the individual to choose the setting for care and services. Assisted living customers share the risks and responsibilities for their daily activities and well-being with a staff geared to helping them enjoy the freedom and independence of private living. Assisted living is licensed by state governments and is known by many different names including the following: residential care, board and care, congregate care, and personal care. Assisted living care is not a substitute for but rather a complement to nursing facility care."
Regnier, Victor	"Assisted living is a long-term care alternative which involves the delivery of professionally managed personal and health care services in a group setting that is residential in character and appearance in ways that optimize the physical and psychological independence of residents."
U.S. Health Care Financing Administration (HCFA)	"Assisted living is one of two categories of Adult Residential Care. Personal care and services, homemaker, chore, attendant care, companion services, medication oversight (to the extent permitted under State Law), therapeutic social and recreational programming, provided in a licensed community care facility, in conjunction with residing in the facility; this service includes 24-hour on site response staff to meet scheduled or unpredictable needs and to provide supervision of safety and security; other individuals or agencies may also furnish care directly or under arrangement with the community care facility, but care provided by these other entities supplements that provided by the community care facility and does not supplant it. Assisted living is distinguished by clients residing in their own living units and routine of care provision and service delivery must be client driven to the maximum extent possible."

(Continued)

TABLE 1.3 Selected Definitions of Assisted Living (*Continued*)	
Association or Researcher	**Definition**
U.S. Department of Housing and Urban Development (HUD)	Assisted living is described as a public facility, proprietary facility, or facility of a private non-profit corporation that is used for the care of the frail elderly and that: 1. Is licensed and regulated by the state and if there is no state law providing for such licensing and regulation by the state, by the municipality or other political subdivision in which the facility is located; 2. Makes available to residents supportive services to assist the residents in carrying out activities of daily living; and 3. Provides separate dwelling units for residents.
Wilson (1990)	Offered a paradigm to describe what she called assisted living (AL) where 1. AL is a setting where a person can create his/her own place; 2. AL is responsive to the needs of individuals at different levels of physical and mental abilities; 3. AL encourages sharing the responsibility with residents and their family members; 4. AL provides autonomy and independence to residents.

Sources: Assisted Living Quality Initiative, 1998; Assisted Living Workgroup, 2003; Lewin-VHI, Inc., 1996; National Center for Assisted Living, 2001; Wilson, 1990.

These selected definitions illustrate that the definitions and concepts of assisted living are not uniform. Depending on the perspective, different dimensions and descriptions are included or excluded. Commonly, stressing the importance of privacy, dignity, and autonomy are seen in these definitions. Privacy is often addressed, and in some cases private rooms and baths are required by definitions of assisted living. Lists of services that must be available are also included, with some distinct statements regarding response to residents' needs around the clock. While some assisted living facilities may offer high quality care in settings that afford maximum privacy and dignity, others lack adequately trained staff and sufficient amounts of care and supervision. This gap is most obvious when philosophy aims to combine privacy, such as locking doors and individual kitchens, with high service levels regardless of changes in health, physical, or cognitive functioning.

RESIDENT CHARACTERISTICS

In order to address quality and safety in assisted living facilities, it is important to know the population of residents residing in and being served within these settings. The research in this area (although limited by methodology) has begun to suggest that residents residing in these facilities are becoming increasingly dependent and frail, which makes issues of quality and safety more critical. Many residents are entering assisted living facilities from the community; one third is admitted from other assisted living facilities, skilled nursing facilities, nursing homes, and hospitals (Morgan, Gruber-Baldini, & Magaziner, 2001). Mollica and colleagues (2007) report that 42 states reimburse for Medicaid eligible residents under Home and Community based waivers and state plans, and as such, these residents require a skilled nursing facility or nursing home level of care. The criteria between states vary, but general skilled nursing facilities or nursing home eligibility is based upon needing assistance with at least three activities of daily living or two with cognitive impairment.

General Resident Profile

The average assisted living resident is often described to be a White female in her mid-80s and widowed (Kane & Wilson, 1993; Morgan et al., 2001; National Center for Assisted Living, 2001). The literature often reports assisted living residents as having similar characteristics to those residing in skilled nursing facilities/nursing homes. McAllister and colleagues (2000) compared assisted living residents and skilled nursing facility/nursing home residents within the same facility, and found that the residents did not differ with respect to age, gender, weight, height, or the number of diagnoses. Multiple studies (Armstrong et al., 2001; McAllister et al., 2000; Rhoads & Thai, 2002; Spore et al., 1995; Williams et al., 1999) described the profiles of residents in assisted living facilities as similar to those of a skilled nursing facility/nursing home resident with the majorities being elderly, White, and widowed females with multiple chronic medical diagnoses and multiple prescribed medications. Catherine Hawes and colleagues (1995) reported that in the 10 years between 1983 and 1993 residents residing in assisted living became increasingly (1) aged (64% in 1993 and 38% in 1983 were 75 and older); (2) cognitively impaired (40% versus 30%); (3) incontinent (23% versus 7%); (4) wheelchair dependent (15% versus 3%); (5) requiring assistance with bathing (45% versus 27%); and (6) taking medications (75% versus 43%). These percentages are most

TABLE 1.4	Assisted Living Residents' Needs for Assistance
Assistance with medications	86%
Assistance with bathing	72%
Assistance with dressing	57%
Assistance with bathroom needs	41%
Assistance with transferring	36%
Assistance with eating	23%

Source: National Center for Assisted Living, 2001.

likely underestimated and have increased even further over the past decade. Further research comparing residents from assisted living to skilled nursing facility/nursing homes has demonstrated that assisted living residents overlap considerably with those receiving long-term care in nursing homes in terms of age, cognitive status, chronic medical illnesses, disability, and care needs (Zimmerman et al., 2003). The National Center for Assisted Living (2001) reported the average needs of today's assisted living residents. These needs are summarized in Table 1.4.

Length of Stay and Reasons for Leaving

The estimate of the average length of stay in an assisted living facility is two and a half to three years (National Center for Assisted Living, 2001). Typical reasons for leaving result from the need for skilled nursing care and death. In 2000, Phillips and colleagues completed a study to understand the reasons for leaving an assisted living facility. Residents sometimes provided more than one reason for leaving an assisted living facility. These results are summarized in Table 1.5.

TABLE 1.5	Assisted Living Residents' Reasons for Leaving
Need for more care	78%
Locations closer to loved ones	14%
Dissatisfied with care	12%
Dissatisfied with price	11%
Other dissatisfaction	11%
Ran out of money	9%
Other or unknown reason	9%

Source: Phillips et al., 2000.

Sources of Payment in Assisted Living

Although Medicaid coverage for assisted living services has increased gradually, assisted living remains a primarily private-pay segment of long-term care. Therefore, the majority of assisted living residents pay with their own funds. Others receive some support from family members and some have private long-term care insurance (AARP, 2004). The lack of public subsidies and often high costs of assisted living often make it unaffordable for persons with low to moderate incomes.

CHALLENGES IN THE ASSISTED LIVING FIELD

The concept of assisted living, as illustrated by the varying definitions, is far less uniform than most realize. In addition, today's assisted living facilities are caring for more physically frail and cognitively impaired residents than ever before. For example, it is not uncommon for assisted living facilities to care for residents with advanced dementia or hospice care needs.

Quality of Care and Safety Concerns

As the interest in assisted living has increased, so have concerns about the quality of care and safety that can be provided to these residents that require special care, staffing, and physical and social environments. In contrast to nursing homes, no federal quality standards exist for assisted living. Additionally, states vary significantly in their licensing requirements, quality standards, monitoring, and enforcement activities (see Chapter 2).

Research and media reports throughout the country and a 1999 report on quality of care and consumer protection issues from the United General Accounting Office (U.S. GAO, 1999) have raised concerns about the quality of care in residential care settings. Older persons receiving necessary care and services in a homelike and residential setting dedicated to preserving dignity and autonomy are attractive and appealing. The determination of what makes it "good" remains an important question.

The U.S. GAO (1999) indicated that assisted living facilities do not always give prospective consumers adequate information as to whether, for how long, and under what circumstances a facility could meet their needs (U.S. GAO, 1999). They further reported that information provided to consumers was often vague, incomplete, or misleading, and that 27% of the facilities reviewed had been cited for five or more quality of care or consumer protection deficiencies during the 1996–1997 time period (U.S. GAO, 1999). The U.S. GAO (1999) report listed four problems commonly associated with assisted living facilities:

1. Providing poor care to residents, such as inadequate medical attention following an accident;
2. Having insufficient, unqualified, and untrained staff, exacerbated by high staff turnover and low pay for direct care staff;
3. Not providing residents with appropriate medications and not storing medications properly; and
4. Not following admission and discharge policies required by state regulations.

Quality Improvement Efforts

One effort to address quality problems was the establishment of the Assisted Living Workgroup (ALW) Formed at the request of the U.S. Senate Special Committee on Aging. The ALW was a national effort of approximately 50 organizations representing consumers, providers, long-term care and health care professionals, and regulators. In 2003, the ALW issued a report with recommendations for improving quality in assisted living. Included in their recommendations were the following components (http://www.theceal.org/ALW-report.php):

1. Introduction
2. Definitions and core principals
3. Accountability and oversight
4. Affordability
5. Direct care services
6. Medication management
7. Operations
8. Resident rights
9. Staffing

To continue and expand the work of the ALW, 11 organizations that participated in the ALW have formed an organizing committee to develop a "Center for Excellence in Assisted Living" (CEAL, 2008). The Center for Excellence in Assisted Living will continue to foster high quality, affordable assisted living by disseminating research and information, and providing technical assistance. The Center for Excellence in Assisted Living's board of directors is composed of representatives from the following national organizations (www.theceal.org):

1. Alzheimer's Association
2. American Assisted Living Nurses Association
3. American Association of Homes and Services for the Aging
4. AARP
5. American Seniors Housing Association
6. Assisted Living Federation of America
7. Consumer Consortium of Assisted Living
8. National Center for Assisted Living
9. NCB Capital Impact
10. Paralyzed Veterans of America
11. Pioneer Network

CONCLUSIONS

This chapter has provided the reader with the context, history, and overview of assisted living facilities. Although assisted living has promised to be a consumer-centered alternative to institutionalized setting for long-term care, quality of care concerns have become increasingly apparent. This chapter illustrates the need for today's assisted living administrators to be well informed and well prepared in the effort to provide high quality long-term services to elderly persons in a challenging and evolving environment.

REFERENCES

American Seniors Housing Association. (1998). *Seniors housing report, 1998.* Washington, DC: American Seniors Housing Association.

Armstrong, E., Rhoads, M., & Meiling, F. (2001). Medication usage patterns in assisted living facilities. *The Consultant Pharmacist, 16,* 65–69.

Assisted Living Federation of America. (2000). *2000 Overview of the assisted living industry.* Washington, DC: Assisted Living Federation of America.

Assisted Living Quality Initiative. (1998). *Building a structure that promotes quality.* Fairfax, VA: Assisted Living Quality Initiative.

Assisted Living Workgroup. (2003). *Assuring quality in assisted living: Guidelines for federal and state policy, state regulations, and operations.* Washington, DC: U.S. Government Printing Office.

Cohen, E. (1974). An overview of long-term care facilities. In E. M. Brody (Ed.), *Social work guide for long-term care facilities* (pp. 11–26). Washington, DC: U.S. Government Printing Office.

Harrington, C., Chapman, S., Miller, E., Miller, N., & Newcomer, R. (2005). Trends in the supply of long-term care facilities and beds in the United States. *The Journal of Applied Gerontology, 20,* 1–19.

Hawes, C., Mor, V., Wildfire, J., Iannacchione, V., Lux, L., Green, R., Greene A., Wilcox, V., Spore, D., & Phillips, C. (1995). *Executive Summary: Analysis of the effect of regulation on the quality of care in board and care homes.* Washington, DC: U.S. Department of Health and Human Services.

Hawes, C., Wildfire, J., & Lux, L. J. (1991). *The regulation of board and care homes: Results of a 50-state survey.* Research Triangle Park, NC: RTI International.

Houser, A. (2007). *Long-term care trends 2007.* AARP Public Policy Institute. Retrieved June 20, 2008, from http://www.aarp.org/research/longtermcare/trends/fs27r_ltc.html

Kane, R., & Wilson, K. (1993). *Assisted living in the United States: A new paradigm for residential care for frail older persons?* Washington, DC: American Association of Retired Persons.

Kemper, P., Komisar, H. L., & Alecixh, L. (2005). Long-term care over an uncertain future: What can current retirees expect? *Inquiry, 42,* 335–350.

Lewin-VHI, Inc. (1996). *National study of assisted living for the frail elderly: Literature review update.* Durham, NC: Research Triangle Institute.

McAllister, D., Schommer, J., McAuley, J., Palm, J., & Herring, P. (2000). Comparison of skilled nursing and assisted living residents to determine potential benefits of pharmacist intervention. *The Consultant Pharmacist, 15,* 1110–1116.

MetLife Mature Market Institute. (2006). *2006 MetLife market survey of nursing home and home care costs.* Hartford, CT: MetLife Mature Market Institute.

Mollica, R., Sims-Kastelein, K., & O'Keeffe, J. (2008). *Residential care and assisted living compendium, 2007.* U.S. Department of Health and Human Services, Office of the Assistant Secretary for Planning and Evaluation, Office of Disability, Aging and Long-Term Care Policy and Research Triangle Institute. Retrieved June 21, 2008, from http://aspe.hhs.gov/daltcp/reports/2007/07alcom.htm

Morgan, L., Gruber-Baldini, A., & Magaziner, J. (2001). Resident characteristics. In S. Zimmerman, P. Sloane, & J. Eckert (Eds.), *Assisted living: Needs, practices and policies in residential care for the elderly* (pp. 144–172). Baltimore, MD: John Hopkins University Press.

National Center for Assisted Living. (2001). *Facts and trends: The assisted living sourcebook, 2001.* Washington, DC: American Health Care Association.

Newcomer, R., & Grant, L. (1990). Residential care facilities: Understanding their role and improving their effectiveness. In D. Tilson (Ed.), *Aging in place: Supporting the frail elderly in residential environments.* Glenview, IL: Scott Foresman.

Phillips, C., Hawes, C., Spry, K., & Rose, M. (2000). *A national study of assisted living for the frail elderly: Residents leaving assisted living - descriptive and analytic results from a national sample.* Beachwood, OH: Myers Research Institute, Menorah Park Center for Assisted Living.

Rhoads, M., & Thai, A. (2002). Potentially inappropriate medications ordered for elderly residents of assisted living homes and assisted living centers. *The Consultant Pharmacist, 17,* 587–593.

Spillman, B., & Black, K. (2006). *The size and characteristics of the residential care population: Evidence from three national surveys.* Washington, DC: U.S. Department of Health and Human Services, Assistant Secretary for Planning and Evaluation, Office of Disability, Aging and Long-Term Care Policy.

Spore, D. L., Mor., V., Hiris, J., Larrat, E. P., & Hawes, C. (1995). Psychotropic use among older residents of board and care facilities. *Journal of the American Geriatrics Society, 43,* 1403–1409.

Williams, B., Nichol, M., Lowe, B., Yoon, P., McCombs, J., & Margolies, J. (1999). Medication use in residential care facilities for the elderly. *The Annals of Pharmacotherapy, 33,* 149–55.

Wilson, K. (1990). *Assisted living: The merger of housing and long-term care services. Long-term care advances.* Durham, NC: Duke University Center for the Study of Aging and Human Development.

Wilson, K. (2007). Historical evolution of assisted living in the United States: 1979 to the present. *The Gerontologist, 47,* 8–22.

Wunderlich, G., & Kohler, P. (Eds.). (2001). *Improving the quality of long-term care.* Washington, DC: National Academy Press, Institute of Medicine.

U.S. General Accounting Office. (1999). *Assisted living: Quality of care and consumer protection issues* (GAO/T-HEHS-99-111).

Zimmerman, S., Gruber-Baldini, A. L., Sloane, P., Eckert, J., Hebel, J., Morgan, L., et al. (2003). Assisted living and nursing homes: Apples and oranges? *The Gerontologist, 43,* 108–117.

Policy, Licensing, and Regulations

Learning Objectives

Upon the completion of Chapter 2, the reader will be able to:

- *Explain the challenges in generically describing assisted living policy, licensing, and regulations.*
- *Cite examples of current changes to state regulation and policy.*
- *Describe state policy related to Medicaid reimbursement for assisted living.*
- *Describe policy and regulations related to assisted living labels, licensure, and philosophy.*
- *Discuss a variety of state regulatory models in assisted living.*
- *Understand the variability of policy and regulations related to resident agreements, admission, retention, and discharge criterion in assisted living.*
- *Describe policy and regulations related to resident rights, services, and special care needs in assisted living.*
- *Discuss the variety of requirements for direct care staff, owners, and administrators in assisted living.*
- *Describe federal statutes that impact assisted living.*

INTRODUCTION

This chapter will address key issues in assisted living policy, licensing, and regulations. Because states are primarily responsible for the monitoring and oversight of assisted living, this chapter provides a broad overview of the models and regulations used by individual states. An assisted living administrator will be required to thoroughly understand the regulations and requirements specific to their individual state, which is beyond the scope of this book. This section will address regulatory models and similarities, and variations in policy and regulations across states. Key concepts typically covered by state regulations are discussed, including assisted living philosophy, room/unit requirements, resident agreements and disclosure requirements, admission and retention criteria, resident rights, services, staff training, medications, and quality assurance. Finally, a summary of federal laws that may pertain to the assisted living industry is included.

The Challenge

Although there are some similarities across states in the licensing, regulations and policy relative to assisted living facilities, these concepts are challenging to generically describe for several reasons. Similar to the assisted living nomenclature and definitions, state regulations and policy are variable and continually changing. Assisted living is a broad and general licensing category in some states and a detailed model in others. Some states (as well as providers) utilize the terms assisted living interchangeably with other titles such as residential care, while others have different licensing categories based upon size, services, and/or philosophy of care. For example, in California, the label assisted living is not used in the state regulations, but it is frequently used by providers. Furthermore, some states have additional licensure requirements that allow for higher levels of care to be provided, such as limited nursing care, specialized dementia care, and hospice care for the terminally ill.

The most comprehensive work in tracking state policy and regulation has been conducted by Robert Mollica with the National Academy for State Health Policy. This research has been continually updated and published for more than a decade, and thus is a primary source of information for this chapter. The National Academy for State Health Policy is an independent academy dedicated to excellence in state health policy. Additional sources of information utilized for this chapter include the Assisted Living Federation of America, National Center for Assisted Living, and the National Senior Citizens Law Center. Furthermore, because there are no specific federal regulations for assisted living facilities, the recommendations of the Assisted Living Workgroup (ALW; 2003) from their report, *Assuring Quality in Assisted Living: Guidelines for Federal and State Policy, State Regulations, and Operations*, are included on important topics such as resident agreements, disclosure medication management, resident rights, and staff training requirements. The ALW was a national initiative of approximately 50 national organizations including providers, consumers, long-term care and health care professionals, and regulators that came together at the request of the U.S. Senate Special Committee on Aging to develop recommendations for federal guidelines for assisted living.

STATE POLICY AND REGULATION

State policy regarding regulations for assisted living facilities continues to evolve. Every year some changes are made, so it is important for the assisted living administrator to be aware of current law, pending legislation, and newly developed or revised regulations. The National Center for Assisted Living (2008), in their report *Assisted Living State Regulatory Review 2008,* provide summary information and examples of the current changes in state policy across the country:

1. Twelve states made major changes to their assisted living regulations in 2007 – many more than in each of the previous 2 years.
2. As in 2006, three states implemented new levels of licensure in part to accommodate increased resident acuity. In 2007, Pennsylvania and the District of Columbia established new "assisted living" licensure alongside existing licensure categories, while Wyoming added new rules allowing secure dementia units under a tiered licensing system. Other states continued refining multi-tiered licensing systems.
3. States continued developing standards for Alzheimer's/dementia populations and adding disclosure requirements.
4. Several states established or tightened criminal background check requirements, made changes to fire safety/emergency preparedness standards, and changed rules concerning food safety and dietary issues.
5. Other areas in which state assisted living regulations changed include staff training, medication management, reporting/record keeping, staffing, infection control, survey procedures, licensure fees, requirements when closing or expanding operations, resident rights, dispute resolution procedures, move-in/move-out requirements, and resident assessments.

Medicaid Reimbursement

Although very limited in availability, many (42) states now have several options for using Medicaid to fund services in assisted living facilities. Public policy and reimbursement issues are discussed further in Chapter 11. As seen in Table 2.1, the majority of states currently utilize Home and Community Based Services waivers [also called 1915(c) waivers] and others utilize state plans, while some utilize both (Mollica et al., 2008) States' ability to expanding the availability of home and community services to Medicaid is an ongoing challenge and often limited by resources.

TABLE 2.1	States Utilizing Medicaid Reimbursement for Assisted Living		
HCBS Waiver		State Plan	HCBS Waivers and State Plan
Alaska	Nebraska	Maine	Arkansas
Arizona	Nevada	Massachusetts	Florida
California	New Hampshire	Michigan	Idaho
Colorado	New Jersey	Missouri	Minnesota
Connecticut	New Mexico	New York	Vermont
Delaware	North Dakota	North Carolina	Wisconsin
Georgia	Ohio	South Carolina	
Hawaii	Oregon		
Illinois	Rhode Island		
Indiana	South Dakota		
Iowa	Texas		
Kansas	Utah		
Maryland	Washington		
Mississippi	Wyoming		
Montana			

Source: Mollica et al., 2008: *Residential Care and Assisted Living Compendium, 2007.*

Labels

The number of states utilizing the label assisted living has continually increased over time. Forty-three states and the District of Columbia now have a licensing category or statute that uses the term *assisted living* (Mollica et al., 2007). For example, some utilized names are assisted living, assisted living facility, assisted living residence and assisted care living facility (National Center for Assisted Living, 2008). Another common label is residential care, which includes terminology such as residential care facility, residential care home, or residential care facility for the elderly. In addition, some states continue to use traditional names such as board and care homes, homes for the aged, and personal care homes. Furthermore, some states utilize more than one label for various types or levels of assisted living and residential care.

Licensure

Although there are some federal laws that impact assisted living facilities, the main public oversight of assisted living facilities is through the enforcement of state regulations. This generally occurs in the form of the initial licensure of facilities, periodic license renewal surveys (inspection visits), and visits in response to consumer complaints or other administrative follow-up. All states have some kind of policy, regulations, or requirements for assisted living facilities.

Philosophy

Twenty-nine states and the District of Columbia (see Table 2.2) now report that provisions regarding assisted living concepts such as privacy, autonomy, and decision making are included in their assisted living regulations (Mollica et al., 2007). This number has increased tremendously from 15 states in 1996 and 22 states in 1998. Overall, this philosophy represents a consumer focused model where the delivery of care is centered on the resident. How the philosophy of assisted living is incorporated into state laws is highly variable. For example, regulations may state the importance of privacy and may require private unit residence while some states have mixed requirements, allowing bedrooms in some settings and individual apartments in others. Other states allow sharing (apartments or bedrooms) by resident choice. According to the *Residential Care and*

TABLE 2.2	States With Regulations That Include an Assisted Living Philosophy	
Alaska	Louisiana	North Dakota
Arizona	Maine	Oklahoma
Arkansas	Maryland	Oregon
District of Columbia	Massachusetts	Rhode Island
Florida	Montana	South Carolina
Hawaii	Nebraska	Texas
Idaho	Nevada	Vermont
Illinois	New Jersey	Washington
Iowa	New Mexico	Wisconsin
Kansas	New York	Wyoming

Source: Mollica et al., 2008: *Residential Care and Assisted Living Compendium, 2007.*

Assisted Living Compendium, 2007 (Mollica et al., 2008), two examples of how states incorporate the assisted living philosophy into their regulations come from Florida and Oregon:

1. **Florida's** statute describes the purpose of assisted living as "to promote availability of appropriate services for elderly and disabled persons in the least restrictive and most home-like environment, to encourage the development of facilities which promote the dignity, privacy, and decision making ability" of residents. The Florida law also states that facilities should be operated and regulated as residential environments, and not as medical or nursing facilities. Regulations require that facilities develop policies to maximize independence, dignity, choice, and decision making.

2. **Oregon**, the first state to adopt a specific philosophy for assisted living, states that: "Assisted living . . . is a program that promotes resident self-direction and participation in decisions that emphasize choice, dignity, privacy, individuality, independence, and home-like surroundings."

A commonly accepted philosophy of assisted living by facilities is offered by the Assisted Living Federation of America (2008). Assisted living Federation of America members commit to a 10-point philosophy of care that includes the follow ideals:

1. Offering cost-effective quality care that is personalized for individual needs.
2. Fostering independence for each resident.
3. Treating each resident with dignity and respect.
4. Promoting the individuality of each resident.
5. Allowing each resident's choice of care and lifestyle.
6. Protecting each resident's right to privacy.
7. Nurturing the spirit of each resident.
8. Involving family and friends, as appropriate, in care planning and implementation.
9. Providing a safe, residential environment.
10. Making the assisted living residence a valuable community asset.

Regulatory Models

States vary in what assisted living is defined to be. Some states consider assisted living to be a *licensed setting* in which many long-term care services are delivered. Fewer define assisted living as a *service* that may be provided in various settings, which do not have to be licensed (Mollica et al., 2007). Furthermore, other states identify assisted living as *a licensed building* in which supportive and health-related services are provided. In an attempt to understand the regulatory models utilized by states, Robert Mollica and colleagues (2007) describe five various models of state regulations, which are not mutually exclusive and are sometimes combined:

1. **Institutional model**
   This model has minimum building and unit requirements; typically, multiple occupancy bedrooms without attached baths, and shared toilets, lavatories, and tub/shower areas. Generally, states permit these facilities to serve people who need assistance with activities of daily living (ADLs). But they either do not allow nursing home eligible residents to be admitted, or do not allow facilities to provide nursing services. Historically, this model did not allow residents who met the criteria for placement in a nursing home to be served. However, as residents have aged in place, some states have made their rules more flexible to allow a higher level of service. For example, some states allow skilled nursing services to be provided in residential care settings for limited periods by a certified home health agency. North Carolina is one of the states using this approach.
2. **Housing and services model**
   This model licenses or certifies facilities to provide a broad range of long-term care services in apartment settings to persons with varying service needs, some of whom may be nursing home eligible. The state allows providers to offer relatively high levels of care; although licensed facilities may set their own admission/retention polices within state parameters, and may choose to limit the acuity of its residents. Depending on the state, some or all of the needs met in a nursing home may also be met in residential care settings. By creating a separate licensing category for this model and retaining other categories, states distinguish these facilities from board and care facilities. Vermont is one of the states using this approach.
3. **Service model**
   This model licenses the service provider, whether it is the residence itself or an outside agency, and allows existing building codes and requirements — rather than new licensing standards — to address the housing structure. This model simplifies the regulatory environment by focusing on the services delivered rather than the physical structure. Approaches for regulating services may also specify the type of buildings, apartment or living space that can qualify as assisted living. Minnesota is one of the states using this approach.

4. **Umbrella model**
   This model uses one set of regulations to cover two or more types of housing and services arrangements: residential care facilities, congregate housing, multi-unit or conventional elderly housing, adult family care, and assisted living. Maine is one of the states using this approach.
5. **Multiple levels of licensing for a single category**
   Some states set different licensing requirements for facilities in a single category, based on the extent of the assistance the facility provides or arranges, and on the type of residents served. For example, Maryland licenses facilities based on the characteristics of residents they serve. The state categorizes low, moderate, and high-need residents based on criteria for health and wellness, functional status, medication and treatment, behavior, psychological health, and social/recreational needs. The state may grant a limited number of waivers to facilities allowing them to serve residents who develop needs that exceed the facility's licensing level.

Another way to consider state regulatory models is to consider the level of care models. Eric Carlson (2005) reviewed laws and regulations of all 50 states in his work with the National Senior Citizens Law Center. To describe the variation in state regulatory models, Carlson (2005) describes two regulatory systems utilized by states:

1. **Single-level system**
   In the single-level system, a state licensing agency licenses only one type of residential care/assisted living. In this model, any residential care/assisted living facility is licensed to accept or retain any resident, as long as the resident does not have a condition that disqualifies him/her from residential care/assisted living generally.
2. **Multi-level system**
   In a multi-level system, residential care/assisted living facilities are licensed to care for residents only up to a particular care need. In this model, a resident typically may not be admitted or retained if the residents needs a level of care that exceeds the specific level at which the facility is licensed.

Sixteen states recognize more than one level of care with a tendency for newer assisted living licensure systems to adopt multi-level of care systems (Carlson, 2005). For example, Florida allows facilities to be licensed for standard assisted living services, limited nursing services, some mental health services, and extended congregate care. Arizona and Montana allow for three levels of care with each level allowing for a higher level of care to be delivered at the assisted living facility. Carlson (2005) makes the important point that even states with "single level" systems (e.g., California) often allow for exceptions within state regulations for specific residents or facilities.

Unit Requirements

The newer models of assisted living facilities became popular with older persons in large part because of the privacy and ability to retain control over personal activities, such as bathing, dressing, eating, and sleeping. The older, more traditional homes, offered shared rooms and bathrooms. Some stakeholders believe that private rooms must be made available to adhere to true assisted living philosophy, while others accept the use of shared rooms as a cost effective alternative. Consequently, there are many types of occupancy styles in assisted living. This is controlled by both consumer demand and state regulations.

To describe the various models relative to facility size and unit types, Zimmerman and Sloane (2007) describe a three-part typology to understand the multiple classifications of assisted living facilities across various states:

1. Facilities with fewer than 16 beds
2. Larger homes of the tradition board and care type
3. New model facilities with 16 beds or more – this new model facility is as (a) having been built in or after 1987 and (b) having two or more private-pay rates, at least 20% of residents who required assistance in transfer, at least 25% of residents who were incontinent, or a registered nurse or licensed practical nurse on duty at all times.

States set occupancy requirements in a variety of ways (Mollica et al., 2007). Some states use the label assisted living for homes that only provide private rooms while other states allow for shared rooms to be offered. Some states have different licensing categories, allowing shared rooms in some settings and requiring private rooms in others. Specifically, Mollica and colleagues (2007) report that currently:

1. Thirty-five states have rules that allow two unrelated people to share a unit or bedroom.
2. Ten states have licensing categories that allow four people to share a room.
3. Three states allow three people to share units.
4. A few states do not specify how many people may share a bedroom.

Resident Agreements/Contracts

In 1999, the U.S. GAO reported that most assisted living facilities provide information about services offered, but do not routinely provide information regarding discharge criteria, staff training and qualifications, services not available from the facility, grievance procedures, and medication policies. The majority of the 721 facilities that responded to the GAO survey stated that they generally provide prospective residents written information about many of their services and costs before they apply for admission. However, only about half indicated that they provide information on the circumstances under which the cost of services may change their policy on medication assistance, or their practice for monitoring residents' needs.

Furthermore, less than half said they provide written information in advance about discharge criteria, staff training and qualifications, or services not covered or available from the facility. The report concluded that the provision of adequate information to prospective and current residents is a major issue that requires additional oversight. This issue has become a key topic in assisted living today, with consumer advocates expressing on-going concern regarding the quality of resident agreements.

States generally have regulations and requirements relating to the resident agreement. There are common requirements such as a description of services and costs of service package, and less common requirements such as services not available, and terms of occupancy. Mollica and colleagues (2007) provided current information of the various states requirements by summarizing the numbers of states with specific provisions within their agreements (see Table 2.3).

The Assisted Living Workgroup (2003) included the following recommendations regarding resident agreements/contracts within the resident rights component of their report, *Assuring Quality in Assisted Living: Guidelines for Federal and State Policy, State Regulations, and Operations*, to U.S. Senate Special Committee on Aging:

1. **Consistency in contracts and marketing**
   All information conveyed by an assisted living residence to prospective residents (e.g., marketing materials, sales presentations, and tours) should be consistent with the contract.
2. **Contracts and agreements: Consistency with applicable law**
   All contract provisions shall be consistent with applicable law. The parties may agree to modify the contract as long as all parties agree to the modification and signify their agreement. Such modification will be consistent with applicable law.

TABLE 2.3 Topics Required in Admissions Agreements	
Topic Required Within Resident Agreement	**Number of States Requiring**
Services included in basic rate	49
Cost of service package	44
Rate changes	30
Refund policy	30
Cost of additional services	28
Admission/discharge	28
Service beyond basic rate	27
Payment/billing	21
Residents' rights	21
Grievance procedures	21
Termination (admission/discharge)	20
Terms of occupancy	13
Advance payments	13
Temporary absences	12
Period covered	11
Accommodations	10
Services not available	7
Other	35

Source: Mollica et al., 2008: *Residential Care and Assisted Living Compendium, 2007.*

3. **Contracts and agreements: Readability and pre-signing review**
   Contracts shall be written in simple language and be understandable. Prior to signature, the prospective resident has the right to review a contract and/or have the contract reviewed by a third party. Prior to the execution of the contract, a representative of the assisted living residence shall offer to read and explain the contract and answer any questions.

4. **Contracts and agreements: Required elements**
   Contracts/agreements should include at a minimum the following information:
   a) the term of the contract
   b) a comprehensive description of the assisted living residence's billing and payment policies and procedures
   c) a comprehensive description of services provided for a basic fee

d) a comprehensive description of the fee schedule for services provided on an a la carte basis or as part of a tiered pricing system that are not included in a basic fee

e) the policy for changing the amount of fees

f) the amount of advance notice the assisted living residence will give before the changing of fees (e.g., 30 days, 60 days). Notices should be readable and understandable by the resident

g) whether the assisted living residence requires an entrance fee, security deposit, and/or other fee(s) at entry, the amount of those fees and/or deposits, and the policies for whether or not fees and deposits are refundable, and procedures for refunding those fees and/or deposits

h) a description of the circumstances under which residents may receive a refund of any prepaid amount such as monthly rent

i) a description of the assisted living residence's policy during a resident's temporary absence

j) the process for initial and subsequent assessments and the development of the service plan based on these assessments, including notification that the resident has the right to participate in the development of the service plan

k) a description of all requirements for assessments or physical examinations, including the frequency and assignment of financial responsibility for such assessments and/or examinations

l) an explanation of the use of third party services (including all health services), how they may be arranged, accessed and monitored (whether by the resident, family or the assisted living residence),whether transportation is available if the services are not provided on-site, any restrictions on third party services, and who is financially responsible for the third party services and transportation costs

m) a description of all circumstances and conditions under which the assisted living residence may require the resident to be involuntarily transferred, discharged or evicted, an explanation of the resident's right to notice, the process by which a resident may appeal of the assisted living residence's decision, and a description of the relocation assistance (if available) offered by the assisted living residence

n) a description of the assisted living residence's process for resolving complaints or disputes, including any appeal rights, and a list of the appropriate consumer/regulatory agencies (if applicable; e.g., appropriate state/local long-term care ombudsman program, the

state regulatory agency, the local legal services program, and other
advocacy bodies/agencies)
o) a description of the procedures the resident or assisted living residence shall follow to terminate the agreement
p) a list of residents' rights as detailed in the statute or regulations
governing assisted living residences is incorporated by reference
and attached

5. **Contracts and agreements: Prohibition on waiver of right to sue**
The contract should not require the resident to waive the right to sue
the assisted living residence under applicable law. The contract may
disclose but not require options for alternative dispute resolution
available to the resident or assisted living residence.

6. **Contracts and agreements: Third party responsibility**
The contract shall disclose clearly that a signature by a third party
(such as a "responsible party") does not indicate acceptance of any
personal financial responsibility for fees, costs, or charges incurred
by the resident, and does not make the third party a guarantor, unless the third party has signed a separate agreement indicating such.
The separate agreement shall include, at a minimum, the following
information:
a) Third party voluntarily agrees to be financially liable for paying the
residents' expenses as agreed.
b) Third party has the right to have this agreement reviewed by an
attorney or other person.
c) Third party has the right to revoke the separate agreement with 30
days notice.

Pre-Admission Disclosures

Furthermore, the Assisted Living Workgroup (2003) included the following recommendations regarding pre-admission disclosure within the resident rights component of their report, *Assuring Quality in Assisted Living:
Guidelines for Federal and State Policy, State Regulations, and Operations,* to
U.S. Senate Special Committee on Aging:

1. **Pre-admission disclosure for specialized programs of care**
Assisted living residences representing in any way that they provide
special care programs for persons with Alzheimer's disease or other
dementias, or any other specific health conditions, shall disclose how
the program and its services are different from the basic services. At
a minimum, the assisted living residence shall disclose the following
information to each prospective resident prior to admission:

a. The assisted living residence's philosophy of the special care program.
b. The process and criteria for placement in, and transfer or discharge from, any specialized unit and/or the assisted living residence.
c. The process for assessing residents and establishing individualized service plans.
d. Additional services provided and the costs of those services relevant to the special care program.
e. Specialized (condition-specific) staff training and continuing education practices relevant to the special care program.
f. How the physical environment and design features are appropriate to support the functioning and safety of residents with the specific condition(s).
g. The frequency and types of activities offered to residents.
h. Options for family involvement and the availability of family support programs.

2. **Pre-admission disclosure on advance directives**
Assisted living residences shall provide residents with information about their rights under state law to make decisions about medical care, including their right to accept or refuse health-related services, the right to formulate advance medical directives, such as a living will, a directive to physicians, or durable power of attorney for health care. The assisted living residence information should disclose its philosophy and policies about implementation of advance medical directives, including, but not limited to, implementation of Do Not Resuscitate order (DNRs) and medical directives that require limitations on delivery of medical services, food, or hydration, and situations in which the assisted living residence is required to summon emergency medical services.

3. **Pre-admission disclosure on end-of-life care**
Assisted living residences shall clearly disclose information to residents about applicable state laws and about the assisted living residence's philosophy and policies regarding delivery of end-of-life care, including delivery of hospice and palliative care services. Disclosure shall include the circumstances, if any, under which a resident with terminal illness or in the process of dying, may be required to leave.

Admission and Retention

In general, states often utilize specific criteria that determine whether or not a person can be admitted to or retained in the assisted living facility. Typically, these include the general condition of the resident, health related conditions, functional conditions, physical function, cognitive function, behavioral problems, and health needs that may require the need for nursing care (Mollica et al., 2007). Mollica (2007) suggests three categories to explain the various state approaches for admission and retention policies, although he notes that these are not always mutually exclusive and that some states allow for exceptions and waivers regarding a variety of conditions. He included states utilizing the various approaches as well as examples:

1. **Full continuum**
   States allow facilities to serve people with a wide range of need and allow for residents to remain in one place as their care needs increase. However, facilities are generally not required to offer all the services a resident may need and are allowed to have their own admission and discharge standards. States using this approach include **Hawaii, Kansas, Maine, Minnesota, Nebraska, New Jersey, Oregon, Arizona, Maryland, Minnesota, New Jersey,** and **Oklahoma**. One example, Oregon generally does not limit whom facilities may serve. The rules contain "move out" criteria that allow residents to choose to remain in their living environment despite functional decline as long as the facility can meet the resident's needs. However, facilities are not required to serve all residents whose needs increase. Providers may ask residents to move if: (1) their needs exceed the level of ADL services available; (2) the resident exhibits behaviors or actions that repeatedly interfere with the rights or well-being of others; (3) the resident, due to cognitive decline, is not able to respond to verbal instructions, recognize danger, make basic care decisions, express need, or summon assistance; (4) the resident has a complex, unstable, or unpredictable medical condition; or (5) the resident has failed to make payment for charges.

2. **Discharge triggers**
   States develop a list of medical needs or treatments that cannot be provided in a facility (often care that requires skilled nursing personnel) and that will result in a resident's discharge from a facility. States using this approach include: **California, Delaware, Florida, Idaho, Illinois, Maryland, Mississippi, Nevada, New Mexico, South Carolina, Tennessee, Virginia,** and **West Virginia**. For example, **Virginia** does not allow residential care facilities to serve people who are ventilator dependent; have Stage III or IV dermal ulcers (unless a Stage III ulcer is healing); need intravenous (IV) therapy or injections directly into the vein except for intermittent care under specified conditions; have an airborne infectious disease in a communicable state; need psychotropic

medications but do not have an appropriate diagnosis and treatment plan; or have nasogastric tubes and gastric tubes (except when individuals are capable of independently feeding themselves and caring for the tube). Other examples of typical discharge triggers utilized by states include requiring 24-hour skilled nursing care, being permanently bedridden, being a danger to self or others, or have unstable medical conditions

3. **Levels of licensure**
   States license facilities based on the needs of residents or the services that may be provided in a specific kind of facility. **Arizona, Arkansas, Florida, Maine, Maryland, Mississippi, Missouri, Utah,** and **Vermont** have two or more levels of licensure based on the needs of residents or the services that may be provided. One example, **Florida** licenses four types of facilities: basic assisted living facilities, limited nursing services (LNS), limited mental health services, and extended-care center (ECC), which is the highest level of care (LOC). ECC facilities serve residents with higher needs and provide more services than the other levels including total help with bathing; nursing assessment more frequently than monthly; measurement and recording of basic vital functions; dietary management; supervision of residents with dementia; health education and counseling; assistance with self-administration and administration of medications; provide or arrange rehabilitative services; and escort services to health appointments.

Resident Rights

Regulation regarding resident rights is included in many states. Resident rights include such concepts as personal rights, disclosure of information regarding services and fees, and marketing practices. A further exploration of the significant challenges related to resident rights in assisted living facilities is found in Chapter 17. The Assisted Living Workgroup (2003) included the following recommendations regarding resident rights in their report, *Assuring Quality in Assisted Living: Guidelines for Federal and State Policy, State Regulations, and Operations,* to the U.S. Senate Special Committee on Aging:

1. **Resident rights**
   Within the boundaries set by law, residents have the right to:
   a. Be shown consideration and respect;
   b. Be treated with dignity;
   c. Exercise autonomy;
   d. Exercise civil and religious rights and liberties;

e. Be free from chemical and physical restraints;
f. Be free from physical, mental, fiduciary, sexual and verbal abuse, and neglect;
g. Have free reciprocal communication with and access to the long-term care ombudsmen program;
h. Voice concerns and complaints to the assisted living residence orally and in writing without reprisal;
i. Review and obtain copies of their own records that the assisted living residence maintains;
j. Receive and send mail promptly and unopened;
k. Private unrestricted communication with others;
l. Privacy for phone calls and right to access a phone;
m. Privacy for couples and for visitors;
n. Privacy in treatment and caring for personal needs;
o. Manage their own financial affairs;
p. Confidentiality concerning financial, medical and personal affairs;
q. Guide the development and implementation of their service plans;
r. Participate in and appeal the discharge (move-out) planning process;
s. Involve family members in making decisions about services;
t. Arrange for third party services at their own expense;
u. Accept or refuse services;
v. Choose their own physicians, dentists, pharmacists and other health professionals;
w. Choose to execute advance directives;
x. Exercise choice about end of life care;
y. Participate or refuse to participate in social, spiritual, or community activities;
z. Arise and retire at times of their own choosing;
aa. Form and participate in resident councils;
bb. Furnish their own rooms, and use and retain personal clothing and possessions;
cc. Right to exercise choice and lifestyle as long as it does not interfere with other residents' rights;
dd. Unrestricted contact with visitors and others as long as that does not infringe on other residents' rights;
ee. Rights that one would enjoy in their own home, such as coming and going.
ff. Residents' family members have the right to form and participate in family councils.

2. Provider responsibilities

    a. Promote an environment of civility, good manners, and mutual consideration by requiring staff, and encouraging residents, to speak to one another in a respectful manner;

    b. Provide all services for the resident or the resident's family that have been contracted for by the resident and the provider, as well as those services that are required by law;

    c. Obtain accurate information from residents that is sufficient to make an informed decision regarding admission and the services to be provided;

    d. Maintain an environment free of illegal weapons and drugs;

    e. Obtain notification from residents of any third party services they are receiving, and to establish reasonable policies and procedures related to third party services;

    f. Report information regarding resident welfare to state agencies or other authorities as required by law;

    g. Establish reasonable house rules in coordination with the resident council.

    h. Involve staff and other providers in the development of resident service plans;

    i. Maintain an environment that is free from physical, mental, fiduciary, sexual and verbal abuse, and neglect.

    j. An assisted living residence may require that providers of third party services ensure that they and their employees have passed criminal background checks, are free from communicable diseases, and are qualified to perform the duties they are hired to perform.

Services

Services provided in an assisted living facility vary both by state admission and retention criteria, and by individual assisted living providers. Typically services that may be offered by assisted living facilities include:

1. 24-hour care and supervision

2. Oversight of personal and supportive services (assistance with activities of daily living and instrumental activities of daily living)

3. Health-related services (e.g., medication management services)

4. Social services

5. Recreational activities

6. Meals and snacks

7. Housekeeping and laundry
8. Transportation

Many states now seek to allow facilities to facilitate aging-in-place and to offer consumers a full range of long-term care options. However, in some cases, most states specify the range of allowable services and a minimum that must be provided, but do not require facilities to provide the full range of allowable services (Mollica et al., 2007). There are varying opinions on what services assisted living facilities should be expected to provide. Some believe that assisted living should remain a social model, and facilities should not be expected to provide services to persons with medically complex conditions or high levels of disabilities. On the other hand, some believe that assisted living facilities should provide additional services to residents as care needs increase in an effort to minimize the need to relocate to a skilled nursing facility or nursing home.

Training Requirements

State regulations generally specify initial training requirements for assisted living administrators as well as direct care staff. However, some states stipulate general requirements, and others include specific topics including the number of hours required (Mollica et al., 2007).

Operator/Administrator Requirements

The Assisted Living Federation of America (2005) completed survey work related specifically to administrator requirements across states. All states except Virginia were included. In the study, it was found that 14 states required licensure, 10 states requires certification, 9 states had training programs, 15 states had education and experience requirements, and 5 states had very few requirements (Assisted Living Federation of America, 2005). Results included the following points of interest: There is much variation within each of the five categories: requirements for administrators are very state specific.

1. About 65% of states mandate licensure, certification, or training programs, but varying amounts of education and experience made up the largest single category (30%).
2. Training programs are not state designed, but programs must be approved by states.
3. Standardized testing is mandatory for licensure and typical for certification.

4. Varying amounts of continuing education is required by about two-thirds of states.
5. Few states require skilled nursing licensure.
6. Licensure states are divided regarding the issue of whether individuals must meet separate education/experience requirements, in addition to participating in state training programs.
7. Two-thirds of states require a minimum age of 21 years.

Direct Staff Requirements

In the report for the U.S. Department of Health and Human Services, Hawes and colleagues (1999) found that the types of training and orientation required for direct care staff varied across assisted living facilities, but overall, relatively little training was required. Seventy-five percent of unlicensed personnel were required to attend some kind of pre-service training. For those that did require training, the most common amount of required training was between 1 and 16 hours. In addition, only 11% of the staff who participated in 4 the required training completed it before the start of work. Staff also reported that they did receive training on the philosophy of assisted living. Seventy-five percent of staff had participated in continuing education activities. Overall, Hawes and colleagues (1999) noted that staff was not well informed about normal aging processes and dementia care.

There is large variation in the staff training requirements and stringency of the requirements among the states (Assisted Living Workgroup, 2003; Carlson, 2005; Hawes et al., 1999; Mollica et al., 2008). Carlson (2005) did extensive work inclusive of all states and reported several characteristics of staff training requirements as follow:

1. Thirty-three states require training in first aid or cardiopulmonary resuscitation or both, but with varying stringency;
2. Thirty-seven states specify training topics;
3. A minority of states require initial training of a certain minimum number of hours with 5 states requiring 12 or fewer hours, 4 states requiring 13-24 hours and 10 states requiring 25 or more hours;
4. Nine states require certain qualifications of the person conducting the initial training for direct-care staff;
5. Six states have some control over the content of the curriculum for initial training;
6. Four states require that a direct care staff member pass a state-developed competency examination; and

7. Twenty-four states require a specific hourly minimum for direct-care staff's continuing education with annual minimum generally falling into a 5- to 15-hour range.

Carlson (2005) makes the important notation that direct care standards for assisted living facilities are far less stringent that those that apply to nursing home staff members, where under the terms of the federal Nursing Home Reform Law, direct care staff must complete at least 75 hours of initial training under the supervision of a registered nurse with a minimum of 2 years experience and at least 1 year nursing experience in long-term care.

Dementia Care

States continue to adopt more regulations with regards to dementia residents in assisted living. Forty-five states now report that they have specific regulatory provisions for facilities serving those with Alzheimer's disease and other dementias, which is an increase from 44 in 2004, 36 in 2002 and 28 in 2000 (Mollica et al., 2008). Two examples of the various additional requirements for facilities serving dementia residents include:

1. **Disclosure**
   These facilities are required to describe in writing how they are different from other facilities. This may include philosophy of care, admission/discharge criteria, the process for arranging a discharge, services covered and the cost of care, and special activities that are available.
2. **Staffing and training**
   Thirty-six states now have requirements for dementia training and staffing for facilities serving people with Alzheimer's disease and other dementias, which may include additional training hours or staffing ratios.

Medication Administration

The issue of medication management and administration is a challenging and key issue for assisted living facilities. In their report, *Assisted Living: Quality of Care and Consumer Protection Issues,* the U.S. General Accounting Office (1999) found "not providing residents with appropriate medications and not storing medications properly" to be a common problem in assisted living facilities. Regulators have also cited medication administration and assistance with self-medication as a major concern (Mollica et al., 2007).

There is much variability in how states address medication issues within their regulations in assisted living facilities. However, several states now report that they are paying closer attention to medication issues, including the tracking of medication problems as the acuity level of residents served increases (Mollica et al., 2007). Some states allow for trained aides to administer medications, and while others allow only trained aides to administer medications or to assist with self-administration of medications. Some states require facilities to have a consulting pharmacist, and several states require licensed nurses to review medication records on a regular basis. Some states are now requiring additional training for direct care staff that administer or assist with self-administration of medications (e.g., California).

The Assisted Living Workgroup (2003) included the following recommendation with regards to medication management in their report, *Assuring Quality in Assisted Living: Guidelines for Federal and State Policy, State Regulations, and Operations*, to U.S. Senate Special Committee on Aging:

The assisted living residence will have and implement policies and procedures for the safe and effective distribution, storage, access, security, and use of medications, related equipment, and services of the residence by trained and supervised staff.

Policies and procedures of the residence should address the following issues:

1. Medication orders, including telephone orders
2. Pharmacy services
3. Medication packaging
4. Medication ordering and receipt
5. Medication storage
6. Disposal of medications and medication-related equipment
7. Medication self-administration by the resident
8. Medication reminders by the residence
9. Medication administration by the residence
10. Medication administration – specific procedures
11. Documentation of medication administration
12. Medication error detection and reporting
13. Quality improvement system, including medication error prevention and reduction
14. Medication monitoring and reporting of adverse drug effects to the prescriber

15. Review of medications (e.g., duplicate drug therapy, drug interactions, monitoring for adverse drug interactions)
16. Storage and accountability of controlled drugs
17. Training, qualifications, and supervision of staff involved in medication management

Quality Assurance Efforts

As the interest in assisted living has increased, so have concerns about quality of care and safety that can be provided to those residents who require special care, staffing and physical and social environments. These concerns have been described in media reports throughout the country and in a 1999 report from the United States General Accounting Office (U.S. GAO, 1999). In 2004, the U.S. GAO issued another report, *Assisted Living: Examples of State Efforts to Implement Consumer Protections*, which describe the quality assurance initiatives in Florida, Georgia, Massachusetts, Texas, and Washington.

Quality assurance strategies described states in the U.S. GAO report (2004) included:

1. Providing technical assistance and follow-up
2. Acting within 10 days on complaints
3. Having clear lines of communication and definition of duties for survey staff
4. Developing clear enforcement procedures that are well understood by state staff meeting with providers to discuss issues
5. Providing training
6. Conducting follow-up visits
7. Maintaining a consumer perspective that focuses on improving care, not just punishing past failures

In addition, states described a number of quality initiatives underway including:

1. Providing training for providers
2. Implementing new training requirements for medication aides
3. Revising the survey process
4. Developing a more formalized consultation program
5. Providing more technical assistance
6. Conducting forums for providers to discuss quality issues
7. Implementing quality assurance and quality initiatives

Furthermore, additional strategies focused on conducting regulatory reviews to bring provisions up to national standards and tighten standards for assessment, training, and level of care, including:

1. Working with providers to develop minimal standards for assessments, service plans, negotiated risk agreements, and disclosure requirements
2. Adding disclosure requirements for dementia care providers
3. Increasing staff training requirements
4. Establishing specific staffing requirements for special care units
5. Increasing requirements for a comprehensive resident assessment

FEDERAL STATUTES THAT IMPACT ASSISTED LIVING

Although states are primarily responsible for the licensing and oversight of assisted living facilities, federal statues also impact the operations of assisted living. Some examples of federal statutes that are important for the assisted living administrator to have knowledge of are offered by the Assisted Living Federation of America (2008):

Americans With Disabilities Act

The Americans With Disabilities Act affects assisted living operators in two primary ways: first, as employers under Title I of that law; and secondly, as "public accommodations" under Title III of that law. Title I of the ADA covers all employers with 15 or more employees, although religious organizations may require all employees, including those with disabilities, to conform to their religious tenets. The principal obligation of employers under Title I of the ADA is to provide "reasonable accommodations" to employees with disabilities which are defined as physical or mental impairments that substantially limit "major life activities" such as walking, breathing, and working—in order to allow them to perform the "essential functions" of a job. In addition, under Title I of the ADA, assisted living employers must refrain from making adverse decisions based on an individual's having a record of a physical or mental impairment, as well as from erroneously regarding an individual as disabled and treating him or her differently on that basis. Finally, the ADA prohibits employers from inquiring whether an applicant has a medical condition or disability prior to extending a conditional offer of employment. Alcoholism is a protected disability under the ADA, although current drug users (as opposed to the rehabilitated) are not covered under the

Act, and the Act does not affect the ability of assisted living employers to test employees for drug use.

Title III of the ADA prohibits discrimination on the basis of disability by 'commercial facilities' and 'places of public accommodation' — such as "social service center establishments" and offices of "service establishments," regardless of size. Title III's prohibitions, however, do not apply to "religious organizations or entities controlled by religious organizations."

Under Title III of the ADA, "commercial facilities" are specifically defined to exclude residential facilities and facilities otherwise covered by or exempted from the requirements of the Fair Housing Act of 1968 as amended by the Fair Housing Amendments Act of 1988. Because the term "dwelling" under the FHAA has been interpreted broadly, the coverage of assisted living facilities as 'commercial facilities' under Title III of the ADA may be correspondingly narrow. However, since certain physically public parts of assisted living facilities, such as lobbies, hallways, sales and management offices, and parking lots, may separately qualify as "places of public accommodation" under Title III of the ADA, assisted living operators can expect the coverage of Title III of the ADA and the FHAA to overlap with respect to such areas. In any event, under either law, assisted living operators will generally be required to make those architectural modifications to facilities that do not constitute "undue hardships."

Moreover, to the extent an assisted living operator offers social services such as dining, counseling, and transportation to its residents, the public areas of an entire facility may independently be deemed a covered "place of public accommodation." As such, if a resident or guest meets the definition of "disabled" under the ADA, he or she will be entitled to reasonable accommodations that will allow him or her to access the facility and its services on a non-discriminatory basis. Assisted living operations must ensure that their delivery of services as well does not result in any of the types of discrimination prohibited under the Title III of the ADA. This generally will mean making reasonable accommodations to ensure that facilities and programs give the disabled equal opportunities to participate and benefit in the most integrated setting appropriate.

Civil Rights Act of 1991

The Civil Rights Act of 1991 consisted primarily of amendments to Title VII of the Civil Rights Act of 1964, which like the ADA, covers assisted living operators employing 15 or more employees. It also affected the prohibition on intentional racial discrimination contained in the Reconstruction Civil Rights Act of 1866 (42 U.S.C. Sec. 1981), which covers assisted living operators regardless of the number of workers they employ.

Prior to the Civil Rights Act of 1991, Title VII of the Civil Rights Act of 1964 had been designed primarily to promote informal resolution of employment discrimination claims, and remedies were generally limited to declaratory judgments, injunctions, orders of reinstatements and/or backpay, and attorneys fees. The most dramatic change caused by the 1991 Act was the replacement of this system with a tort-like compensation scheme for intentional employment discrimination including compensatory damages for emotional pain and suffering, punitive damages, and jury trials. Though it expanded the range of remedies available under Title VII, Congress also capped damages, however, at levels rising in 3 increments from $50,000 to $100,000, $200,000 and $300,000, for employers with up to 100, 200, 500, and over employees, respectively. These caps notwithstanding, the 1991 Act still significantly raised the financial stakes and risks for assisted living operators litigating federal employment discrimination claims.

In addition, the 1991 Act specifically overruled several Supreme Court decisions that had narrowed the scope of the Reconstruction Civil Rights Act and Title VII. In particular, Congress reversed a 1989 Supreme Court decision that had limited the reach of the Reconstruction Civil Rights Act, and expanded the kinds of acts prohibited by that law to encompass intentional discrimination in virtually any aspect of the employment relationship. Second, Congress adopted the broad interpretation of "adverse impact" discrimination announced by the Supreme Court in a landmark 1971 case — Griggs v. Duke Power Co. — thereby legislatively reversing another 1989 Supreme Court decision that briefly appeared to make it more difficult for plaintiffs to prevail in challenges to employment practices with disproportionate negative effects on classes of employees protected under Title VII. Finally, the 1991 Act also helped plaintiffs by partially reversing another 1989 decision of the Supreme Court — Price Waterhouse v. Hopkins — and newly allowing plaintiffs to 'prevail' and receive declaratory judgments, injunctions, and attorneys fees even if an employer could establish that a decision adverse to an employee would have been made for legitimate reasons, any actual discriminatory motivation notwithstanding.

Rehabilitation Act of 1973

Section 504 of the Rehabilitation Act of 1973 will apply to assisted living operators that receive federal financial assistance, and Section 503 of that Act will also apply to the rare operator that contracts with the federal government for more than $10,000 in personal property or "nonpersonal" services annually. Generally speaking, if a facility directly or indirectly receives Medicaid funds, it will likely be deemed the "recipient" of federal financial "assistance."

If an assisted living operator is covered by Section 504, it will effectively have no obligations than it already had under Titles I and III of the ADA. Thus, for all practical purposes, unless the operator is exempt from the ADA for some reason, Section 504 of the Rehabilitation Act will not impact its operation. If an assisted living operator also becomes covered under Section 503 of the Rehabilitation Act, however, wholly apart from any obligations it may have under Titles I or III of the ADA, it will also have an obligation to take affirmative action to employ the disabled.

Family and Medical Leave Act

The Family and Medical Leave Act requires assisted living operators with 50 or more employees to provide up to 12 weeks of unpaid leave for family and medical reasons to employees who have worked for them for at least 12 months and a total of 1,250 hours during the previous 12-month period. Employers must maintain employees' pre-existing group health insurance benefits while they are on FMLA leave, and must restore employees to the same or equivalent positions when their leave ends.

Employees can take FMLA leave for the birth of a child, adoption of a child, placement of a foster child, to care for a spouse, child or parent with a "serious health condition," or to care for a minor child who is unable to care for himself or herself due to a physical or mental disability as defined under the ADA. The statute also provides for leave for employees with "serious health conditions," defined as an "illness, injury, impairment or physical or mental condition that results in: (1) an overnight inpatient stay at a hospital, hospice, or residential medical care facility; (2) absence from work or other regular daily activities and continuing treatment for more than 3 days; or (3) continuing treatment for a chronic or long-term condition that if not treated would incapacitate the family member for more than 3 days."

An employee may take FMLA leave on a continuous or intermittent basis if medically necessary — such as when the employee or the employee's family member has an episodic illness. Though the law requires the employee to give the employer 30 days notice of needed FMLA leave when possible, fundamentally, the employee must simply make a reasonable attempt to schedule leave so as to minimize the disruption of the employer's operation. Moreover, employers may choose to designate paid leave as concurrent FMLA leave when taken by an employee qualifying for FMLA leave.

Fair Housing Amendments Act

The Fair Housing Amendments Act of 1988 altered Title VIII of the Fair Housing Act of 1968 in two main ways: first, it expanded the prohibitions contained in the Fair Housing Act to include discrimination in the sale or rental of "dwellings" on the basis of disability; and second, it enhanced the procedural enforcement options available for private litigants, as well as the Department of Housing and Urban Development (or its designated equivalent state or local agency, such as the City of Dallas), as they pursue relief under the Fair Housing Act.

Many of the residents of assisted living facilities qualify as 'disabled' within the meaning of FHAA. Thus, the expansion of the Fair Housing Act to cover the disabled is having a complex effect on the assisted living industry. For example, on the one hand, the FHAA has put a new arrow in the quiver of assisted living operators faced with state and local regulations — such as zoning restrictions — that can interfere with or prevent the construction of new (or expansion or operation of existing) facilities. On the other hand, however, the FHAA may result in new architectural burdens with respect to interior residential facilities, and may also create new potential liability for operators attempting to comply with state regulations that govern, for example, the placement of patients in assisted living (as opposed to long-term care) facilities.

The changes in the enforcement procedures contained in the FHAA also significantly increase the financial risk faced by assisted living operators sued under the Fair Housing Act. In particular, in addition to lengthening the period of time during which complaints of discrimination can be bought, in stark contrast with the prior $1,000 cap on punitive damages under the former law, the FHAA newly allows plaintiffs to recover unlimited punitive damages, and increases the ability of plaintiffs to recover attorneys fees in suits brought under the Fair Housing Act. Finally, the FHAA significantly enhances the ability of the federal government or its state or local agents to enforce the provisions of the Fair Housing Act in administrative proceedings and to recover fines for violations.

Fair Labor Standards Act (FLSA)

The Fair Labor Standard Act of 1938 is the primary federal law setting minimum wage, overtime pay, equal pay, recordkeeping, and child labor standards for employers in the assisted living industry. An assisted living employer will qualify as an "enterprise" covered under the FLSA — and its non-exempt employees will be covered — if it has a gross annual sales volume of $500,000 or more, and two or more of its employees "handle," "sell" or "work on" goods or materials that have been "moved in or produced for commerce by any person." Depending on the precise nature of the services they provide, however, some assisted living operators may qualify for special exemptions from certain of the FLSA's requirements. These include, for example, exemptions related to individuals employed to provide companionship to the aged, "live-in" domestics, and workers residing on-site at their workplace.

As of September 1, 1997, the federal minimum wage is $5.15 per hour. Employers with unionized employees may not negotiate agreements that waive employees' statutory rights under the FLSA. Thus, collective bargaining agreements may only contain provisions that are more beneficial to employees than what such employees would otherwise receive under the FLSA.

Many of the questions and complexities that arise under the FLSA derive from the rules governing what constitutes compensable "hours worked" under that law, and employer errors in interpreting these rules may be particularly significant since (especially where full-time employees are concerned) they can result in unpaid overtime liability. Waiting time, on-call time, breaks, sleep time, meal periods, training, and travel time are all governed by detailed rules requiring separate analyses based on the facts and circumstances of employment.

In addition, with certain limitations, the FLSA allows assisted living employers to institute certain "alternative" work schedules. For example, under 29 U.S.C. Sec. 270(j), employers "engaged in the operation of . . . establishment[s] . . . primary engaged in the care of the . . . aged" can adopt a so-called "8-80" payroll system whereby employees are scheduled to work 80 hours on a 14-day basis rather than 40 hours on a 7-day basis.

Occupational Safety and Health Act

The Occupational Safety and Health Act of 1970 sets a national minimum standard for workplace safety. Section 18 of OSHA encourages states to develop and operate their own job safety and health programs, and OSHA approves and monitors state plans and provides up to 50% of an approved plan's operating costs. Some states, however, including Texas, do not maintain their own plan, and enforcement and the applicable statutes and regulations in such states are federal.

Assisted living employers have two general duties under OSHA: first, to furnish employees with employment (and a place of employment) that is free from recognized hazards that are likely to cause death or serious physical harm; and second, to comply with the detailed occupational safety and health standards promulgated under OSHA. Moreover, assisted living employers with 11 or more employees during the previous calendar year must keep records of occupational injuries and illness in the form of an OHSA Log 200.

OSHA compliance officers are authorized to inspect and investigate (at reasonable times and in a reasonable manner) places of employment for compliance with OSHA regulations, and are empowered to obtain injunctions, issue citations, and assess penalties for non-compliance through administrative proceedings.

CONCLUSIONS

This chapter has provided the reader with an overview of state policy, licensing and regulations for the assisted living industry. It is quite apparent that the states vary tremendously in regards to the licensing and monitoring of assisted living facilities. Although federal regulations do not currently exist, the reader has been offered national guidelines and recommendations stemming from the work of prominent national organizations. Examples of federal statutes that impact assisted living facilities have been described. This chapter illustrates the need for today's assisted living administrators to be well informed with regards to individual state laws and regulations and remain updated as requirements are commonly changed and frequently modified.

REFERENCES

Assisted Living Federation of America. (2005). *Special report: Executive director/administrator requirements: Survey of state practices.* Assisted Living Federation of America. Retrieved March 31, 2005, from http://www.alfa.org/membersonly/articles/Exec_Dir_Req_Spec_Rpt.pdf

Assisted Living Federation of America. (2008). *Federal statutes that impact assisted living.* Retrieved July 10, 2008, from http://www.alfa.org/i4a/pages/index.cfm?pageid=3516

Assisted Living Federation of America. (2008). *What is assisted living?* Alexandria, VA: Assisted Living Federation of America. Retrieved June 21, 2008, from http://www.alfa.org/i4a/pages/index.cfm?pageid=3285#philosophy

Assisted Living Workgroup. (2003). *Assuring quality in assisted living: Guidelines for federal and state policy, state regulations, and operations.* Washington, DC: U.S. Government Printing Office.

Carlson, E. (2005). *Critical issues in assisted living: Who's in, who's out and who's providing the care.* Washington, DC: National Senior Citizen's Law Center.

Hawes, C., Phillips, C., & Rose, M. (1999). *A national study of assisted living for the frail elderly: Results of a national survey of facilities.* Washington, DC: U.S. Department of Health and Human Services.

Mollica, R., Sims-Kastelein, K., & O'Keeffe, J. (2008). *Residential care and assisted living compendium, 2007.* U.S. Department of Health and Human Services, Office of the Assistant Secretary for Planning and Evaluation, Office of Disability, Aging and Long-Term Care Policy and Research Triangle Institute. Retrieved June 21, 2008, from http://aspe.hhs.gov/daltcp/reports/2007/07alcom.htm

National Center for Assisted Living. (2008). *Assisted living state regulatory review 2008.* Washington, DC: National Center for Assisted Living. Retrieved June 21, 2008, from http://www.ncal.org/about/2008_reg_review.pdf

U.S. General Accounting Office. (1999). *Assisted living: Quality of care and consumer protection issues* (GAO/T-HEHS-99-111).

U.S. General Accounting Office. (2004). *Assisted living: Examples of state efforts to implement consumer protections* (GAO-04-684).

Zimmerman, S., & Sloane, P. (2007). Definitions and classification of assisted living. *The Gerontologist, 47,* 33–39.

Organizational Overview

With Contributing Author: Sarah Dillon

Learning Objectives

Upon the completion of Chapter 3, the reader will be able to:

- *Understand the concept of aging in place in the context of assisted living.*
- *Describe the variation in assisted living according to the size of the facility and services provided.*
- *Explain the differences between multiple service models in assisted living.*
- *Describe organization patterns in assisted living, both by size and service model.*
- *Understand the various business models in assisted living.*
- *Describe assisted living facilities that cater to the needs of special populations.*

INTRODUCTION

This chapter will consider key issues related to organizational management in the assisted living industry. First, the concept of *aging in place* is discussed in the context of models of care and levels of services within assisted living. Facility size (i.e., number of beds) is highly variable among assisted living facilities. Some common size variations will be outlined, and also considered is how these size variations affect the organizational structure. An overview of common organizational models and patterns is described. Modern organizational designs, such as those with specific affiliation, are also included. This chapter provides the reader with an overview of common organizational considerations for assisted living facilities.

Aging in Place — A Consideration

"Aging in place" is a subject of much dialogue and debate among various assisted living stakeholders. As assisted living continues to evolve, questions such as, who is an appropriate resident for a certain facility, and how long a resident can remain have become complicated. Should residents be allowed to remain in assisted living regardless of their care needs? Should they be allowed to die there? The concept of aging in place is a key concern for assisted living administrators as models of care and levels of services are discussed. "Aging in place" is a term used in marketing by those in the rapidly evolving senior housing industry, which includes assisted living.

"Growing older without having to move" is frequently offered as a definition of aging in place. In comparison, the definition of aging in place offered by of M. Powell Lawton (1990), a leader in aging research, described aging in place as a multidimensional phenomenon for seniors: "Aging in place represents a transaction between an aging individual and his or her residential environment that is characterized by changes in both person and environment over time with the physical location of the person's being the only constant." In Lawton's definition there is a dynamic between the person and the environment. Lawton further explains that three types of changes occur as aging in place progresses. First, there are the psychological changes of aging. Second, there is change to the physical environment due to natural physical wear, and the behaviors of other people. Third, there are changes that occur during the process of aging in place based upon alterations made to the environment to create a more supportive and private atmosphere.

The assisted living ideal allows the physical place to stay the same, and implies that necessary services to meet an older person's needs be brought to them. Older persons usually move into supportive environments with the hope of avoiding other subsequent moves, and that the facility will be able to provide for their changing needs over time. The facility's ability to do this is an important aspect of security for older people. Aging in place is limited by several things in assisted living including state regulation and facility discretion. The models of care, in regards to admission and retention criteria, discharge triggers, and the availability of hospice/end-of-life care, are all important to consider.

Jacquelyn Frank (2001) described the difficulties faced by providers of assisted living. She offered the following questions for consideration. *Who are suitable candidates for assisted living? When is it time for a resident to leave?* These are important questions for the assisted living administrator to consider. While minimizing the need to move and providing prolonged residence are frequent goals of an assisted living facility, "never having to move" is a promise that should not be made.

Size

Nationally, the average assisted living community has 58 units. However, assisted living facility size varies greatly and facilities may be much smaller or larger (The National Center for Assisted Living, 2009). In some states, different size facilities have varying regulations and names, as explained in Chapter 2. Furthermore, for the assisted living administrator, job satisfaction may vary according to facility demographics, such as size (Gilchrist, 2009).

Services

As noted in the previous chapters assisted living facilities typically offer services including personal care and assistance with activities of daily living, social and recreational activities, meals, medication management, housekeeping, laundry, and escort services. Some facilities offer additional health services, such as intermittent nursing care oversight. These services may be offered directly or through a third party contractor. Under the direct services model, services are provided by the in-house staff. Under the contracted service model, outside agencies provide services to residents. Examples of contracted services include home health care and hospice services.

SERVICE MODELS

There is no standardized service model in assisted living. There are advantages to this, such as flexibility for industry and consumers, wide span of services (at facility's option), and a wide range of structures (site-based and imported services, bundled and unbundled charges and services). There are also disadvantages to this variety. For example, there is less clarity. A consumer's ability to plan is reduced and the accountability of the facility can be unclear, creating regulatory oversight complexities. More extensive information of assisted living models of care are found in Chapter 13. Here four common examples of service models in assisted living are offered to illustrate the variety. These examples were chosen because they illustrate common models, but the reader should be aware that other models exist.

Board and Care

Small group homes which provide care for seniors and frail elders have many names. Depending on location, they may be called board and care homes, assisted living, residential care homes for the elderly, personal care, adult foster care, adult group homes, adult family homes, or boarding care homes. These residences characteristically offer room and board in a small environment, typically housing 10 persons or fewer. These homes are commonly located in residential neighborhoods and offer a less institutional alternative. A home-like environment is of high priority. Although these facilities sometimes offer somewhat less independence and privacy, they often house persons with more cognitive impairments, chronic health conditions, and impairments with activities of daily living as opposed to larger models. Home health care and hospice services are sometimes available from third party vendors. The ability of a resident to age in place in a board and care home is variable, depending on regulations and individual operator philosophies. Because of the smaller number of residents, these homes often have very few staff. For example, an owner or administrator may also be a direct caregiver and have only one or two additional employees.

Hospitality Model

Some assisted living facilities offer apartment-style living and hotel-type services with limited personal care assistance. Services provided are meals, housekeeping, transportation, and security. Personal care services such as toileting, getting up from a chair, or assistance eating are limited. Residents have a high-degree of independence, but may not be able to stay if their care needs worsen. Hospitality model assisted living facilities can be very appealing to consumers because of the high level of privacy that can be provided. Private units with private bathrooms and kitchenettes are common amenities. This type of model may experience higher resident turnover rates, because of the lower level of care provided. Depending on size, this type of facility will have varying number of staff. Hawes and colleagues (2003) classified an assisted living facility to bear a low service status if it did not have an RN on staff and did not provide nursing care with its own staff, but did provide the following:

- 24-Hour staff oversight
- Housekeeping
- At least 2 meals a day

■ Personal assistance, defined as help with at least two of the following: medications, bathing, or dressing

New Model

New model assisted living facilities have typically more than 60 beds. Hawes, Phillips, and Rose (2000) described the newer model facilities as "high service and high privacy." The criteria for being a high service facility was that at least the following were provided:

■ 24-Hour staff oversight
■ Housekeeping
■ At least 2 meals a day
■ Personal assistance, defined as help with at least two of the following: medications, bathing, or dressing
■ At least one full-time registered nurse (RN) on staff
■ Nursing care (monitoring or services) with its own staff

In the report, *High Service or High Privacy Assisted Living Facilities, Their Residents and Staff: Results from a National Survey (2000)*, Hawes and colleagues made several conclusions regarding high service assisted living facilities (ALFs) nationwide: (1) the high privacy or high service ALFs provide this care in a setting that has many components valued by consumers, particularly in terms of privacy and environmental autonomy; (2) most high service or high privacy ALFs offered a wide array of services; (3) the issue of whether such services can meet residents' unscheduled needs is more complex; (4) the degree to which such facilities enable residents to age in place is clearly mixed unless one limits the concept to one of "*aging in place without significant decline in physical or cognitive functioning*"; and (5) assisted living is still a largely private-pay sector and, among the high service or high privacy ALFs, one that is largely unaffordable for most moderate and low income older persons unless they spend down their assets or receive help from relatives.

Specialized Dementia Care Model

A growing specialty area in assisted living facilities is dementia care. The market demand for dementia care has continued to grow. Specialized facilities exist, as well as specialized units within assisted living facilities. Special care units may promote a physical environment, activities, staff training, and program philosophy which address the special care needs of individuals with memory loss and related behavioral problems. Specialized dementia units often have a secure environment and a specialized physical design layout. To enhance the quality of life of persons with dementia, these specialty units will often include additional interventions and philosophies such as:

- Holistic assessment
- Regular formal assessments
- Refer to other professionals as appropriate
- Care planning involving resident, family, and staff
- Provide person-centered care
- Provide opportunities for residents to express themselves
- Medication and non-pharmacological treatment
- Training and management of staff
- Provide positive and safe environment

ORGANIZATIONAL PATTERNS BY SIZE AND MODEL

Assisted living facilities generally have traditional areas of work including the following:

- Marketing
- Admissions
- Direct Care

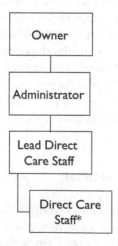

*Number of Direct Care Staff variable based upon number and needs of residents

FIGURE 3.1   Sample organizational pattern for a smaller facility (board and care).

- Dietary
- Laundry
- Housekeeping
- Maintenance

However, depending on the size and model of the facility, staffing levels and organizational patterns will vary greatly. Figure 3.1 illustrates a sample organizational pattern for a smaller, board and care type of facility. Figure 3.2 illustrates a sample organizational pattern for a mid-sized or hospitality model facility, and Figure 3.3 illustrates a sample organizational pattern for a larger or new model facility.

BUSINESS MODELS

For-Profit Versus Non-Profit

Both for-profit and non-profit investors will want to see a well managed operation. For-profit investors look for low costs, which means more profit for the organization. Non-profit investors, on the other hand, are actually investing in a cause, so they want to see as much money as possible go toward that cause, not toward overhead. As an administrator, you should keep in mind that any plan you put together should build the case that you can operate the facility well and deliver what you claim to offer.

Profit Investors

For profit investors want to see a profitable business that offers a safe, high return on their money. You'll need to demonstrate there's a market for your product or service that's willing to pay for it out of their own pockets. If you're starting a facility, for example, investors want assurance that in your location, there's enough demand at the price you charge to make a good business. Furthermore, since for-profit investors want their money back, the business must either generate a lot of cash or be a good acquisition candidate. The emphasis is on profit, so much so that in some cases, companies may change their line of business in order to reach their goals.

Non-Profit Investors

Non-profit investors are usually funded by foundations or people who want to see the organization provide a community service. They are concerned about what you will accomplish and how you'll get the results

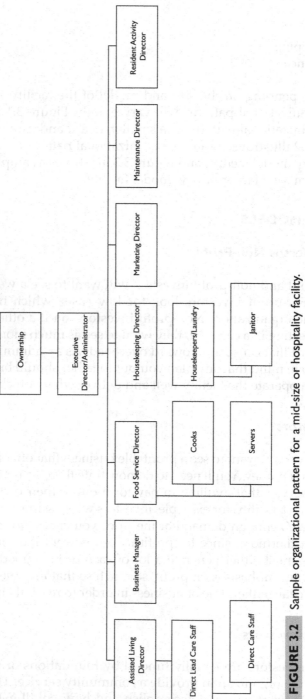

FIGURE 3.2 Sample organizational pattern for a mid-size or hospitality facility.

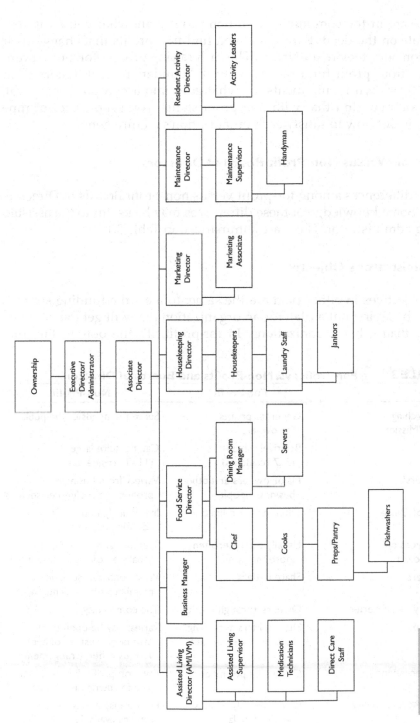

FIGURE 3.3 Sample organizational pattern for a large or new model facility.

they want in the community. In a non-profit plan, what you do is concentrate on the deed. Rarely will you find non-profits that change their mission once they're underway. The cash raising process for a non-profit differs from profit fund raising as well. Foundations and donors often have their own requirements for what goes into a non-profit proposal, and you may find that with non-profit status, you spend a lot of time figuring out how to satisfy each organization's requirements.

For-Profit Versus Non-Profit Board of Directors

Some differences among for-profit versus non-profit Boards of Directors exist. Some knowledge of these differences may be useful to the assisted living administrator. These are summarized in Table 3.1.

Administrator's Objective

The objectives in either plan are the same: to meet the funding source's needs by laying out a plan for an organization that will get the job done better than other organizations. In for-profit, it's the bottom line that

TABLE 3.1	For-Profits vs. Non-Profits and Boards of Directors	
	For-Profit	**Non-Profit**
Overarching Goal/Mission	Generate profits for owners	Serve the needs of the public
Size	Relatively small (3–7 residents)	Can be quite large (11–35 residents)
Membership	Major owners and other business people	Variety from business, professional, volunteer sectors
Term of Office	Often no term limits	Increasingly, non-profits are adopting term limits
Employees on the Board	Usually the case; often more than one	Typically, only the CEO and usually ex officio (non-voting)
"Owners"	Shareholders	Varies: public, association members, donors, church, etc.
Primary Beneficiaries	Owners, through profits	The community
Elections	Shareholders according to # of shares owned	Varies: May be open to all members, trustees only, or various other arrangements
Compensation	Often paid per meeting	Few non-profit directors are paid for being on the board
Public Accountability	Discloses only what is required by law	High transparency — tax returns available on line

counts, and your facility's plan will be geared around that. In non-profits, it's what you do that matters, so you should set a business plan to meet that need.

SPECIFIC AFFILIATIONS

Assisted living facilities may sometimes cater to the specific needs of special populations. Although these facilities do not discriminate against any person and still must comply with state regulations, they may offer services that are designed to benefit a distinct population where common

Religious

Catholic Health Services

A middle ground between independent living and nursing homes, Catholic Health Services' assisted living facilities aim to foster as much autonomy as the resident is capable of. Assisted living provides a balance of residential living, medical and recreational services, and assistance with day-to-day living activities.

Pastoral and spiritual care services are integral to the health care and services of the Catholic Health Services organization. Pastoral and spiritual care offers healing, sustaining, guiding, reconciling, and counseling services. Pastoral Care is provided to patients, their families, and staff; giving spiritual support with respect for each person's faith, tradition, and spiritual perspective, and functioning in an interdisciplinary manner with other health care colleagues.

Because the human person is by nature spiritual, pastoral care seeks to honor and facilitate the search for meaning and integrity in the experiences of life including sickness, death and bereavement, by offering presence, compassion, listening, support and education.

Source: www.catholichealthservices.org

FIGURE 3.4 Catholic assisted living model.

values, language, food, and customs are promoted. Examples include affiliations such as religious, ethnicity, gender, or lesbian/gay/bisexual/transgender as seen in Figures 3.4 through 3.7.

Ethnic

Kokoro Assisted Living

Kokoro Assisted Living is a non-profit housing community dedicated to helping seniors to live in dignity and comfort. Kokoro seeks to promote and enhance the independence, well-being, and security of older people through the provision of housing and assisted living services in a Japanese culture-centered environment.

Over seventeen years ago, the idea of Kokoro Assisted Living began. In 1990, Pine Methodist Church formed a committee known as the Japanese American Skilled Nursing Home Project Committee to augment the culturally sensitive services available to older adults. The committee found that Nisei (second generation Japanese Americans) preferred to remain in their homes for as long as possible, and that there was a strong need for in-home services. In 1995, the committee joined with the Japanese American Religious Federation (JARF) to form the JARF Senior Housing Task Force. After extensive research, the task force changed its focus to assisted living. In 1996, JARF Senior Housing Task Force bid for the ability to develop a piece of land on the corner of Bush and Laguna Street in San Francisco's Japantown. They won the bid and purchased the land for one dollar. In order to move to the next stage of financing, construction and management of the project, a separate corporate entity was created, to be known as the Japanese American Religious Federation Assisted Living, Inc. (JALFI). JALFI named the project, "Kokoro," a Japanese term that communicates the combined notions of heart, mind and inner spirit as it reflects the true vision of the project.

Source: www.kokoroassistedliving.org

FIGURE 3.5   Japanese assisted living model.

Gender

University Mound Ladies Home

Mission: Our mission is to provide high-quality, affordable assisted living for women.

We serve women from diverse cultural, linguistic backgrounds in a beautiful, home-like

environment.

We offer an alternative to board-and-care facilities for women who want a higher level of

socialization. We strive to promote aging in place, including palliative and hospice care.

History: The University Mound Ladies Home has evolved over the past 125 years to

meet the changing needs of older women in San Francisco. Here's a look back at how far

we've come.

The original Lick Old Ladies Home, established in 1884 with a $100,000 bequest from

James Lick, was a large, three-story wooden building on 25 acres of land at the present

location.

In 1932, the Home's present Colonial Revival building was constructed at 350 University

Street. The Ladies Home's Matron lived on the premises, and the chief nurse and her

husband, two kitchen helpers, and the chef lived in rooms on the second floor.

Today's University Mound Ladies Home represents a collaboration between eldercare

professionals and laypeople, assisted by area universities and city government, all

seeking to fully realize the vision of this treasured institution: to provide older women

with affordable, compassionate care in a beautiful, homelike setting.

Source: www.ladieshome.org

FIGURE 3.6 Gender-specialty assisted living model.

Lesbian/Gay/Bisexual/Transgender

Rainbow Vision

Rainbow Vision Properties is the dream that all of our hearts made, come true. The team that drives the vision combines a unique set of skills around leadership in the LGBT community, senior housing, community building and design.

Every aspect of Rainbow Vision is a celebration of community. We are a place where your neighbors are your family and everyone belongs. The experience of people being together and sharing in the same values and activities is what creates a community.

Source: www.rainbowvisionprop.com

FIGURE 3.7 LGBT assisted living model.

FUTURE LANDSCAPE

Looking forward to the future, the Green House Project is one example of a new model of assisted living philosophy being adopted and integrated by assisted living communities across the nation (Figure 3.8).

THE GREEN HOUSE® model creates a small intentional community for a group of elders and staff. It is a place that focuses on life, and its heart is found in the relationships that flourish there. A radical departure from traditional skilled nursing homes and assisted living facilities, The Green House model alters facility size, interior design, staffing patterns, and methods of delivering skilled professional services. Its primary purpose is to serve as a place where elders can receive assistance and support with activities of daily living and clinical care, without the assistance and care becoming the focus of their existence. Developed by Dr. William Thomas and rooted in the tradition of the Eden Alternative, a model for cultural change within nursing facilities, The Green House model is intended to de-institutionalize long-term care by eliminating large nursing facilities, and creating habilitative, social settings.

Source: www.ncbcapitalimpact.org

FIGURE 3.8 Green House project.

CONCLUSIONS

This chapter has provided the reader with an overview of organizational patterns and models in the assisted living industry. Variety exists among organizations greatly due to varying sizes and service models. Typical organizational patterns for common models are illustrated. Examples of specific affiliation models show that assisted living is emerging and advancing to serve a diverse population with varying needs. This chapter illustrates the need for today's assisted living administrators to be well informed and remain attuned to the evolving needs, practices, and models in the industry.

REFERENCES

Catholic Health Services. (2009). *Assisted living facilities.* Retrieved June 2, 2009, from http://www.catholichealthservices.org/?id=11&sid=1

Frank, J. (2001). How long can I stay? The dilemma of aging in place in assisted living. *Journal of Housing for the Elderly, 15,* 5–30.

Gilchrist, E. (2009). *Job satisfaction and communication competence of assisted living facility managers as related to facility and employment demographics.* Paper presented at the annual meeting of the NCA 94th Annual Convention, TBA, San Diego, CA. Retrieved June 1, 2009, from http://www.allacademic.com/meta/p256999_index.html

Hawes, C., Phillips, C., & Rose, M. (2000). *High service or high privacy assisted living facilities, their residents and staff: Results from a national survey.* Washington, DC: U.S. Department of Health and Human Services.

Hawes, C., Phillips, C., Rose, M., Holan, S., & Sherman, M. (2003). A national study of assisted living facilities. *The Gerontologist, 43,* 875–882.

Kokoro Assisted Living. (2009). *An assisted living community.* Retrieved June 10, 2009, from http://www.kokoroassistedliving.org/templates/System/details.asp?id=39813&PID=475397

Lawton, M. P. (1990). Knowledge resources and gaps in housing for the aged. In D. Tilson (Ed.), *Aging in place: Supporting the frail elderly in residential environments.* Glenview, IL: Professional Books on Aging, Scott, Foresman and Company.

National Center for Assisted Living. (2009). *Assisted living facility profile.* Retrieved June 1, 2009, from http://www.ncal.org/about/facility.cfm

NCB Capitol Impact. (2009). *The Greenhouse replication initiative.* Retrieved June 1, 2009, http://www.ncbcapitalimpact.org/default.aspx?id=146

Rainbow Vision Properties Inc. (2009). *Vision realized.* Retrieved June 1, 2009, from http://www.rainbowvisionprop.com/company.html

University Mound Ladies Home. (2009). *Affordable, compassionate assisted living for women since 1884.* Retrieved August 10, 2009, from http://www.ladieshome.org.

CHAPTER **4**

Recruiting and Hiring Staff

Learning Objectives

Upon the completion of Chapter 4, the reader will be able to:

- *Describe the assisted living workforce.*
- *Discuss the challenges of workforce recruitment in assisted living.*
- *Understand a variety of factors that influence workforce recruitment in long-term care.*
- *Identify the steps in the recruitment and hiring process.*
- *Recognize the importance of written job requirements and job descriptions.*
- *Identify the legal issues surrounding recruitment and hiring.*

INTRODUCTION

This chapter addresses critical issues in the recruitment and hiring of personnel for an assisted living facility. Background information is included, such as a description of the assisted living workforce and the challenges of workforce recruitment. Factors that influence workforce recruitment are discussed. For example, issues such as the economy, pay and benefits, working conditions, education, and training are discussed to provide an understanding of the complexity of today's long-term care workforce. The five steps on the recruitment process (i.e., planning, searching, screening, selection and hiring, and maintaining an applicant pool) are then described in detail with examples to assist the reader in understanding the included concepts.

The Assisted Living Workforce

Providing formalized long-term care in an assisted living facility requires an adequate, skilled, and diverse workforce. Paraprofessionals (i.e., unlicensed, direct care staff) represent the largest component of personnel in long-term care and will likely make up the majority of an assisted living facility's staff. All facilities employ a licensed or certified administrator and many larger facilities also employ licensed nurses (i.e., registered nurses, licensed vocational nurses). Other employed or typical personnel include those who work in various support departments such as business (e.g., accounting, marketing), dietary (e.g., cooks, dieticians), personal support (e.g., activities, social services), laundry, housekeeping, and maintenance. Other professionals necessary for the provision of long-term care include physicians, social workers, therapists, pharmacists, podiatrists, dentists, and mental health providers. These other professionals are typically third party contractors that provide services to the residents, and are not employed by the assisted living facility.

Challenges of Workforce Recruitment

The recruitment and hiring of quality personnel is a growing challenge for assisted living facilities. Assisted living facilities face the same workforce issues as other long-term care facilities. This is especially true for paraprofessionals (i.e., direct care staff) due to low wages and benefits, hard working conditions, and work that is stigmatized by society (Stone & Weiner, 2001).

The Institute for the Future of Aging Services (2007), in their report to the National Commission for Quality Long-Term Care, described three main concerns relative to today's long-term care workforce:

1. There is a well-documented shortage of competent professional and paraprofessional personnel to manage, supervise and provide long-term care services in facility-based and home care settings—the result is high turnover, large numbers of vacancies, and difficulty attracting new employees.
2. The instability of today's long-term care workforce has contributed to:

   a. service access problems for consumers and in many cases, has seriously compromised their safety, quality of care, and quality of life;
   b. excessive provider costs due to the need to continuously recruit and train new personnel, and use temporary higher-cost contract staff;

c. extreme workloads for both nurses and paraprofessional staff, inadequate supervision, less time for new staff to learn their jobs, and high accident and injury rates exceeding those in the construction and mining industries.

3. As a result of a growing demand from aging baby boomers and a shrinking of the traditional caregiver labor pool, the future will be immeasurably worse without decisive action by both the public and private sectors.

Paraprofessional workers or direct care staff makes up the majority of the long-term care workforce (Stone & Weiner, 2001). As with many caregiving jobs, the majority of direct care staff are women. There is a significant geographic variation in the race and ethnicity profile of direct care workers. In some areas, more minority workers are available and willing to work in long-term care. Direct care workers most often have some economic disadvantages, such as low levels of education and low household earnings. These "frontline" workers engage in very demanding and important work, but the occupation itself is relatively low paying.

FACTORS INFLUENCING WORKFORCE RECRUITMENT

The Economy

The current state of the economy and labor market influence directly impacts assisted living facilities' ability to recruit and hire staff. For example, if unemployment is low (in a strong economy), persons who considered a job in long-term care may have other options available. If the labor market is less competitive, it may be easier to attract personnel.

Pay and Benefits

Pay and benefit considerations are critical for attracting personnel. This is especially problematic with the paraprofessional workforce in long-term care because wages and benefits are typically quite low considering the level of responsibility expected, difficult workloads and high injury rates. The actual level at which salaries would have to be set to attract adequate personnel for assisted living facilities is unknown. The assisted living facilities' ability to provide health care insurance and other benefits, such as vacation time and other fringe benefits, may improve their ability of attracting potential applicants.

Working Conditions

The way in which an assisted living workplace is organized and managed affects the working conditions. The utilization of mentoring, coaching and collective involvement of staff in decision making is a way to create positive working conditions. Nurses and aides often complain about managers who lack respect for the knowledge and skills they bring to the job and refuse to share information.

Image of the Industry

Workforce recruitment in long-term care is often difficult because of the image of the industry. Although assisted living facilities may not be as affected as nursing homes in this regard, ageism in society coupled with media reports of poor care quality, scandals, and abuse can bias the view of the public. Frontline worker jobs in long-term care are sometimes viewed by the public as unpleasant and poor paying.

Education and Training

The professional and paraprofessional workforce often lacks the necessary training to address the special health and medical care needs of the frail elderly. Standards for direct care staff training are often minimal and not specific. Few nurses or physicians specialize in geriatrics. Long-term care is not a traditional component of a nursing curriculum. Administrator requirements vary by state, but are often inadequate.

Transportation

The ease of which potential employees can commute to the facility will impact the geographic area from which employees can be recruited. The availability of an efficient public transportation system will improve the ability to hire employees who do not drive. This may be especially true in regards to direct care staff.

THE RECRUITMENT PROCESS

Recruitment is the process of sourcing, screening, and selecting people for a job or vacancy within an organization. Figure 4.1 lists the main components of the recruitment process that will then be discussed in detail.

```
1. Planning

2. Searching

3. Screening

4. Selection and Hiring

5. Maintaining Applicant Pool
```

FIGURE 4.1 Steps in the recruitment process.

Planning

Planning recruitment efforts begins with forecasting employment needs. The assisted living administrator is responsible for projecting the needs (e.g., number of residents, levels of care) of the facility, and identifying the personnel requirements necessary to meet those needs. Advanced planning for employment needs are critical to the success of the facility.

Projections

Advanced knowledge of trends in the industry can assist in the planning of recruiting employees. As noted earlier, consider the factors that influence workforce availability (i.e., labor market and economy, wages and benefits, education and training, image of the industry, transportation). The Department of Labor and the Employment Security Commission (within individual states) may also be a source of information to consider in the planning phase.

Job Requirements

Defining job requirements is a necessary and essential step in the planning of recruitment. In assisted living facilities, some job requirements are mandated by state regulation (e.g., criminal background checks, education and experience). Job requirements for direct care staff are minimal, and training is often completed on the job (see Chapter 5 for training topics for direct care staff). Requirements for the administrator are specific to each state (see Table 4.1 for a summary of current state requirements).

TABLE 4.1	State Requirements for the Assisted Living Administrators	
State	**Initial Licensure**	**Continuing Education**
Alabama	Licensed by the assisted living administrator Licensure Board.	6 hours per year.
Alaska	Administrator must be at least 21 years of age, complete an approved training course, relevant experience and adequate education and training. A criminal background investigation is required.	18 hours per year.
Arizona	Managers must be at least 21 years of age and certified assisted living facility managers.	6-12 hours per year depending on scope.
Arkansas	Administrator must be at least 21 years of age, have a high school diploma or a GED, complete a state criminal background check, and be a certified assisted living facility administrator through approved program.	6 hours per year.
California	Administrators must complete a 40-hour initial Certification Training Program from an approved training vendor and pass a written test. Additional college education is required depending on the capacity of the facility.	40 hours every 2 years; must include 8 hours in dementia education.
Colorado	Administrator must have the equivalent of 30 hours of training in 15 required topics and 15 hours of training pertinent to the care needs of the residents served by the facility.	Not specified.
Connecticut	No administrator is required. The supervisor of assisted living services must be a registered nurse specified education and experience.	Not specified.

(Continued)

TABLE 4.1	State Requirements for the Assisted Living Administrators (*Continued*)	
State	**Initial Licensure**	**Continuing Education**
Delaware	A nursing home administrator license is required with reduced requirements for facilities with four beds or fewer.	Per state law for nursing home administrators.
District of Columbia	Variable depending on facility license. Residence director or administrator must be at least 21 years of age. Education and experience variable depending of facility type and size.	Not specified.
Florida	Administrators must have a high school diploma or GED, complete a core training program, and pass a competency test.	12 hours every 2 years.
Georgia	Not specified.	16 hours per year.
Hawaii	Administrator must have at least two years of relevant experience. The completion of an assisted living facility administrator's course is required.	Not specified.
Idaho	Administrators must be licensed by the state.	12 hours per year.
Illinois	Administrator must be a high school graduate or equivalent and at least 21 years of age.	6 hours per year if providing dementia care.
Indiana	Administrators must have specified required education (BA or higher; AA in health care or long-term health care study program) plus completion of required training program.	40 hours every 2 years.
Iowa	The administrator must be at least 18 years of age.	2 hours per year if providing dementia care.

(Continued)

TABLE 4.1   State Requirements for the Assisted Living Administrators (*Continued*)

State	Initial Licensure	Continuing Education
Kansas	Operators must be 21 years of age, possess a high school diploma or equivalent, and hold a Kansas license as an adult care home administrator, or engage in an operator training program.	50 hours every 2 years.
Kentucky	Not specified.	Annual in-service education required.
Louisiana	Administrators must be at least 21 years of age.	12 hours per year.
Maine	Administrators must be at least 21 years of age with additional education and experience requirements depending on level of care.	12 hours per year
Maryland	Assisted living manager must be at least 21 years of age and possess a high school diploma or equivalent and complete an approved 80-hour training program.	Not specified.
Massachusetts	Manager of a facility must be at least 21 years of age; hold a Bachelor's degree or have equivalent experience, including supervisory and management skills.	10 hours per year plus addition for specialized care.
Michigan	Variable depending on facility type – specified education, training, experience and competencies.	Variable by facility type; up to 16 hours per year.
Minnesota	Not specified.	Not specified.
Mississippi	Operators must be at least 21 years of age, be a high school graduate or have passed the GED and not be a resident of the licensed facility. Two days training with licensing agency. Abuse clearance required.	Not specified.

(Continued)

TABLE 4.1	State Requirements for the Assisted Living Administrators (Continued)	
State	**Initial Licensure**	**Continuing Education**
Missouri	Variable by facility type. Must be a licensed nursing home administrator or a manager who is at least 21 years of age without history of offense in long-term care setting. Medication and dementia training.	Attend one department approved workshop per year.
Montana	Variable by facility levels. Administrator license or valid nursing home administrator license, or have completed all of the self-study modules of "The Management Library for Administrators and Executive Directors."	16 hours per year plus additional 8 depending on facility level.
Nebraska	Administrators must be 21 years of age or older. Completed initial, department-approved training that is at least 30 hours and includes six specific topic areas. Hospital licensed nursing home administrators are exempt from this training requirement.	12 hours per year unless exempt by licensure.
Nevada	Administrators must be licensed by the Nevada State Board of Examiners for Administrators of Facilities for Long-Term Care. Trained in first aid and CPR. Plus additional 3 years relevant experience for Alzheimer's facility.	8 hours per year.
New Hampshire	Administrator shall (1) be at least 21 years of age; (2) not have been convicted of a misdemeanor or felony; and (3) have three letters of reference. Additional education and experience requirements according to facility size.	12 hours per year.

(Continued)

TABLE 4.1	State Requirements for the Assisted Living Administrators (*Continued*)	
State	**Initial Licensure**	**Continuing Education**
New Jersey	Administrators must be at least 21 years of age and possess a high school diploma or equivalent. Administrators must also either hold a current New Jersey license as a nursing home administrator or be a New Jersey certified assisted living administrator.	30 hours every 3 years.
New Mexico	Administrators must be at least 21 years of age, possess management and administrative skills, have a high school diploma or equivalent, and are financially solvent.	Not specified.
New York	Administrators generally must be at least 21 years of age and have varying levels of education and experience based in part on the number of residents in the facility.	60 hours every 2 years.
North Carolina	Adult care home administrators must be certified by the state, which requires completion of a 120-hour administrator-in-training program.	30 hours every 2 years.
North Dakota	None specified.	12 hours per year.
Ohio	Administrators must be 21 years of age and be licensed as a nursing home administrator or have 3,000 hours of direct operational responsibility or complete 100 credit hours of relevant post-high school education.	9 hours per year.

(Continued)

TABLE 4.1	State Requirements for the Assisted Living Administrators (*Continued*)	
State	**Initial Licensure**	**Continuing Education**
Oklahoma	An administrator must either hold a nursing home administrator's license, a residential care home administrator's certificate of training, or a nationally recognized assisted living certificate of training and competency approved by the Department of Health.	16 hours per year.
Oregon	The administrator is required to be at least 21 years of age, have specified education and experience. Additionally, all administrators must: (1) Complete a state-approved training course of at least 40 hours.	20 hours per year.
Pennsylvania	An administrator must meet specified education and experience requirements; be at least 21 years of age, complete an orientation program approved and administered by the Department and pass Department-approved competency based training test.	24 hours per year.
Rhode Island	The Department of Health Facilities shall issue an initial certificate for an administrator of an assisted living residence for a period of up to one year if the applicant meets all of the specified educational, training, and experience requirements. A written examination may be required.	32 hours every 2 years.
South Carolina	Administrators must have an associate's degree, at least one year of experience, and be licensed by the South Carolina Board of Long-Term Care Administrators.	18 hours per year.

(Continued)

TABLE 4.1	State Requirements for the Assisted Living Administrators (*Continued*)	
State	**Initial Licensure**	**Continuing Education**
South Dakota	Administrators must be licensed health care professionals or hold a high school diploma or equivalent and complete a training program and competency evaluation.	Not specified.
Tennessee	Administrators must hold a high school diploma or equivalent must not have been convicted of a criminal offense involving abuse or neglect of elderly. An administrator must be certified by the Board for Licensing Health Care Facilities (nursing home administrators exempt).	24 hours every 2 years.
Texas	Specified educational requirements according to facility size. Managers must complete a 24-hour course in assisted living management within their first year of employment.	12 hours per year.
Utah	Administrators must be 21 years of age and successfully complete criminal background screening. Educational and certification requirements vary by facility type.	None specified.
Vermont	The director must have completed a state-approved certification course or specified experience or education.	20 hours per year.
Virginia	Variable by facility type. For facilities licensed for residential living care only, an administrator must be a high school graduate or have a GED, and specified experience or education. For facilities licensed for assisted living care, additional educational and experience requirements apply. After January 2009, licensure will be required.	20 hours per year.

(*Continued*)

TABLE 4.1	State Requirements for the Assisted Living Administrators *(Continued)*	

State	Initial Licensure	Continuing Education
Washington	The administrator must be at least 21 years of age and not a resident of the boarding home. Very specific combinations of education, training, and experience qualify a person to be a boarding home administrator.	10 hours per year.
West Virginia	For large facilities, the administrator must be at least 21 years of age and hold an Associate's degree or its equivalent in a related field. For small facilities, the administrator must be 21 years of age and have a high school diploma or GED. Requirements vary by facility type.	8 hours per year.
Wisconsin	Variable by facility type. Must be at least 21 years of age; education and experience vary by facility type. Specified training varies by experience level. Administrators must have a clean criminal background check.	12 hours per year.
Wyoming	The manager must be at least 21 years of age; pass an open book test on the state's assisted living licensure and program administration rules, and meet specific additional education and experience requirements.	16 hours per year.

Source: National Center for Assisted Living (2008), *Assisted Living Regulatory Review 2008.*

Remember, state requirements are only minimal standards, and assisted living facilities may consider higher standards regarding job requirements for personnel.

When defining job requirements, the assisted living administrator must understand the responsibilities involved with the job, the tasks involved with the job, and the background (i.e., education and experience) necessary to complete the job. In addition, consider the personal characteristics that may be required (e.g., interpersonal skills, decision-making skills, motivation), the culture of the facility, and managerial style of the administrator.

Job Descriptions

Well-developed job descriptions are imperative to the planning phase of recruitment. Job descriptions are often utilized to establish salary ranges, define performance expectations, and evaluate performance, but they can also be very useful in a successful recruitment plan. Job descriptions contain detailed information on the skills, knowledge, abilities, and experience that a candidate should possess for a specific job. Keep in mind that state regulations sometimes include specifics on what must be included in job description of assisted living personnel. Figure 4.2 illustrates a list of information typically included in a job description.

---

1. Position title, name of the specific unit (if indicated), and name of the facility.

2. Duties, essential job functions, and responsibilities of the position.

3. Education, training experience, and licensure requirements.

4. Knowledge, skills, and abilities necessary to perform assigned duties.

5. Reporting relationships (i.e., hiring manager, reporting manager).

6. Hours and location of work.

7. Pay grade and salary ranges (optional).

8. Background characteristics required.

9. Personal characteristics required.

10. Continuing education and training required to maintain competence.

11. Other specifications of the position, such as legal requirements.

FIGURE 4.2 Information to be included in job description.

Searching

The search process will vary depending on the type of position being filled. For example, strategies that may be appropriate for the recruitment of an administrator, may be very different from the recruiting of direct care staff. Recruitment plans should be developed accordingly, and incorporate strategies that have worked in the past, as well as allow for new ideas. If a facility has a very limited candidate pool, the development of a continuous recruitment plan may be appropriate. There are both internal and external sources for recruitment. Of course, the facility should choose the method that is likely to produce the best results.

Internal Sources

Recruitment from individuals from within an organization can be beneficial for several reasons. Internal recruitment often allows for internal growth opportunities and may also result in greater retention, as well as improved staff morale and loyalty. Internal recruitment may be less expensive, less time consuming, and less disruptive to a facility. Internal recruitment may be facilitated by posting notices of a job opening within the organization prior to the information being published outside of the organization. Figure 4.3 lists some ideas for internal recruitment. For example, postings may be distributed by memorandum e-mail, voice mail, newsletters, bulletin boards, or announcements at staff meetings. The development of internal career ladders (i.e., a path in which in employee may hope to progress within a facility) may also be an important internal source of recruitment.

```
1.  Bulletin Board Notices

2.  Staff Meeting Announcements

3.  Internal email

4.  Development of Career Ladders
```

FIGURE 4.3 Internal sources for recruitment.

1. Advertisements in professional journals, newspapers, professional newsletters, and internet postings.

2. Personnel placement service provided by national or state agencies.

3. Events, such as educational sessions or community outreach programs.

4. Community job fairs.

5. Educational Institutions. Consider recruitment visits to colleges and universities, as well as possible internships for qualified students.

6. Referrals from employees, residents, families, assisted living facilities, and provider organizations.

FIGURE 4.4   External sources for recruitment.

External Sources

External recruitment sources expand the number of potential candidates. This can be beneficial because it decreases the reliance on seniority as a primary basis for promotion, as well as bring new talent and experience to the facility. Potential methods for recruiting candidates from external sources are seen in Figure 4.4.

Screening

Applicant screening involves the elimination of unqualified applicants from the recruitment pool. To start, it is easiest to eliminate those with valid reasons for exclusion such as inadequate education or experience, or failure to pass a criminal background check. Reviewing job applications, resumes, and reference checks are common ways to learn about applicants. It is important to consider professionalism, experience, enthusiasm, and a desire to work with elderly persons when reviewing applications.

If multiple applicants are identified as candidates, consider an initial screening interview. This interview can be briefly conducted to assess the suitability of a candidate for a position. A telephone interview may be appropriate especially if the candidate lives far from the facility, or to save time.

Selection and Hiring

There are many aspects to consider during the selection and hiring process. For example, you will need to consider the legal aspects, the interview process, and background verification. Additionally, deciding to hire and then offering the job is a part of this process.

Legal Aspects

There are a number of federal laws that employers must consider and follow when hiring employees (U.S. Department of Labor, 2008). In general, these laws prohibit discrimination in employment decisions based on race, color, religion, sex, age, ethnic/national origin, disability, or veteran status. The U.S. Department of Labor administers and enforces laws affecting the hiring of employees under the age of 18, veterans, and certain foreign workers. The U.S. Department of Labor is also responsible for laws that ensure that federal contractors and grantees provide equal employment opportunity to applicants and employees. Three important examples of legal concerns (U.S. Department of Labor, 2008) which may affect the hiring process include:

1. Equal Employment Opportunity. EEO laws prohibit specific types of employment discrimination. These laws prohibit discrimination on the basis of race, color, religion, sex, age, national origin, or status as an individual with a disability, or protected veteran.
2. Hiring People with Disabilities. The U.S. Department of Labor (DOL) enforces laws prohibiting discrimination against individuals with disabilities, and allowing payment of special minimum wage rates to certain individuals with disabilities.
3. Hiring Foreign Workers. The U.S. Department of Labor's (DOL) responsibilities regarding foreign workers includes certification of positions for temporary and permanent employment of aliens, as well as hiring and wage issues. Foreign labor certification programs permit U.S. employers to hire foreign workers on a temporary or permanent basis to fill jobs essential to the U.S. economy. These programs are generally designed to ensure that the admission of foreign workers into the United States on a permanent or temporary basis will not adversely affect the job opportunities, wages, and working conditions of U.S. workers.

Keep in mind that there are many other legal aspects of employment law that you must follow both in hiring and maintain personnel. A full description is beyond the scope of this book, but as an administrator you must become familiar with all applicable state, federal and local laws.

Interviews

The goal of the interview process is to successfully match the best available candidate to a specific position. Successful interview should allow for a prediction of future performance of candidates.

The individual interview is the most common type of interview. Individual interviews are simple, easier to schedule, and allow for a consistent perspective. They may be less intimidating to the candidate, and therefore easier to more accurately evaluate the applicant, as well as allow the applicant an opportunity to ask questions.

Another type of interview is a group interview where members of a team interview the candidate individually and then pool results, or interview the candidate as a group. This is more commonly utilized when attempting to hire a nurse or administrator than with direct care personnel. The team approach can be advantageous because it can offer multiple perspectives. Group interviews are much more time consuming and may be more intimidating for a candidate. However, group interviews can foster an ideal of teamwork, and a shared sense of responsibility.

A successful interview is an effective interview. Characteristics of an effective interview process are illustrated in Figure 4.5.

Interview methods are variable. Some interviews are more structured while others are non-directive, and allow the candidate more freedom to both answer and ask questions. While a structured interview may have very specific questions, less structured interviews may ask broader, open-ended questions, and allow for more engagement with the candidate. Figure 4.6 gives some example interview questions.

Understanding unlawful questions and inquiries is critical to the interview process. Figure 4.7 lists subjects inappropriate for interviews.

Background Verification

If a candidate is of serious consideration for a position, the accuracy of all information provided by the candidate should be verified. It is important to obtain a signed request for references so that information may be obtained, especially from previous employers. In addition, the following are important sources of background verification:

1. Providing information to the candidate about the facility, the agenda for the interview, and the job description.
2. The interview should be carefully planned. Allow adequate time for each part of the process.
3. Interviewers should be prepared. Information previously submitted by the candidate should be reviewed in advance of the interview.
4. Carefully planned questions should be developed in advance. Open-ended questions allow for more dialogue and a better understanding of the applicant's suitability. Take special care to maintain compliance with laws and regulations regarding suitable questions.
5. In order to create a means of comparison, a core group of questions should be established that will be asked of all candidates.
6. The interviewer should maintain focus of the criteria for the position and the qualifications of the candidates. Remember, the goal is to match the best candidate with the open position.
7. The interviewer should give the candidate a realistic perspective of the job, including favorable and unfavorable information.
8. Standards for performance and methods of evaluation should be carefully explained to the candidate. A discussion of professional growth should be included.
9. Provide the candidate with a description of employee benefits associated with the job. For example, health insurance, vacation leave, and retirement benefits.
10. Include a discussion of both initial salary and salary ranges.
11. A description of the likely work schedule should be reviewed with the candidate. Expectations regarding weekends and holidays is especially important in a long-term care facility.
12. If possible, include a tour of the facility.
13. A follow-up letter should be sent regardless if the candidate is hired or not. Thank the applicant and indicate any next steps. Well-organized communication improves the recruitment process.

FIGURE 4.5 Characteristics of an effective interview process.

1. Personal Traits / Motivations:
   a. What motivates you to do best work?
   b. Provide an example of when you went "out of your way" to get a job done.
   c. What do you think the advantages of this type of work are?
   d. What do you think the disadvantages of this type of work are?
   e. How do you define doing a good job?
   f. What makes a job enjoyable for you?
   g. Under what conditions do you work best?

2. Goals:
   h. Tell me what success means to you.
   i. Do you consider yourself successful?
   j. Do you set goals for yourself and how do you do that?
   k. Tell me your 5 year goal.

3. Communication:
   l. Tell me how you best communicate.
   m. Tell me about a work situation you had that required excellent communication skills.
   n. How would you grade your ability to communicate with management, customers, and peers?

4. Flexibility:
   o. How important is communication and interaction with others on your job?
   p. How many departments did you deal with?
   q. What problems occurred?
   r. In what areas do you typically have the least amount of patience at work?

5. Stress:
   s. You have worked in a fast paced environment. How did you like the environment?
   t. What kinds of decisions are most difficult for you?
   u. What is the most difficult work situation you have faced?

6. Skill Level:
   v. What are your present job responsibilities?
   w. What are your greatest strengths on the job?
   x. What areas need improvement?
   y. Provide me with an example of an on the job problem you were able to solve.
   z. How would you describe your professional competence?

FIGURE 4.6 Example interview questions.

1. Age

2. National origin

3. Religion

4. Race

5. Marital or family status

6. Childcare arrangements or childbearing plans

7. Arrest records (although criminal background checks are required)

8. Financial information.

9. Military discharge status

10. Any general information that would point out handicaps or health problems unrelated to job performance.

FIGURE 4.7   Inappropriate interview subjects.

1. Criminal background checks are often included in state regulations and should be completed on all staff working in an assisted living facility. State and federal clearances are typically obtained through a fingerprint process.
2. Credit ratings are sometimes obtained, especially if the job requires financial responsibility. The employer must advise applicants that a credit report will be requested. If the candidate is rejected based upon the credit report, the name and address of the credit reporting agency must be given to the candidate in writing.
3. Physical examinations are required for assisted living facility personnel. Tests for communicable diseases such as tuberculosis are included. Pre-employment physicals should be done after a job offer has been made to avoid any issues with discriminations. The physical examination will establish the physical capability of the applicant to perform the job. Recently, tests for illicit drugs are sometimes included in the physical examination.

Deciding to Hire

The decision to hire is complex. Once the candidates have been interviewed, the administrators must make an objective evaluation of each candidate. Review the important aspects such as education and training, previous experience, job accomplishments, skills and knowledge, and personal attributes. The development of a rating system is sometimes a useful means to make objective hiring decisions. Despite efforts to maintain objectivity, evaluating candidates can still be subjective. Avoid being overly impressed with experience or maturity, or allowing personal biases influence your assessment. Each candidate should be reviewed on a case by case basis and decide if their skills and qualifications meet your facility's needs.

Offering the Job

Once the decision to hire has been made, the candidate should be informed. All information, such as proposed salary, job title, description, and start date should be clearly communicated verbally and in writing. If possible, a personnel handbook should be included that describes the facility's personnel policies. The process involved in the facility's hiring procedures, such as work eligibility forms, tax withholding forms, and other required paperwork must then be completed.

Maintaining Applicant Pool

Maintaining an applicant pool can be useful for future needs of the facility. If immediate selection is not anticipated, but the applicant is desirable, keep a file of applications and resumes. Keep applicants informed of their status indicating that they have not been selected for a current interview, but that their application will be kept on file for future needs.

CONCLUSIONS

A critical issue for today's assisted living facilities is the recruitment and hiring of capable staff who understand the needs of elderly residents. The administrator of the facility is responsible for identifying personnel who are committed to high quality long-term care. This chapter has identified some of the challenges that the administrator will face relative to workforce recruitment and hiring. A five-point recruitment process has been described in detail, including planning, searching, screening, selection and hiring, and maintaining an applicant pool. Possible approaches and examples were given to assist the reader in the application process of this job.

REFERENCES

Institute for the Future of Aging Services. (2007). *The long-term care workforce: Can this crisis be fixed? Problems, causes and options.* Washington, DC: American Association of Homes and Services for the Aging and the Institute for the Future of Aging Services. Retrieved July 15, 2008, from http://www.futureofaging.org/publications/pub_documents/LTCCommissionReport2007.pdf

National Center for Assisted Living. (2008). *Assisted living state regulatory review 2008.* Washington, DC: National Center for Assisted Living. Retrieved June 21, 2008, from http://www.ncal.org/about/2008_reg_review.pdf

Stone, R., & Weiner, J. (2001). *Who will care for us? Addressing the long-term care workforce crisis.* Washington, DC: The Urban Institute and the American Association of Homes and Services for the Aging. Retrieved July 15, 2008, from http://aspe.hhs.gov/daltcp/reports/ltcwf.pdf

United States Department of Labor. (2008). *Compliance assistance: Hiring issues.* Washington, DC: U.S. Department of Labor. Retrieved July 15, 2008, from http://www.dol.gov/compliance/topics/hiring-issues.htm

Training Staff

With Contributing Authors: Sandi Flores and Clara Allen

Learning Objectives

Upon the completion of Chapter 5, the reader will be able to:

- *Understand the importance of staff training in assisted living.*
- *Describe the value of orientation for assisted living employees.*
- *Recognize best practices in orientations of assisted living employees.*
- *Explain the training requirements of direct care staff in assisted living.*
- *Identify best practices and models in the training of assisted living direct care staff.*
- *Describe the use of learning circles as a model of training.*

INTRODUCTION

This chapter addresses critical factors in the training of staff in assisted living facilities. Administrators must insure that all staff are adequately trained. This chapter begins with a discussion of the importance of staff training and addresses some current concerns regarding training in assisted living facilities. Recommendations from national experts on the orientation for all assisted living staff, are included. States vary in the training requirements for direct staff and these variations are described for the reader. Finally, some model training program systems and materials are included from a leader in the training and education for assisted living facilities. The chapter concludes with a description of "The Learning Circle," a group training process that may be useful for assisted living administrators as training programs are developed.

The Importance of Staff Training

The importance of staff training long-term care facilities is often under-emphasized. There is a common misconception that long-term care requires less skills and knowledge than acute care. However, long-term care is complex and specialized, requiring distinct skills and knowledge.

Knowledgeable and skilled employees are the greatest asset to the assisted living facility, but training employees is challenging due to the costs and increased staff time, and workload involved in training new employees. Pressures to contain costs may sometimes reduced training budgets. At the same time, employees are faced with increasing resident acuity, changing demands and regulatory requirements. As a result, staff may lack the experience, knowledge, or skills to complete tasks expected of them. Generally, long-term care employees will recognize the importance of maintaining and developing critical skills and expertise, and will turn to their employers for appropriate resources, guidance, and assistance. If these resources are not provided, frustration grows and the consequence is often lower quality of care and increased turnover.

Training requirements are an important aspect component of quality assurance and quality improvement. The U.S. GAO (1999) identified insufficient and undertrained staff, low pay rates and high staff turnover as major contributors to quality of care problems in residential care/assisted living. Carlson (2005) raised concerns regarding the experience and training of direct care staff. While state laws and regulations consistently require certain minimum training to be provided to direct care staff, the specifics of the training is often left to the individual facilities. He cites numerous reports of the consequences of this inadequacy in training including incidence of staff failing to administer prescribed emergency medication for a diabetic, and failure of facility staff to recognize signs of acute infection resulting in the death of a resident (Carlson, 2005).

It is critical that assisted living staff be trained in a wide variety of areas to help them fulfill their job responsibilities. However, because assisted living communities may serve different populations, providers do need a certain amount of flexibility to determine the training needs of their staff. *The Assisted Living Federation of America (ALFA) supports training requirements that reflect the responsibilities of each particular position. Specialized training in dementia must be provided for staff caring for residents with these needs. Cardiopulmonary resuscitation (CPR) and First Aid training is encouraged for all staff, and at a minimum one CPR/First Aid trained person must be available in each community at all times* (Assisted Living Federation of America, 2009).

ORIENTATION FOR ASSISTED LIVING EMPLOYEES

The Assisted Living Workgroup (2003) provided the following recommendations based upon practice and research in long-term care facilities regarding orientation for all assisted living employees in their report, *Assuring Quality in Assisted Living: Guidelines for Federal and State Policy, State Regulations, and Operations,* to U.S. Senate Special Committee on Aging:

1. Within 14 days of employment, all assisted living staff shall successfully complete an orientation program designed by the facility to provide information on:
   a. The care philosophy of the assisted living facility.
   b. The understanding of dementia.
   c. The understanding of the common characteristics and conditions of the resident population served.
   d. Appropriate interaction with residents and family members.
   e. Customer service policies, including resident rights and recognizing and reporting of signs of abuse and neglect.
   f. Fire and life safety, emergency disaster plans, and emergency call systems.
   g. The use of facility equipment required for job performance.
   h. The facility's employment/human resource policies and procedures.
2. All staff shall have specific orientation relevant to their specific job assignments and responsibilities.
3. Contract staff should receive an orientation on topics relevant to their job tasks, including orientation of the facility's fire, life safety, emergency disaster plans, and emergency call systems.

DIRECT CARE STAFF

Direct Care Staff Training Requirements

In the report for the U.S. Department of Health and Human Services, Hawes and colleagues (1999), found that the types of training and orientation required for direct care staff varied across assisted living facilities, but overall, relatively little training was required. Of the unlicensed personnel, 75% were required to attend some kind of pre-service training. For those that did require training, the most common amount of required training was between 1 and 16 hours. In addition, only 11% of the staff who took the required training completed it before the start of work.

TABLE 5.1	Staff Training Requirements by State	
State	**Initial**	**Annual**
Alabama	Topics	Topics
Alaska	Topics	12 hours
Arizona	Topics/hours*	12 hours
Arkansas	Topics	6 hours
California	10 hours/topics	4 hours/topics
Colorado	Topics	Topics
Connecticut	10 hours/topics*	6 hours
Delaware	Topics	12 hours
District of Columbia	40 hours	12 hours
Florida	26 hours*	Not specified
Georgia	Topics	16 hours
Hawaii	Topics	6 hours
Idaho	16 hours	8 hours
Illinois	Topics	8 hours
Indiana	Topics	Topics/hours*
Iowa	Plan on file	Not specified
Kansas	Topics	Topics
Kentucky	Topics	Not specified
Louisiana	Topics	Annual plan
Maine	Complete course	8 hours/2 years
Maryland	Topics*	Topics
Massachusetts	7 hours/topics	10 hours/topics
Michigan	Topics	Not specified
Minnesota	Competency test	Not specified
Mississippi	Topics	Quarterly
Missouri*	1 hour/topics	Not specified
Montana	Topics/16 hours*	Not specified
Nebraska	4 hours	12 hours
Nevada*	4 hours	8 hours
New Hampshire	Topics	Topics
New Jersey	Complete course	20 hours/2 years*
New Mexico	Complete course	Topics
New York	40 hours*	12 hours

(Continued)

TABLE 5.1	Staff Training Requirements by State (*Continued*)	
State	**Initial**	**Annual**
North Carolina	80-hour course	Not specified
North Dakota	Topics	Topics
Ohio	Training course	6 hours/topics
Oklahoma*	8 hours	8 hours
Oregon	Topics	Not specified
Pennsylvania	Topics	12 hours
Rhode Island*	10 hours/topics	Not specified
South Carolina	Topics	General
South Dakota	Topics	Topics
Tennessee	Not specified	Not specified
Texas	16 hours	6 hours/topics
Utah	Topics	Topics
Vermont*	Topics	20 hours
Virginia	Topics	8 hours
Washington	Topics/competency test	Not specified
West Virginia	Topics	Topics
Wisconsin	Topics	Not specified
Wyoming	Topics	Not specified

Note. Rules specifying a number of hours also include topics that are covered. Rules listing only topics do not specify how many hours of training are needed.

* STATE NOTES:

AZ: Hours/topics vary by level of licensing.

CT: Aides must pass a competency exam.

FL: Core training for staff is 26 hours. Additional hours are required for specific tasks or settings (e.g., medication assistance).

IN: Nursing staff, 8 hours per year; non-nursing staff, 4 hours per year.

MD: For Medicaid waiver programs, 8 hours on medication administration is also required.

MO: Complete course for medication administration. Additional topics required for assisted living staff.

MT: Topics are listed for category A and 16 hours of training in services provided by category B facilities.

NV: Three hours additional training every 3 years for staff who assist with medications.

NJ: 20 hours every 2 years; medication aides, 10 hours every 2 years.

NY: Topics are specified in the Department's curriculum.

OK: For residential care homes.

RI: Medicaid waiver: 1 hour orientation; 12 hours annual.

VT: For residential care homes.

Source: Mollica et al., 2008: *Residential Care and Assisted Living Compendium, 2007.*

Alabama	Massachusetts	Oregon
Arizona	Michigan	Pennsylvania
Arkansas	Minnesota	Rhode Island
California	Mississippi	South Carolina
Colorado	Missouri	South Dakota
Florida	Montana	Texas
Idaho	Nebraska	Utah
Illinois	Nevada	Virginia
Indiana	New York	Vermont
Iowa	North Carolina	Washington
Kansas	North Dakota	Wisconsin
Maine	Ohio	Wyoming
Maryland		

Source: Mollica et al., 2008: *Residential Care and Assisted Living Compendium, 2007.*

FIGURE 5.1 States with additional training requirements for facilities serving residents with dementia.

Staff also reported that they did receive training on the philosophy of assisted living. Seventy-five percent of staff had participated in continuing education activities. Overall, Hawes and colleagues (1999) noted that staff were not well informed about normal aging processes and dementia care.

There is large variation in the staff training requirements and stringency of the requirements among the states (Carlson, 2005; Hawes, 1999; Mollica, Sims-Kastelein & O'Keeffe, 2008; National Center for Assisted Living, 2008). Carlson (2005) did extensive work inclusive of all states and reported several characteristics of staff training requirements:

1) Thirty-three states require training in first aid or cardiopulmonary resuscitation or both, but with varying stringency
2) Thirty-seven states specify training topics
3) A minority of states require initial training of a certain minimum number of hours with 5 states requiring 12 or fewer hours, 4 states requiring 13-24 hours and 10 states requiring 25 or more hours
4) Nine states require certain qualifications of the person conducting the initial training for direct-care staff
5) Six states have some control over the content of the curriculum for initial training
6) Four states require that a direct care staff member pass a state-developed competency examination
7) Twenty-four states require a specific hourly minimum for direct-care staff's continuing education with annual minimum generally falling into the 5- to 15-hour range

ORIENTATION AND RESIDENT RIGHTS
Proper conduct when interacting with residents and family. How to dress appropriately when at work. Confidentiality and reporting. How to follow regulations regarding resident rights.

ASSISTING WITH ADLs
How to identify and meet resident needs for assistance with ADLs. Successful tips for giving a bath. How to provide incontinent and perineal care. Best techniques for transfer and ambulation. Providing oral and denture care.

DELIVERING PERSONAL CARE AND STANDARD PRECAUTIONS
An introduction to safe infection control pratices. How and when to wash hands. Proper cleansing and disinfection techniques. Handling of sharps containers. Information provided according to CDC guidelines.

PSYCHOSOCIAL CARE
Understand psychosocial care needs. Seeing the resident as a whole person and an individual.
Implementing interventions for effective psychosocial care. Strategies and tips for successful activity programs. Making life meaningful for your residents.

SPECIAL NEEDS OF THE ELDERLY
Possible changes that may occur in our resident's bodies as they age. Adapting care to address the needs of elder adults. How aging affects the heart, skin, lungs, and other body systems. Planning care for residents who have suffered a stroke. Recognizing signs and symptoms of dementia.

UNDERSTANDING MENTAL ILLNESS: SCHIZOPHRENIA
An introduction to understanding the complexities of schizophrenia, including signs and symptoms, daily care strategies, behaviors, aging issues, and common medications and their side effects.

BIPOLAR DISORDER
This video, featuring mental health specialist John Simmons, RN, PHN, BC, explains common myths and misbeliefs, signs and symptoms of bipolar disorder, daily care strategies, behaviors, common medications, and suicidal ideations.

BLOODBORNE PATHOGENS:
HIV, HEPATITIS, AND STANDARD PRECAUTIONS
Complies with OSHA training requirements. This video reviews the key basics regarding bloodborne pathogens, including what are bloodborne pathogens, preventing transmission, universal precautions, and more. This video is perfect for every member of your staff.

FIGURE 5.2 Resident care training DVDs. *(Continued)*

HAND WASHING

Hand washing is one of the most important steps in infection control. This video is quick and to-the-point, demonstrating for your staff how and when to wash their hands.

CARING FOR PERSONS WITH LUNG DISEASE

This video explores the daily challenges faced when caring for someone with COPD and other forms of lung disease. The story is told directly from the viewpoint of a person with lung disease, sharing tips and techniques for effective care measures.

RECOGNIZING DIVERSITY

Racial and cultural differences do exist in residential communities. You can make a difference through educated and compassionate care staff. This video addresses how diversity can affect caregiving, including religious, cultural, and sexuality issues.

DIABETES

This video reviews key concepts related to caring for residents with diabetes, including the definition of diabetes, types of diabetes, preventing complications, and assisting with the use of insulin.

RECOGNIZING AND REPORTING ELDER ABUSE

This video guides staff in the promotion of resident choice, privacy, and prevention of abuse. Neglect, exploitation, and mistreatment are defined. Staff will learn about reporting requirements as well as recognition of abuse.

SPECIAL CARE NEEDS: OXYGEN, OSTOMY, CATHETER, AND SKIN BREAKDOWN

This video provides the caregiver with real-world, step-by-step tips on caring for residents with these challenging health conditions and needs. State regulations require that caregivers receive appropriate training when providing care to residents. This video provides an excellent resource to assist you in meeting those requirements.

YOUR FIRST DAY AT WORK

Get your staff on the floor quickly and safely. This video discusses clocking in and out, resident supervision, key control, use of pagers and walkie-talkies, reporting, and documentation.

FALL PRECAUTIONS IN ASSISTED LIVING

This video addresses the essentials regarding falls in the assisted living facility in a format easily understood by direct care staff, including types of injuries caused from falls, fall risk factors, prevention strategies, responding to falls, and when to call 911.

CARING FOR BEDRIDDEN RESIDENTS

This video reviews key care concepts when caring for bedridden residents, including preventing skin breakdown and other complications, turning and positioning, and much more.

FIGURE 5.2   *(Continued)*

MONITORING RESIDENTS FOR CHANGES IN CONDITION
Unreported changes in a resident's condition is a major source of liability for assisted living and residential care providers. Use this video to train your staff in identifying the key indicators of change that may be seen in your residents and how to respond appropriately.

WHEELCHAIRS AND OTHER AMBULATORY AIDES
This video teaches your staff how to assist residents with their ambulatory aides and safe transfer techniques. Also explained are practices that should be avoided, such as pushing residents while sitting on their walker bench.

PRESSURE ULCERS
In this video your staff will learn about the stages of pressure ulcers and important strategies to minimize the risk of skin breakdown in your residents.

END OF LIFE
Understand what your resident is experiencing at the end of life. Prepare yourself and your staff to handle the emotional and physical burdens experienced by everyone close to the resident.

FOOD SAFETY IN RESIDENTIAL CARE
This video demonstrates safe-food handling techniques, including safe-food preparation, safe-food storage, cooling foods for storage, labeling foods, handwashing, cleaning and disinfection practices, proper food temperatures, using a thermometer, and foodborne illness.

EMERGENCY PROCEDURES
This video will prepare your staff to respond to fires and other emergency situations in your community. Topics addressed include fire safety, responding to emergencies, evacuations, and step-by-step use of fire extinguishers.

VITAL SIGNS
Do you expect your caregivers to take vital signs? If so, use this video to help train staff in the appropriate techniques. During this video, Sandi Flores, RN, reviews step-by-step procedures for taking blood pressure, temperature, pulse, respirations, and weight. Documenting and reporting vital signs are also addressed.

INFECTION CONTROL
This video introduces your staff to the key principles of infection control, including hand washing, use of gloves, disinfection procedures, and other essential information.

ACTIVITIES: ENCOURAGING RESIDENT PARTICIPATION
A successful activity program is an essential part of the care and services provided in your community. This video reviews activity planning, evaluating resident needs and preferences, and also offers creative suggestions to maximize resident participation in your activity program.

Source: Advanced Healthcare Studies, 2009 (www.advhs.com)

FIGURE 5.2

Carlson (2005) notes that direct care standards for assisted living are far less stringent that those that apply to nursing home staff members where under the terms of the federal Nursing Home Reform Law, direct care staff must complete at least 75 hours of initial training under the supervision of a registered nurse, with a minimum of 2 years' experience and at least 1-year nursing experience in long-term care.

Although states' regulations specify initial and ongoing training requirements for staff and administrators, the level of specificity varies (Mollica et al., 2008). While some states specify only general requirements, others specify topics to be covered, the number of training hours required, the completion of approved courses, or some combination of topics, hours and courses. Table 5.1 summarizes the initial and annual direct care staff requirements of all states and Figure 5.1 lists states that have dementia specific training for direct care staff.

Ensuring the appropriate training of your medication aides is one of your greatest areas of responsibility as an assisted living and residential care provider. Our comprehensive medication training kit, developed with nationally recognized assisted living expert Sandi Flores, RN, will make it easier for you to complete this vital training in your community.

The kit includes:

1. Five Medication Training DVDs
   • Introduction to Medication Management
   • Medication Orders and Working With Pharmacies
   • Medications and Documentation
   • Assistance With Medication Administration
   • Side Effects, Adverse Reactions, and Medication Errors
   • California providers also receive Understanding California Medication Regulations

2. A 150-page training manual including an easy-to-follow instruction guide.

3. Competency and training verification forms.

4. A thorough exam to test your employee's comprehension of key medication management principles.

5. A certificate of completion to duplicate and present to your staff upon successful completion of the program.

Source: Advanced Healthcare Studies, 2009 (www.advhs.com)

FIGURE 5.3   Assisted living medication training kit.

COUMADIN MANAGEMENT IN ASSISTED LIVING

This video will prepare your staff (both nurses and medication aides) to safely handle Coumadin in your facility, including dosing regimens, documentation, side effects, and laboratory testing.

REDUCING MEDICATION ERRORS: USING THE MAR

This video, which features numerous on-screen demonstrations with detailed explanations, provides concrete methods your staff can use to reduce medication errors. In this video we focus on effectively utilizing the medication administration/assistance record (MAR), including how to add medications to a MAR, how to correct errors, and documenting refusal.

REDUCING MEDICATION ERRORS: PRN MEDICATIONS

During this video your staff will learn essential techniques for the safe handling of PRN (as needed) medications, including how to use a PRN record, when to give a PRN medication, as well as physician orders for PRN medications.

REDUCING MEDICATION ERRORS: MEDICATION

This video, which features numerous on-screen demonstrations, covers essential aspects of managing narcotic medications, including storage and security, handling physician orders, end of shift counts, and documentation.

INTRODUCTION TO MEDICATION MANAGEMENT

This video covers the fundamentals of medication management including the six rights, storage, and security.

MEDICATION ORDERS & WORKING WITH PHARMACIES

This video covers: how to read a physician order, handling orders, ordering medications from the pharmacy, and changes in medication orders.

MEDICATIONS AND DOCUMENTATION

Successful medication management depends on accurate and thorough documentation. Help prepare your staff using this training video.

ASSISTANCE WITH MEDICATION ADMINISTRATION

This video reviews hands-on procedures for assisting with medications, including oral medications, liquids, topical medications, and more.

SIDE EFFECTS, ADVERSE REACTIONS, AND MEDICATION ERRORS

Elderly adults are at increased risk for adverse reactions and side effects. This video will prepare your staff to monitor for and respond to the dangerous situations.

Source: Advanced Healthcare Studies, 2009 (www.advhs.com)

FIGURE 5.4 Medication management DVDs.

Training Direct Care Staff

The assisted living facility will develop a direct care staff training program that satisfies the specific state regulatory requirements and suits the needs of the environment and residents served. The following are examples of topics which are important to include in direct care staff training:

Direct Care Issues

- Principles of assisted living
- Personal/direct care skills
- Meeting the needs of consumers/residents
- Appropriate, related to tasks/duties
- Hygiene
- Housekeeping/sanitation
- Nutrition/food preparations/diets
- Social/recreation activities
- Dementia/Alzheimer's care
- Mental health/emotional/behavioral needs
- Restraints

Our Dementia Care Staff Training Kit can be used to help you stay in compliance with your state regulations regarding dementia care and staff-training. This comprehensive kit includes:

1. Twelve Staff Training DVDs
   - Introduction to Dementia Care • Dementia Care: Tips for ADLs
   - Food Service in Dementia Care • Dementia Care: Health Complications
   - Medications in Dementia Care • Sexuality and Promoting Dignity
   - Dementia Care: Hydration • Dementia Care: Sundowning
   - Dementia Care: Wandering • Dementia Care: Aggression
   - Activities and Communication • End of Life Care

2. Instructor Guides
The Instructor Guides include training outlines and suggested discussion topics to make conducting in-services easier for administrators and managers.

3. Quizzes
Each training module includes a quiz to verify staff understanding of the information presented. A quiz key is included as well.

4. Documentation Forms
This kit also includes forms and certificates to be placed in the employee's file.

Source: Advanced Healthcare Studies, 2009 (www.advhs.com)

FIGURE 5.5   Dementia care training kit.

INTRODUCTION TO DEMENTIA CARE

As the demand for dementia care in the assisted living/residential setting increases, so does the need for better staff training. Featuring recognized dementia care experts, this video covers the most common dementia care questions in clear, understandable terms.

Key topics addressed include:
- What is dementia?
- What is Alzheimer's disease?
- Why does my resident act this way?
- How can I make personal care easier?
- How can I communicate better?
- What can I do when my resident does not eat?

DEMENTIA CARE: TIPS FOR ADLs

This video addresses the special care techniques needed to successfully provide ADL care to residents with dementia.

DEMENTIA CARE: HEALTH COMPLICATIONS

Three health complications – pneumonia, swallowing disorders and aspiration – often lead to death in persons with dementia. This video will prepare your staff to prevent, identify, and intervene successfully.

DEMENTIA CARE: WANDERING

Elopement and wandering are significant concerns for any provider caring for residents with dementia or other memory impairment. Your staff will learn about the causes of wandering, types of wandering, resident care strategies, and elopement prevention.

THERAPEUTIC INTERVENTIONS, ACTIVITIES, AND COMMUNICATION

This video addresses the vitally important "non-medical" interventions used in dementia care, including activities, successful communication, sensory stimulation and more.

DEMENTIA CARE: SEXUALITY ISSUES AND PROMOTING INDEPENDENCE

Seeing and treating each resident as an individual is what distinguishes outstanding care. During this video your staff will learn how to learn more about each resident and how to handle the sensitive issues of sexuality and independence.

DEMENTIA CARE: AGGRESSIVE BEHAVIORS

Aggressive behaviors can be frightening to both staff and other residents. In this video your staff will learn causes and most importantly, interventions for aggressive behaviors.

DEMENTIA CARE: EFFECTS OF MEDICATIONS ON PERSONS WITH DEMENTIA

Residents with dementia can be particularly sensitive to medications and at risk for inappropriate use. This video will assist your staff in understanding the effects and side effects of commonly used psychotropic medications.

FIGURE 5.6 Dementia DVDs. (*Continued*)

DEMENTIA CARE: HYDRATION
This video addresses signs and symptoms of dehydration, the effects of dehydration, effective strategies to ensure proper hydration, and dementia-specific care issues.

DEMENTIA CARE: SUNDOWNING
Residents with dementia may become more agitated, confused, and disoriented in the evening hours, in a syndrome referred to as sundowning. This video will provide you and your staff with practical tips and techniques for managing this challenging condition.

FOOD SERVICE IN DEMENTIA CARE
Is your resident agitated or overwhelmed at mealtime? This video explores techniques and strategies to gear food and nutrition service to the needs and abilities of your resident. See actual real world, effective techniques demonstrated to optimize the food service experience in your community.

Source: Advanced Healthcare Studies, 2009 (www.advhs.com)

FIGURE 5.6

Health-Related Issues

- Basic nursing skills
- Prevention/restorative skills
- Medication administration/assistance

Knowledge Areas

- Resident rights
- Aging process/gerontology
- Working with the needs of elderly
- Death and dying
- Psycho-social needs
- Assessment skills
- Care Plan development
- Communication skills
- Knowledge of community services

Safety and Emergency Issues

- CPR
- First Aid
- Fire, safety, emergency procedures
- Infection prevention/control

Process Issues

- Agency/facility policies
- Regulation/law
- Reporting abuse/neglect
- Complaint procedures
- Record keeping
- Confidentiality
- Legal/ethical issues
- Survey process

Direct Care Staff Training: Model Education and Training Programs

Sandi Flores, RN, and colleagues, in their work with Advanced Health-care Studies, LLC, have created multiple model staff training materials (i.e., training programs, manuals and DVDs) (http://www.advhs.com).

SERVICE PLANS

Successful resident care starts with individualizing services to the resident and having a plan in place. State regulations require that each resident in your facility have a current service plan on file. This video demonstrates effective service planning strategies, how to work with the family, the role of hospice and the physician, and licensing compliance.

INCIDENT REPORTING

Incident reports are required by state regulations and when done properly, can be an important part of your risk management strategy. This video will cover when to report an incident, what to document, how to fill out an incident report form, and when multiple reports might be necessary.

DOCUMENTATION: SAFE AND SOUND NARRATIVE CHARTING

This training will improve your care staff's ability to document effectively. The purpose of narrative charting and risk management approaches are included in this video.

INTRODUCTION TO MARKETING

Your marketing plan and analysis is a necessity in developing and implementing appropriate service offerings in your assisted living program. This video will explore how to pinpoint the areas to which you should focus your marketing plan.

LEADERSHIP SKILLS

Perfect training for the small facility manager or team leaders in large communities. Excellent for staff new to leadership positions and for current lead staff to enhance their skills.

Source: Advanced Healthcare Studies, 2009 (www.advhs.com)

FIGURE 5.7 Leadership and management DVDs.

Get in compliance with OSHA training requirements! Employee training is a critical component of OSHA compliance that benefits both the employer and employee. Your employees benefit from safety and health training through fewer work-related injuries, and reduced stress and worry caused by exposure to hazards. You benefit from regulatory compliance, reduced workplace injuries, increased productivity, lower costs, higher profits, and a more cohesive and dependable workforce. To help you stay in compliance and avoid costly OSHA fines, this training kit includes:

1. Six Staff Training DVDs
   • General Safety • Back and Lifting Safety
   • Bloodborne Pathogens • Personal Protective Equipment
   • Workplace Violence • Fire, Electrical, and Chemical Safety

2. Instructor Guides
The Instructor Guides include training outlines and suggested discussion topics to make conducting in-services easier for administrators and managers.

3. Quizzes
Each training module includes a quiz to verify staff understanding of the information presented. A quiz key is included as well.

4. Documentation Forms
OSHA regulations require thorough documentation of all training provided. Our kit includes forms and certificates to document training.

Source: Advanced Healthcare Studies, 2009 (www.advhs.com)

FIGURE 5.8 OSHA training kit.

Advanced Healthcare Studies is considered a leader in educational and training materials in assisted living, a useful resource for the assisted living administrator. Figures 5.2 through 5.10 illustrate some of these model materials.

FACILITATING STAFF TRAINING THROUGH LEARNING CIRCLES: A MODEL FOR TRAINING

Learning circles are used in facilities nationwide and are changing the way management, staff, and residents communicate among one another. The purpose is to create an environment where people feel free to share their ideas and opinions without being criticized or reprimanded. This helps build trust among the participants which serves to strengthen relationships. Organizations that have been successful in implementing culture change attest to the value of learning circles. For example, Mea-

Our complete Disaster Manual includes everything you need to complete your disaster preparedness planning and policy and procedure development, including sample policies and procedures, forms, and training materials that include:

Disaster Manual
1. Chain of command and communication policies and procedures.

2. Forms and procedures for maintaining lists of emergency contacts.

3. Disaster procedures for:
• Fires • Wild fires • Earthquakes • Hurricanes • Tornadoes • Floods
• Power failures • Elevator failures • Bomb threats

4. Evacuation procedures.

5. Plans for your community to be self-reliant for at least 72 hours following an emergency or disaster, including power failure.

6. Procedures for resident care during a disaster.

7. Numerous forms and checklists to help your staff be safe in a disaster, including:
• Emergency contacts • Emergency information request letter • Identification of emergency shut-offs and controls • Resident roster • Visitor and staff sign-in sheet • Disaster supplies checklist
• Many more...

Staff Training DVD
Also included is our *Emergency Procedures* staff training DVD that covers how to use a fire extinguisher, evacuations, fire safety, and much more.

Resource CD
The entire Disaster Manual, including all policies and forms, is also supplied in a CD-ROM to allow you to edit, customize, and make copies as needed.

Source: Advanced Healthcare Studies, 2009 (www.advhs.com)

FIGURE 5.9 Disaster manual for assisted living and residential care.

dowlark Hills Retirement Community in Manhattan, KS, holds Learning Circles daily to address concerns and work through problems, and at White Community Hospital in Aurora, MN, Learning Circles are used between departments to strengthen relationships. Learning circles can be utilized in various ways, such as part of education and in-servicing, a practice at Meadowood, in Worchester, PA, or as a way for residents, caregivers and available family members to determine the day's activities, as done at Northern Pines Community in Big Fork, MN (Norton, 2003). The following is a description of a learning circle.

Our popular policy and procedure manual is written specifically for the assisted living and residential care provider. With policies that include:

I. Admission and assessment

2. Hospice care

3. Reassessment

4. Death of a resident

5. Psychiatric crisis

6. Coumadin and lab management

7. Pre-placement appraisals

8. Staff supervision

9. Medication management

10. Documentation, and much more...

In addition to the policies and procedures, there is a staff orientation and training section that includes written training on basic skills for caregivers; handling medications; record keeping and documentation; disease processes; resident rights; and dementia care. Each section includes written quizzes and projects. The full manual is also included on CD-ROM to allow you the option of customizing and reprinting any section of the manual as necessary.

Source: Advanced Healthcare Studies, 2009 (www.advhs.com)

FIGURE 5.10   Assisted living policy and procedure manual.

The learning circle is a leveling technique that encourages quiet people to speak, talkative people to listen, and everyone to share in making decisions (Figure 5.11). Participants observe, interpret, and experience not only their own feelings about an issue, but also broaden their perspective by considering the many viewpoints around them. Learning Circles are most effective when they become a way of life in the long-term care facility, and when everyone take a turn facilitating.

Because this technique helps in fostering a sense of trust and connection between participants, it would also be a useful intervention to promote a more cohesive community. There are too many examples of cases where family members sued an assisted living facility, and the underlying reason being their impression that the organization does

1.	Participants sit in a circle without tables or other obstructions blocking their view of one another. Participants can include any combination of workers, residents, families, and other community members.
2.	The ideal number of participants is 10 to 15. If the facilitator believes the discussion will provoke strong feelings of sadness, depression, grief, or anger, it is helpful to limit the number to 5 to 10.
3.	One person is chosen to be the facilitator. He or she poses the question or topic to the circle, gives encouragement, and keeps the circle moving in an orderly fashion.
4.	The process begins when the facilitator poses the question or issue.
5.	A volunteer in the circle responds with his or her thought about the topic.
6.	The person sitting to the right or left of the first respondent speaks next, followed one by one around the circle until everyone has spoken on the subject without interruption. Participants may choose to pass rather than speak. After everyone else in the circle has taken a turn, the facilitator goes back to those who passed, and allows each another opportunity to respond. Only after everyone has had a chance to speak is the floor open for general discussion.

FIGURE 5.11 Procedure for learning circle.

not care, or is not being honest. Techniques such as learning circles can be employed at family council meetings, resident council meetings, or community meetings involving residents, staff and family members (L. Norton, 2003).

CONCLUSIONS

This chapter has addressed the important topic of staff training in assisted living facilities. A variety of topics have been covered to assist the administrator in understanding the importance of staff training, its context within the industry, and recommendations from national experts in the field. Multiple training programs and materials have been included that may be useful for the administrator while staff training programs are developed.

REFERENCES

Advanced Healthcare Studies. (2009). *Staff training and compliance tools for providers*. Retrieved May 18, 2009, from http://www.advhs.com

Assisted Living Federation of America. (2009). *Core principles*. Retrieved March 31, 2005, from http://www.alfa.org/alfa/ALFA_Core_Principles1.asp?SnID=1067116361# training

Assisted Living Workgroup. (2003). *Assuring quality in assisted living: Guidelines for federal and state policy, state regulations, and operations*. Washington, DC: U.S. Government Printing Office.

Carlson, E. (2005). *Critical issues in assisted living: Who's in, who's out and who's provid-ing the care.* Washington, DC: National Senior Citizen's Law Center.

Hawes, C., Phillips, C., & Rose, M. (1999). *A national study of assisted living for the frail elderly: Results of a national survey of facilities.* Washington, DC: U.S. Department of Health and Human Services.

Mollica, R., Sims-Kastelein, K., & O'Keeffe, J. (2008). *Residential care and assisted living compendium, 2007.* U.S. Department of Health and Human Services, Office of the Assistant Secretary for Planning and Evaluation, Office of Disability, Aging and Long-Term Care Policy and Research Triangle Institute. Retrieved June 21, 2008, from http://aspe.hhs.gov/daltcp/reports/2007/07alcom.htm

National Center for Assisted Living. (2008). *Assisted living state regulatory review 2008.* Washington, DC: National Center for Assisted Living. Retrieved June 21, 2008, from http://www.ncal.org/about/2008_reg_review.pdf

Norton, L. (2003). The power of circles: Using a familiar technique to promote culture change. In A. Weiner & J. Ronch (Eds.), *Culture change in long-term care* (pp. 285–292). Binghamton, NY: The Hawthorne Press Inc.

U.S. General Accounting Office. (1999). *Assisted living: Quality of care and consumer protection issues* (GAO/T-HEHS-99-111).

Retaining Employees and Empowerment

Learning Objectives

Upon the completion of Chapter 6, the reader will be able to:

- *Discuss workforce retention as a critical issue in assisted living.*
- *Define staff turnover.*
- *Recognize the consequences and risks associated with staff turnover.*
- *Understand how to calculate staff turnover rates.*
- *Describe the factors associated with staff turnover and retention.*
- *Identify multiple, specific staff retention strategies.*

INTRODUCTION

This chapter addresses the critical issue of workforce retention in the assisted living industry. The current trends and increasing need for quality workforce retention in long-term care set the tone for the chapter. First, staff turnover is described and defined. The reader will also learn the consequence of staff turnover and the factors which influence this turnover and retention. The remainder of the chapter is organized into subsets of specific retentions strategies: (1) Wages and Benefits; (2) Working Conditions; (3) Recognition; (4) Scheduling Options; (5) Supportive Management; (6) Opportunities for Growth; and (7) Staff Empowerment. Examples and ideas are presented as possibilities and considerations for the assisted living administrator to incorporate into creating both a unique and useful retention strategy.

Workforce Retention in Assisted Living: A Critical Issue

The retention of qualified and adequate staff is becoming a recognized challenge for assisted living facilities. Recent national surveys report that the annual rates of staff turnover range from 21% to 135% reaching a national average of 42% (American Association of Homes and Services for the Aging, 2002; National Center for Assisted Living, 2001). The growing population of elderly persons coupled with current and projected workforce shortages (Stone & Weiner, 2001) increases the likelihood of high staff turnover rates in the future.

Paraprofessionals (i.e., direct care staff) who provide hands-on care are identified as the most difficult staff to retain because many factors, including low wages and benefits, hard working conditions, heavy workloads, and a job that has been stigmatized by society, make worker retention difficult.

Employee retention, and all of the elements associated with job satisfaction, should become a primary focus of human resources management in the assisted living facility. The challenges of retention tend to be ongoing. However, keeping your employees satisfied will lower your risk of losing staff to the increasing number of opportunities available in long-term care today. The more strategic planning efforts you make toward recruitment, the better prepared the facility will be. A well thought out and planned retention strategy will improve the facility's chance for success. Because long-term care administrators are often consumed with day to day operations of the facility, employee retention is sometimes overlooked. However, taking the time to identify and determine retention challenges may provide valuable information to plan strategic interventions that will improve retention.

STAFF TURNOVER

Defining Staff Turnover

Turnover refers to the number of staff that leave employment at the facility for any reason. Retention means keeping valued employees. To understand the facility's retention challenges, the administrator should review turnover. All facilities will experience turnover, but the extent of the turnover can seemingly be minimized with effective retention strategies. Keep in mind that when turnover is not excessive, there can be the some benefits. New staff often bring fresh energy and ideas that may bring new optimism to your long-time staff. However, at some point turnover becomes disadvantageous because it is expensive both in time and reputation and will affect resident care.

Turnover itself, depending on type, may be negative or positive. *Negative turnover* is the loss of qualified employees, while *positive turnover* is the result of strong employees being promoted within the facility or less desirable employees leaving. The administrator's strategies should aim to minimize negative turnover and promote and maintain positive turnover.

Consequences of Staff Turnover

The adverse effects of staff turnover in long-term care facilities have long been identified. Consequences of staff turnover include increased facility costs, lower job satisfaction and lower resident quality of care (Castle & Engberg, 2005). The exact cost of staff turnover in assisted living facilities is unknown; however the costs are substantial considering recruitment, hiring and training costs. Because staff turnover interrupts continuity of resident care, workload increases and resentment of staff may build when additional responsibilities must be met. The most serious negative consequence of high staff turnover rates is the potential for negative health outcomes relative to poor quality of care. Research has long identified this concern in nursing homes, and staff turnover has been associated with quality of care in assisted living facilities as well. For example, U.S. General Accounting Office (1999), in the report *Assisted Living: Quality of Care and Consumer Protection Issues,* having insufficient, unqualified and untrained staff, exacerbated by high staff turnover and low pay for direct care staff, was cited as one of the four main quality of care concerns.

Calculating Turnover Rates

Consider creating a baseline of staff turnover rates. If possible, compare turnover rates to other similar facilities in your geographical area. For larger facilities, you may also contemplate comparing individual units to one another within the facility. The baseline will assist you identifying and predicting staff turnover rates so that the best retention strategies can be implemented.

One common way to define and calculate staff turnover rates is to determine an annual turnover rate. Annual turnover rates are calculated by dividing the difference between the number of individuals (e.g., direct care staff) employed during a fiscal year, and the number employed at the end of the year which multiplied by 100 produces a rates. Figure 6.1 illustrates how to calculate annual staff turnover. Terminations include all reasons for leaving the facility such as resignation, retirement, or firing. This percentage should be calculated for each position, each unit, as well as the entire facility.

Sum of terminations in 1 year / the sum of established positions x 100

Example: 16/50 x 100 = 32%

FIGURE 6.1   How to calculate turnover rates.

Once you have calculated turnover rate for each position in your facility, consider the problem areas. Are there large differences between units? Are certain positions more vulnerable to turnover? If one unit has consistent long-term staff and another does not, what issues may be affecting that particular unit? For example, is there a difference in the care levels of the residents? Asking these types of questions may assist you in identifying issues and challenges that will influence your retention strategy.

It is important to remember that annual turnover rates are not always accurate due to the high number of staff that leaves employment in long-term care facilities within the first 180 days of employment. One-hundred percent turnover does not necessarily mean that every single employee leaves employment in the course of one year. It may mean that for every employee who stays the full year, for example, two or more came and one left a similar job at the same facility. Castle (2006), well known for research in nursing home staff turnover, has offered an alternative definition of turnover as the total number of staff (measured in full-time equivalents) who leave employment during a 6-month period divided by the total number of staff (measured in full-time equivalents) who were employed during this period. This calculation should include all shifts, part-time staff, and voluntary and involuntary turnover.

Identifying Risk of Staff Turnover

The administrator should pay close attention to the number of employees that are at risk for leaving employment at the present time. Sometimes, staff are seeking new opportunities because the facility cannot adequately meet their personal needs. On occasion, appropriate intervention can result in retention of a valued employee. Several warning signs of potential staff turnover are seen in Figure 6.2.

If you do not know your employees well, you may have difficulty noticing these types of warning signs. Get to know your staff and illicit assistance from direct supervisors. They are important resources for identifying quality employees who are considering leaving.

1. Visibly unhappy

2. Complaints about workload or peers

3. Life events (e.g., childbirth, death in family, divorce, returning to school)

4. Unexplained absences

5. Increased use of sick time

6. Rejection for promotion or wage increase

7. Reduced interest in job

8. Change in job performance

9. Favorite peers or mentors leaving employment

FIGURE 6.2 Warning signs of potential turnover.

Factors Associated With Turnover and Retention of Direct Care Staff

To better address workforce retention, an understanding of the factors associated with staff turnover is essential. Although many factors associated with staff turnover and retention may beyond the direct control of the assisted living facility, the understanding of both *intrinsic factors* (i.e., those factors specific to the individual employee) and *extrinsic factors* (i.e., those factors not specific to the individual employee) associated with staff turnover will aid the administrator in developing strategies to improve retention over time (see Figures 6.3, 6.4, and 6.5). These factors greatly impact job satisfaction, a primary factor in staff turnover.

RETENTION STRATEGIES

Retention strategies should be developed with a specific plan for the individual facility. This plan should address potential losses of highest risk positions and persons within your unique facility. The following strategies are presented as interventions for the assisted living

1. **Age**: Younger workers are less likely to remain on the job, while workers over the age of 30 are more likely to stay (Parsons, Simmons, Penn, & Furlough, 2003; Riggs, 2001).

2. **Education**: Workers with more than a high school education are more likely to turnover (Parsons et al., 2003; Riggs, 2001). More educated workers may choose to leave their job to pursue additional education.

3. **Marital status:** Workers who are the sole source of income for themselves and dependents are less likely to turnover (Parsons et al., 2003).

4. **Social support:** Workers with reliable social support systems, such as transportation and childcare, are less likely to turnover (Riggs, 2001).

5. **Lack of job preparation:** Workers with a lack of hands-on training and inadequate skills are more likely to turnover (Lescoe-Long, 2000).

6. **Employment tenure:** Workers with a history of shorter prior job tenure may be more likely to turnover (Parsons et al., 2003).

7. **Values and attitudes:** Workers who value being needed and demonstrate a positive affect toward older adults are more likely to stay on the job. On the other hand, those more oriented to rewards such as salary are more likely to turnover (Lescoe-Long, 2000; Parsons et al., 2003; Riggs, 2001).

FIGURE 6.3 Intrinsic factors associated with turnover and retention.

1. *Multiple employment opportunities*
2. *Inadequate job training*
3. *Excessive workload*
4. *Poor continuity of care*
5. *Lack of respect*
6. *Wages and benefits*

FIGURE 6.4 Extrinsic factors associated with turnover.

---

1. *Clean, safe work environments*

2. *Higher staff ratios*

3. *Union contracts for workers*

4. *Low rates of professional staff turnover*

5. *Positive relationships with residents, peers and supervisors.*

6. *Employee recognition.*

FIGURE 6.5   Extrinsic factors associated with retention.

administrator to consider in developing a plan, but other solutions should be explored and incorporated into your plan. You will need to tailor your plan to address the resources available at the facility and options available to you and your staff.

Wages and Benefits

Wages

When feasible, consider wage increases. Consider longevity, as well as merit increases for staff. Inform staff of costs associated with benefits (e.g., provide benefits costs to employees).

Benefits

Provide health, dental, vision and life insurance. Consider the development of pension plans and profit sharing for all employees. Consider sponsoring a 401k plan with an employer contribution. Assist staff with payroll deduction options.

Sick Time

Allow for a specified number of paid sick days per year. For employees that use no sick time, allow for a paid wellness day. Consider a bonus or wage increase for employees with no absences.

Working Conditions

Attendance Policies

Develop fair and consistent attendance policies. Create a system to track all unscheduled absences. Consider exempting physician excused absences. Develop steps of discipline related to inconsistent attendance. Reward good attendance with bonuses, extra days off, and hourly incentives for no late arrivals, for no absences, and for not leaving early any time during the week.

Respect

Create an environment that respects all members of the health care team. Encourage staff, families and residents to provide positive feedback related to job performance. Develop growth opportunities and advancement for all staff positions.

Morale

Acknowledge the hard work of the staff. Have a casual dress day or themed day. Consider a "staff appreciation" day for specific positions. Vary assignments if appropriate. Incorporate humor into the workplace.

Performance Objectives

Performance objectives should be clear and measurable and included in the job description. When conducting performance evaluations, utilize the job description as a reference point. Consider peer performance evaluations as well.

Consistency

Policies and procedures should be written. Have a well developed appropriate disciplinary system that is enforced consistently across disciplines and shifts. Flexibility is important in special circumstances. Consistently consider the whole picture.

Supplies/Equipment

Ensure adequate supplies for the entire facility. Safety and assistive equipment is important to keep up to date and in working condition. Provide personal protective equipment and ergonomic equipment as necessary. Consider new technologies that may aid staff in providing high quality care.

Orientation Programs

Develop excellent and efficient training programs. Consider implementing a mentoring program and pairing staff to promote teamwork. Be sure to include introductions to all staff by name and job title. See Chapter 5 for further information on training.

Work Environment

Provide adequate lounge space for breaks and mealtime. Consider heating and air conditioning, ample comfortable seating, vending machines, refrigerator, microwave and toaster. Allow access to a telephone for personal calls. Set up a communication system for staff (e.g., bulletin board). Provide secured lockers. Sponsor occasional treats to acknowledge a job well done (e.g., pizza party).

Assignments

When possible, allow for permanent shift assignment. Consider part-time or permanent "float" position, and offer permanent assignments as a longevity bonus.

Shift Differential

Weekend, evening and night shift differential should be established. Offer bonuses for covering extra shifts.

Recognition

Recognize the Value of Each Employee

Know your staff and call them by name. Let the staff see you daily on the unit and thank them for their work. Promote the value of the staff to all employees, residents and families. Listen to the concerns of the staff. Involve staff with interview processes. Help out with residents by answering call lights or assisting with employee-specific tasks. Consider having employees from one department spend a day with an employee from another department.

Special Recognition/Appreciation

Create an award system, such as an award pin or "Employee of the Month" bulletin board. Compliment staff and allow others to hear your compliment. Publically acknowledge anniversary dates. Some considerations include notes or cards, food and treats, gift certificates, merit bonuses, or wage increases. Consider ideas that also provide good public relations, such as facility shirts or jackets. Attend staff meetings and care conferences. Acknowledge longevity annually and present special awards at 5 year increments in honor of an employee's loyalty. Honor staff in the facility newsletter. Present special "gifts" such as gift cards or certificates to acknowledge special achievements.

Food

Have an employee picnic or banquet. Use the opportunity to provide recognition awards. Promote the involvement of resident families by asking their participation in a holiday or tea party. Order take-out food spontaneously to acknowledge a difficult job well done.

Activities

Involve staff in resident specific activities. For examples, invite staff to have their children attend a Halloween party. Have an employee gift exchange at holiday time.

Just Say "Thank You"

Take every opportunity to just say "thank you." Post thank you notes for other staff and residents to see. Acknowledge individuals. Have lunch with staff when you can.

Employee of the Month

Establish an official "Employee of the Month" process that incorporates a committee of peers and other staff. Make each selected employee of the month eligible for an "Employee of the Year." Consider acknowledgment with a plaque, dinner, recognition in newsletters and monetary bonuses.

Display Special Postings

Consider having bulletin boards in the staff lounge area. Acknowledge births, engagements, wedding or other special events. Welcome back employees from a vacation or other leave. Recognize the accomplishments of employees' children such as academic or athletic achievements and honors.

Utilize Employees in Facility Public Relations

Include employees in your facility's promotional pamphlets and brochures. Put individual or group pictures of employees by your facility's front door.

Monthly Prize Drawings

Place the names of employees who worked extra shifts into a monthly prize drawing. Simple gifts such as a gift certificate or phone card are often much appreciated.

Merit Increases

Acknowledging longevity with bonuses, hourly increase or extra time off is critical. Consider awarding an extra day off for perfect attendance. Reward staff involved with the training and orientation of new employees.

Scheduling Options

Flexible Scheduling

Make establishing a set schedule for full-time employees a priority. Allow employees to switch days with approval. Accept special requests prior to the completion of the schedule. Consider allowing job sharing positions and establishing an internal pool. Try to maintain set days off for senior staff.

Self-Scheduling

Ask employees their preferred work days while keeping staffing requirements in mind. Guide employees in the scheduling process, but allow for them to work together to complete a schedule. Provide incentives for employee flexibility as a reward.

Weekend Options

Establish a standard weekend and holiday rotation. Explore offering bonuses for employees willing to work on their weekend off. Create a standard weekend differential for wages. Consider higher rates for those willing to work every weekend.

Plan for Absences

Create a system where employees are "on call" to cover absences. Reward extra work with acknowledgement and a cash bonus or extra time off later. If an employee is called in with short notice, award with additional reward. Can the facility provide a free meal for staff who are working overtime?

Increased Staffing

Know your facility's busiest times. Try to have more staff available during the busiest times. Determine what duties may be delegated to other employees (however, ensure compliance with regulations).

Support Staff and Volunteers

Utilize volunteers to assist with tasks that they are able. Consider hiring support staff to assist with simple tasks such as passing ice water, changing linens or sitting one-to-one with clients.

Vacation Scheduling

Post a vacation schedule for employees to be able to see the possible times available to them. Have a policy that indicates that employees must sign up at least 30 days in advance for vacation. Consider seniority and sign up dates when approving requests for vacation time off. Try to accommodate vacations based on seniority.

Supportive Management

Supervisors are the human connection between your employees and the success of the facility. Supervisors must balance the competing demands of the work environment and are responsible for creating a positive work environment. Employees working with supportive supervisors will have likely have:

1. Higher job satisfaction
2. Lower level of stress
3. Feel more secure
4. Have more organizational commitment
5. Have greater productivity
6. Provide higher quality of care
7. Be willing to work on solutions to problems
8. Have lower turnover

Employees who are dissatisfied with their direct supervisors will consider opportunities for new employment before choosing to face problems and create solutions.

Supportive managers are imperative to employ. Supportive managers engage in two-way communication with all of their staff. They share information and seek the opinions and advice of their staff. Supportive managers provide positive feedback and recognize the assets of each individual. They facilitate the work of their staff by providing good working conditions, such as adequate training and supplies. Supportive managers mentor their employees and encourage autonomy and independent work. They recognize that employees also have a life outside of the workplace and allow for flexible scheduling to accommodate the needs of their staff.

Opportunities for Growth

Professional Development

Provide on-sight educational in-services relative to professional development (see Chapter 7 for additional information). Consider topics that would be mutually beneficial for the employees and the facility such as teamwork, conflict resolution, cultural awareness, improving organizational skills, and communication skills. Seek input from employees on topics of interest.

Education related to dealing with difficult behaviors should be included, especially in facilities that provide care to dementia residents. Invite a professional psychologist, social worker, or geriatric nurse to provide on-site in-services.

Skills for Personal Growth

Invite guest speakers to discuss topics important for life skills and coping. For example, educational in-services on stress management, parenting, finance, and motivations may be helpful. Create partnerships with local community organizations that may be willing to offer discounts for employees. Provide assistance for costs as a reward or benefit. Develop support groups that might meet before or after work.

Off-Site Education

Offer tuition support for off-site educational programs. Allow an employee to attend an off-site program as a reward for good performance.

Scholarships

Provide scholarships for continued education in any health care field. Seek contributions for the scholarship fund and support staff fund raisers for the scholarship.

Written Materials

Publish a newsletter and include useful information for the staff. Subscribe to geriatric newsletters and journals for employees to share. Provide a staff library.

Tuition Assistance

Provide tuition assistance and link payback to longevity and continued service. Formalize tuition assistance as a benefit. Promote partnerships for discounted tuition for students.

Employee Assistance Programs

Provide referrals for counseling services. Partner with churches and community agencies for staff support services. Provide informational material in staff lounges on topics such as parenting, divorce, alcohol and drug abuse, wellness, and financial planning.

Career Ladders

Develop career ladders for all positions. Develop criteria for each level within each careered ladder. Offer training for specialized units. Promote from within the facility when possible.

Recruitment

Seek the assistance of employees in your recruitment efforts. Ask employees to participate. Provide shadowing opportunities. Recognize the staff's participation in the recruitment process.

Post Open Jobs

Post all job openings and keep it updated. Search for qualified individuals from within your facility.

Trainer Acknowledgments

Pay a higher rate for trainers as part of career ladders. Consider a bonus at the end of a successful training program.

Peer Review

Encourage employees to participate in the development of standards for in-services, attendance, scheduling, routines, and policies. Allow for peer input at job performance reviews.

Promote Health and Wellness

Have intermittent health screenings available. Have wellness programs available both on- and off-site. Provide health insurance. Negotiate discounts for employees at local gyms. Provide employees access to on-site exercise equipment. Identify employees who are willing to facilitate walking or exercise groups.

Other Incentives

Treats

Provide free coffee or tea in the employee lounge. Provide a refrigerator and microwave for staff use. Sponsor an ice cream social or pizza party on occasions. Sponsor celebratory meals in honor of staff recognition awards.

Transportation

Assist employees to create carpools. Arrange for pick-up of staff at certain locations on a set schedule with a shuttle service. Arrange for discounted purchases of bus passes. Transportation is a critical issue for today's long-term care workforce.

Uniforms

If possible pay an allowance for uniforms. Negotiate discounts for employees at local uniforms shops. Is volume ordering feasible? Can uniforms be provided?

Child Care

Have a list of child care providers for employees with children. Support employee efforts to assist each other with child care issues. Is it feasible to create and in-house daycare with reduced fees for employees?

Meals

Allow employees to purchase meals at facility cost. Consider free meals especially for staff working extra shifts. Provide inexpensive vending items.

Teams

Sponsor employee sports teams. Purchase shirts printed with the facility logo.

Discounts

Seek discounts for employees with all vendors associated with the facility. In addition, try to negotiate discounts at local grocery stores, department stores, and local services such as drycleaning.

Staff Empowerment

Empowerment is the process of enabling individuals to think, behave, take action, control work, and decision making in autonomous ways. It is empowering to take control of one's own destiny. The empowerment of employees can result in increased initiative, innovation, involvement, enthusiasm, and efficiency. Empowerment involves enabling employees to make decisions on their own, involving employees to take responsibility for improving things, and encouraging employees to take an active role in their work.

Bowen and Lawler (1992) offer a common definition of empowerment as: *"the sharing with frontline employees four organizational ingredients: 1) information about the organization's performance; 2) rewards based on the organization's performance; 3) knowledge that enables employees to understand and contribute to organizational performance; and 4) power to make decisions that influence organizational direction and performance."*

Hahklotubbe (2005) suggests that long-term care facilities often overlook the concept employee empowerment and hence are missing a key component of both employee productivity and job satisfaction. His research linked empowerment to morale and productivity in long-term care environments, and identified employee empowerment as being frequently ignored as way to potentially improve quality of care.

Because job satisfaction is linked with retention, understanding and promoting employee empowerment is crucial for the assisted living facility. There are some considerations that the administrator may take into account in an effort to promote employee empowerment.

Overall Picture

Help your employees understand the overall picture of the facility. Educate employees by sharing you mission, strategic plans, public relations, and financial status. Teach customer service. Explain how public image and reputation is linked to facility success. Stress the importance of their role in creating success for the organization.

Input on Care Decisions

All employees should be asked for and encouraged to provide input to supervisors and managers. The input of direct care staff in the formation of care plans is critical. Seek the participation of direct care staff in resident specific concerns such as behavioral or feeding problems.

Input on Policies and Procedures

Request and accept input from employees for changes to policies and procedures.

Input on Quality Assurance/Improvement

Include employees from all levels in your quality assurance/improvement teams. Include issues such as training and orientation, retention, staffing policies, documentation tools, and scheduling. Ask for employee assistance, and ask staff to share their problems and successes. Invite and encourage all staff levels to be involved in staff meetings.

Committees

Invite all employees to serve on other committees such as food/dining, infection control, and ethics. Provide paid time for employees to attend those meetings and provide reports to employees who cannot attend.

Planning

Ask employees to assist in goal planning for specific departments. Encourage staff to have their own goals as well. Ask for their opinion on purchases of supplies and equipment.

Benefits

Request input from employees about benefit concerns. When possible, allow options and choices. Periodically review the benefit package and adjust accordingly.

Residents

Encourage suggestions regarding residents, such as room assignments and scheduling. Frontline staff will have valuable information on residents, such as resident conflicts and current problems. Seek ideas for improving care. Assist employees in the improvement of communication skills. Ask open-ended questions that promote the sharing of ideas. Communicate directly with employees about resident care, such as personal care and activities. Seriously consider the ideas of the staff with respect.

Meetings With the Administrator

Schedule regular meetings with all staff to discuss facility information and share feedback. Sponsor informational meetings and share corporate ideas and plans.

Newsletter

Have an employee newsletter. Encourage employees to author articles. Give them thoughtful ideas. For example, ask them to write about a recent positive employee experience.

CONCLUSIONS

This chapter has illustrated the importance of retaining and empowering quality employees in the assisted living facility. The reader has learned the definitions, risks, and factors associated with and adverse consequences of staff turnover in long-term care facilities. Job satisfaction is the most important factor in retaining quality staff. Job satisfaction is influenced by many factors, including wages and benefits, working conditions, respect, and morale. Retention strategies have been described and illustrated with examples that the reader may want to be considered in the development of a successful retention plan.

REFERENCES

American Association of Homes and Services for the Aged. (2002). *Assisted living salary and benefits report*. Washington, DC: American Association of Homes and Services for the Aged.

Bowen, D., & Lawler, E. (1992). The empowerment of service workers: What, why, how and when. *Sloan Management Review, 33*, 31–45.

Castle, N. (2006). Measuring staff turnover in nursing homes. *The Gerontologist, 46*, 210–219.

Castle, N., & Engberg, J. (2005). Turnover and quality in nursing homes. *Medical Care, 43*, 616–626.

Hahklotubbe, D. (2005). Empowerment and long-term care: A contradiction in terms. In D. Yee-Melichar & A. Boyle (Eds.), *Aging in contemporary society: Translating research into practice* (pp. 165–185). Ann Arbor, MI: XanEdu Publications.

Lescoe-Long. (2000). Why they leave: A new approach to staff retention. *Nursing Homes Long-Term Care Management, 10*, 70–75.

National Center for Assisted Living. (2001). *Facts and trends: Assisted living sourcebook 2001*. Washington, DC: National Center for Assisted Living.

Parsons, S., Simmons, W., Penn, K., & Furlough, M. (2003). Determinants of satisfactions and turnover among nursing assistants: The results of a statewide survey. *Journal of Gerontological Nursing, 29*, 51–58.

Riggs, C. (2001). A model of staff support to improve retention on long-term care. *Nursing Administration Quarterly, 25*, 43–54.

Stone, R., & Weiner, J. (2001). *Who will care for us? Addressing the long-term care workforce crisis.* Washington, DC: The Urban Institute and the American Association of Homes and Services for the Aging. Retrieved July 15, 2008, from http://aspe. hhs.gov/daltcp/reports/ltcwf.pdf

U.S. Senate Special Committee on Aging. (2003). *Assuring quality in assisted living: Guidelines for federal and state policy, state regulations, and operations.* Washington, DC: U.S. Government Printing Office.

Continuing Education

With Contributing Author: Sandi Flores

Learning Objectives

Upon the completion of Chapter 7, the reader will be able to:

- *Define continuing education.*
- *Identify the importance of continuing education as a key component of professional staff development.*
- *Describe a variety of methods for delivering continuing education.*
- *Understand the regulatory requirements surrounding continuing education in assisted living.*
- *Learn about several model continuing education programs.*
- *Recognize online continuing education as an innovative way to provide continuing education for professionals.*

INTRODUCTION

This chapter focuses on continuing education, a key component of professional staff development for both assisted living administrators and direct care staff. Continuing education is defined, and its importance is discussed. A variety of modalities utilized for continuing education are explained. Regulations for continuing education requirements are summarized by states for both assisted living administrators and direct care staff. The chapter then continues with descriptions of model continuing education programs from leading professionals in the industry. In addition, a model of online training courses is included to highlight course descriptions and useful resources.

CONTINUING EDUCATION

Continuing education is an integral part of professional development (Puetz, 1981). Although it is often a requirement for certification or licensure renewal, it should not be viewed as just a necessity. As discussed in Chapter 6, professional development is the key to retaining valuable employees. Most professional groups, such as physicians, nurses, teachers, and engineers, aim to improve the quality of their professional performance by continuing professional development, often in the form of continuing education classes (Todd, 1987). Long-term care professionals, specifically assisted living administrators and staff, also benefit from continuing education.

Continuing education is an all-encompassing term within a broad spectrum of post-secondary learning activities and programs. Recognized forms of post-secondary learning activities within the domain include: degree credit courses, non-degree career training, workforce training, formal personal enrichment courses, self-directed learning (such as through Internet interest groups, clubs or personal research activities), and experiential learning as applied to problem solving.

Within the domain of continuing education, professional continuing education is a specific learning activity generally characterized by the issuance of a certificate or continuing education units for the purpose of documenting attendance at a designated seminar or course of instruction. Licensing bodies in a number of fields impose continuing education requirements on members who hold licenses to practice within a particular profession. These requirements are intended to encourage professionals to expand their knowledge and stay up-to-date on new developments. Depending on the field, these requirements may be satisfied through college or university coursework, extension courses, or conference and seminar attendance.

Methods for Delivering Continuing Education

The method of delivery of continuing education can include traditional types of classroom lectures and laboratories. However, continuing education makes heavy use of distance learning, which not only includes independent study, but which can also include videotaped/CD-ROM material, broadcast programming, online/internet delivery, and online interactive courses.

In addition to independent study, the use of conference-type group study, which can include study networks (in many instances, can meet together online) as well as different types of seminars/workshops, can be used to facilitate learning. A combination of traditional, distance, and conference-type study, or two of these three types, may be used for a particular continuing education course or program.

Vital Need for Continuing Education

The U.S. Department of Health and Human Services (2000), in the publication, *Healthy People 2010*, included over 75 objectives related to health education and professional development. Furthermore, the landmark report for the Pew Health Professions Commission, listed 21 specific competencies necessary for all professionals in the changing health care environment with seven competencies directly related to education and professional development (Allegrante, Moon, Auld, & Gebbie, 2001). The demographics of the aging population highlight the need to anticipate an increase in need for both long-term care services and professionals (U.S. Department of Health and Human Services, 2000). Certainly, assisted living professionals will continue to be an integral part of meeting the needs of the aging population.

Continuing Education: What Administrators Say

Cristina Flores (2005), in a California study, surveyed certified assisted living administrators to identify their perceived need for additional knowledge in specific areas of practice. Areas in which *maximum need for knowledge* was identified by most participants included:

- Health and aging
- Mental health and aging
- Behavioral/dementia management
- Activity programs
- Marketing
- Regulatory updates
- Management and staffing
- Elder abuse

Areas in which *moderate need for knowledge* was identified by most participants included:

- Public policy for the aged
- Death and dying
- Hospice regulations
- Dementia regulations
- Meeting the cultural needs of residents
- Biology of aging
- Nutrition and aging
- Health care and service
- Pharmacology
- Exercise physiology
- Women's health and aging

TABLE 7.1	Annual Staff Training Requirements by State
State	**Annual**
Alabama	Topics
Alaska	12 hours
Arizona	12 hours
Arkansas	6 hours
California	4 hours/topics
Colorado	Topics
Connecticut	6 hours
Delaware	12 hours
District of Columbia	12 hours
Florida	Not specified
Georgia	16 hours
Hawaii	6 hours
Idaho	8 hours
Illinois	8 hours
Indiana	Topics/hours
Iowa	Not specified
Kansas	Topics
Kentucky	Not specified
Louisiana	Annual plan
Maine	8 hours/2 years
Maryland	Topics
Massachusetts	10 hours/topics
Michigan	Not specified
Minnesota	Not specified
Mississippi	Quarterly
Missouri	Not specified
Montana	Not specified
Nebraska	12 hours
Nevada	8 hours
New Hampshire	Topics
New Jersey	20 hours/2 years
New Mexico	Topics
New York	12 hours
North Carolina	Not specified
North Dakota	Topics

(Continued)

TABLE 7.1	Annual Staff Training Requirements by State (*Continued*)
State	**Annual**
Ohio	6 hours/topics
Oklahoma	8 hours
Oregon	Not specified
Pennsylvania	12 hours
Rhode Island	Not specified
South Carolina	General
South Dakota	Topics
Tennessee	Not specified
Texas	6 hours/topics
Utah	Topics
Vermont	20 hours
Virginia	8 hours
Washington	Not specified
West Virginia	Topics
Wisconsin	Not specified
Wyoming	Not specified

Rules specifying a number of hours also include topics that are covered. Rules listing topics only do not specify how many hours of training are needed. *Source*: Mollica et al., 2008: *Residential Care and Assisted Living Compendium, 2007.*

There were no areas in which a *minimal or no need for additional knowledge* was identified by most participants.

REGULATORY REQUIREMENTS

The requirements for continuing education are fueled by government legislature, professional organizations standards and requirements. Societal pressures for improved quality of care and regulatory agencies, such as state agencies are responsible for the oversight of assisted living facilities. These types of demands give rise to the need for quality continuing education courses.

As noted throughout this book, regulations vary state by state. Table 7.1 summarizes the annual direct care staff training requirements (i.e., continuing education) by state and Table 7.2 summarizes the annual continuing education requirements for assisted living administrators by state.

TABLE 7.2	Annual Continuing Education for Assisted Living Administrators by State
State	**Annual**
Alabama	Contain a minimum of 12 equivalent hours of continuing education per year for licensees issued a Category I assisted living administrator license. Contain an additional 6 equivalent hours of continuing education per year for licensees issued a Category II assisted living administrator license.
Alaska	Training requirements are as follows: each administrator shall complete 18 clock hours of continuing education annually.
Arizona	A certified adult care home manager seeking renewal shall submit an application for biennial renewal of certificate, accompanied by the prescribed fee, showing address and current employment, and shall submit evidence of completion of 24 hours of continuing education credit per year.
Arkansas	All staff and contracted providers having direct contact with residents and all food service personnel shall receive a minimum of 6 hours per year of ongoing education and training to include in-service and on-the-job training designed to reinforce training.
California	Administrators are required to complete at least 20 hours of continuing education per year from an approved vendor. 8 hours of dementia training is also required every 2 years upon certification renewal.
Colorado	None specified.
Connecticut	Must complete 12 hours of continuing education per year.
Delaware	Continuing education programs consisting of Board approved seminars, resident or extension courses, conferences and workshops totaling 48 classroom hours or more, in specific subject areas are required for biennial licensure of a license.
District of Columbia	12 hours annually.
Florida	Administrators and managers shall participate in 12 hours related to assisted living every 2 years.
Georgia	All persons, including the administrator or on-site manager, who offer direct care to the residents, must satisfactorily complete a total of at least 16 hours of continuing education each year, in applicable courses approved by the Department.
Hawaii	None specified.
Idaho	Applicants for annual recertification/renewal shall be required to have a minimum of 12 hours of continuing education courses within the preceding 12 month period.

(Continued)

TABLE 7.2	Annual Continuing Education for Assisted Living Administrators by State (*Continued*)
State	**Annual**
Illinois	Each manager and direct care staff member shall complete a minimum of 8 hours of ongoing training, applicable to the employee's responsibilities, every 12 months after the starting date of employment.
Indiana	Licensed Health Facility administrators must obtain at least 40 hours of continuing education during each 2 year licensing period.
Iowa	Not specified.
Kansas	Not specified.
Kentucky	Not specified.
Louisiana	The Director shall participate annually in at least 12 hours of continuing education in the field of geriatrics, assisted living concepts, specialized training in the population served and/or supervisory/management techniques.
Maine	Licensed Residential Care Administrators shall be required to accrue 12 hours of Board-approved CEUs between July 1 and June 30 of each year.
Maryland	An assisted living manager employed in a program that is licensed for 5 or more beds shall be required to complete 20 hours of Department-approved continuing education every 2 years.
Massachusetts	A minimum of 10 hours per year of ongoing education and training is required for all employees, with at least 1 hour spent on dementia/cognitive impairment topics.
Michigan	*Homes for the Aged:* None indicated *Adult Foster Care:* Licensee and administrator training requirements. (1) A licensee and an administrator shall complete the following educational requirements specified in subdivision (a) or (b) of this sub-rule, or a combination thereof, on an annual basis: (a) Participate in, and successfully complete, 16 hours of training designated or approved by the department that is relevant to the licensee's admission policy and program statement. (b) Have completed 6 credit hours at an accredited college or university in an area that is relevant to the licensee's admission policy and program statement as approved by the department
Minnesota	Not specified.
Mississippi	Quarterly training.
Missouri	Not specified.
Montana	Not specified.

(Continued)

TABLE 7.2	Annual Continuing Education for Assisted Living Administrators by State (*Continued*)
State	Annual
Nebraska	Each year of employment, a facility administrator must complete 12 hours of ongoing training in areas related to care and facility management of the population served.
Nevada	Receive annually not less than 8 hours of training related to providing for the needs of the residents of a residential facility.
New Hampshire	Administrators must complete a minimum of 12 hours of continuing education per year relating to resident plan of care; characteristics of client disabilities; nutrition, basic hygiene, and dental care; first aid; medication management; dementia; resident assessment; aging; and resident rights.
New Jersey	In order to be eligible to renew a current certification, an assisted living administrator shall complete at least 20 hours, every 2 years, of continuing education regarding assisted living concepts and related topics, as specified and approved by the Department of Health and Senior Services.
New Mexico	Not specified.
New York	Sixty hours every 2 years.
North Carolina	The administrator must verify that he earns 15 hours a year of continuing education credits related to the management of domiciliary homes and care of aged and disabled persons in accordance with procedures established by the Department of Health and Human Services.
North Dakota	Twelve hours of continuing education annually.
Ohio	Each administrator shall receive at least 12 hours per calendar year of continuing education beginning with the second full calendar year of employment. Continuing education shall be relevant to their job responsibilities.
Oklahoma	Administrators shall have 16 hours of job-related training annually.
Oregon	Twenty hours of continuing education every year. Up to 20 of those hours may be taken online.
Pennsylvania	Administrators shall have at least 24 hours of annual training related to the job duties.
Rhode Island	Sixteen hours annually.
South Carolina	A community residential care facility administrator must have 18 hours of continuing education.
South Dakota	None indicated.

(Continued)

TABLE 7.2	Annual Continuing Education for Assisted Living Administrators by State (*Continued*)
State	**Annual**
Tennessee	Biennial renewal of certification is required. During the period, prior to renewal, of at least 24 classroom hours of continuing education courses approved by the board.
Texas	All managers must show evidence of 12 hours of annual continuing education.
Utah	During each 2 year period commencing on June 1 of each odd numbered year, a licensee shall be required to complete not less than 40 hours of qualified professional education directly related to the licensee's professional practice.
Vermont	Administrators must complete 20 hours of continuing education per year in courses related to assisted living principles and the philosophy and care of the elderly and disabled individuals.
Virginia	The administrator shall attend at least 20 hours of training related to management or operation of a residential facility for adults or client specific training needs within each 12-month period. When adults with mental impairments reside in the facility, at least 5 of the required 20 hours of training shall focus on the resident who is mentally impaired.
Washington	Individuals subject to a continuing education requirement must complete at least 10 hours of continuing education each calendar year (January 1 through December 31) after the year in which they successfully complete basic or modified basic training.
West Virginia	Ten hours each year.
Wisconsin	Each administrator and each resident care staff employee of the CBRF shall receive at least 12 hours per calendar year of continuing education beginning with the second full calendar year of employment.
Wyoming	Not specified.

Source: www.aladvantage.com

MODEL CONTINUING EDUCATION PROGRAMS

David Hahklotubbe, MA, has developed seven model continuing education classes for assisted living administrators and staff. Descriptions of the courses he has developed and improved over time are seen in Figure 7.1 (www.hahktc.com). Another example of model continuing education programs includes the work of Sandi Flores, RN, and colleagues (www.communityed.com). Figure 7.2 illustrates eight important continuing education classes developed under her direction.

1. You Have Openings, You Need This Marketing Class
An in-depth look into the principles of marketing, sales and business development. Most operators of long-term care communities are equipped to provide quality care, but do not have the education, ability, or interest in managing the sales and marketing side to their businesses. The overall impact on neglecting the marketing of their services are far reaching, utilizing System's Theory, we can see that a lack of marketing effects Budgets for Staffing, Quality of Care for Residents, Perception in the Community, Lifespan of the Business, Capital Upgrades, and The Perception that the general public will form of Long-Term Care Living. Designed to: First, help empower students with tools to recognize that marketing is a necessary component to running a quality care home; Second, to assist the student with recognizing what services are marketable; Thirdly, how to create a successful marketing plan, accentuating their individual points of difference; Fourth, to understand the importance of execution, maintenance, and constant penetration into the market; Lastly, tips and tricks of utilizing referral sources effectively – who to steer clear from.

2. The Best Dementia Class You Will Ever Take
Designed as an overview of various Dementias, Alzheimer's Disease and other Memory Impairments. It identifies the most recurring difficult behaviors to manage in persons suffering from these impairments. It introduces an intervention which treats the difficult behavior as a system rather than as a random occurrence. The behaviors focused on are: Anxiety, Agitation, Hallucinations, Wandering, "Wanting to go home," Paranoia, Dressing/Bathing, Inappropriate Sexual Behaviors, Sleeping Problems, Incontinence, and Eating Issues. It allows the students to become comfortable applying the techniques through studying fictitious case studies and then acting out the management techniques in a group role-playing format. Lastly, this course has a segment dedicated to Sundowner's Syndrome. There is no reason why learning about dementia can't be fun!

3. The Best Activities Class You Will Ever Take
Content: Designed as an in-depth overview of various approaches to activities for those suffering from Dementia, Alzheimer's Disease and other related cognitive impairments. It identifies the most recurring difficult behaviors to manage with a special spotlight on the role of activities in managing Sundowner's Syndrome. It shows how activities can be utilized to redirect or even prevent behaviors from occurring. It introduces assessment techniques for both the care staff and the client. It applies the system approach toward managing behavior, introduces different levels of activities designed to stimulate and redirect certain behaviors. It addresses the physical/psychological and emotional components to each activity. It spotlights knowing when to abandon an activity and when to move on to the next. It introduces activities as a marketing tool. It discusses and maps out how to create an activity calendar. Lastly, and most fun, failure-free activities created by HAHK are introduced, participated in, and led by students.

4. The Staffing Class You Hope Your Competitors Aren't Taking
Designed to assist the management team in acquiring, empowering and retaining quality personnel. Group activities designed to tackle common staffing issues utilizing real-life mistakes as functional case studies. The concept of **empowerment** and how it fits in long-term care is discussed. The students learn techniques and strategies on how to employ the

FIGURE 7.1　Seven model courses for administrators and direct care staff.

empowerment concept into their facilities. The systems approach is discussed in terms of cyclical rewards from employing the concept. In-depth discussions about how empowerment has a direct relationship with morale, productivity and effectivity are explored. Techniques for building effective teams from the ground up by successful staffing are given. The fact that training and education are necessary ingredients in retention is covered. Finally, management paradigm change and the results of being a pro-active/hands-on manager are shared.

5. Successfully Managing Your Biggest Challenge: Families of Your Clients
Designed as an in-depth, hands-on tutorial of how to manage familial psychodynamics. Understanding the pressure, emotional stress, and the bevy of other influences on the behavior of the family members of clients in long-term care. The class begins with an empathic exercise and leads into discussion about common psychological issues that afflict families. Clinical definitions of common psychological issues are presented as a foundation. Discussion about how these psychological issues can influence behavior and the types of behavior that are commonly manifested is shared. Most importantly, a discussion about how to avoid the behaviors from occurring is presented. Finally, there is great emphasis on a cutting edge concept of "Viewing a Complaint as a Gift." Role plays and fictitious case studies are used to create an interactive environment. Lastly, a profound exercise on the power.

6. Burnout: If You and Your Staff Are Immune to it, You Don't Need This Class
The foundation is laid by providing the grim statistics of how burnout affects the physical, emotional, and financial well-being of the long-term care provider. Systems theory is applied to how burnout ultimately affects the quality of life of our clients and staff. The clinical definition of burnout is provided as well as relaxing group activities designed to empower the student with the ability to identify burnout, identify the source, and how to implement a program to manage and prevent it. Specific, effective, stress management, and prevention techniques are discussed and engaged in. Applied activities include: purposeful breathing, smudging (spiritual Native American cleansing), releasing the demons through drumming, visualization and aroma therapy. The discussion of creating ritual and forming "Good Habits" is discussed. The goal of this class is to educate while relaxing, recharging and rejuvenating. The dress code is "relaxed" (sweats, pajamas, and slippers are recommended).

7. Maintaining Compliance Through Safe Food Handling Practices (ServSafe®)
Designed as an in-depth look into safe food handling and satisfying dietary requirements. This course is nationally recognized and required certification training for compliance with the Department of Health. This course covers principles and detailed instruction on preparing, storing, and serving food to paying clientele. In addition, a segment has been added to cover the dietary needs of clients of long-term care. This course is accompanied by an optional exam which provides the opportunity to those who wish to be in complete compliance by having a ServSafe ® certificate in their building. This course is approved for 8 hours of CEU as well as satisfying Department of Health Curriculum duration is 8 hours; exam time is an additional 1 hour. It is highly recommended that the student take the exam and receive the ServSafe® Certificate, however, it is not required.

Source: Hahk Training and Consulting (http://www.hahktc.com)

FIGURE 7.1   *(Continued)*

I. Regulation Compliance Review

This course provides participants with a review of the regulations that generate the most serious and common licensing citations for adult residential facilities and residential care facilities for the elderly. Additionally, participants will examine ways to proactively remain in compliance with each of the regulations discussed, including suggestions from successful administrators. Recent regulatory changes or updates will also be discussed. Videos are included of representatives answering key administrator concerns.

2. Leadership Skills for Today's Administrators

The success of any assisted living or residential care community is dependent upon the skills of its administrative team. This course focuses on two key areas necessary to be a successful administrator: leadership and staffing. Effective leadership is the result of great leadership skill. Participants will have an opportunity to identify their leadership skills and develop an action plan. Next, as many businesses know, a good company is only as good as their employees. Skills for recruiting, interviewing, and hiring employees will be presented. Participants will also learn how to motivate great staff to excel, as well as how to work with difficult employees. This course will prepare effective administrators to become proactive leaders who are supported by outstanding staff.

3. Food Service in Residential Care

This program is designed to provide administrators with the fundamentals they need to provide outstanding food service in residential care. As we all know, food service and the dining experience is the highlight of the day for many of our residents. Meal times provide both nutritional and social needs for our residents. This course discusses what is important in the social aspects of our residents' dining experience. Prevention of food borne illness is addressed as well as how to establish a safe food program. Participants will obtain in-depth knowledge on meeting the nutritional needs of our clients.

4. Enhancing Resident Care

This course will focus on direct resident care issues with an emphasis on enhancing resident quality of life. Discussions will address common physical limitations, such as visual impairments, hearing deficits, and mobility limitations. Assisting with ambulation, including a review of ambulatory aides, such as walkers and wheelchairs, with a focus on safe and appropriate use of the devices will be discussed. The commonly overlooked issue of oral care will also be addressed, and the important role of direct care staff will be a focus throughout the course.

5. Dementia Care: Progress Report

It is important for residential care and assisted living administrators to have a working knowledge of current information and research related to Alzheimer's disease. This course will review the most recent Progress Report on Alzheimer's Disease from the National Institute on Aging. Topics addressed will include causes and progression of Alzheimer's Disease (AD); lifestyle interventions; and emerging treatments.

FIGURE 7.2   Eight model courses for administrators and direct care staff.

6. Mind, Body, and Spirit in Dementia Care
Residents with dementia have emotional and spiritual needs that should be met and go beyond simply attending to their basic physical care. This dementia care program encourages maintaining a positive care environment that embraces the unique care needs, rather than view care as a constant burden or challenge. Practical approaches to the variety of personal care needs, including bathing, grooming, feeding, and assisting with medications will be covered. Safety concerns and risk management strategies will address the special care concerns. Meeting the needs of the resident's family will also be covered.

7. Emergencies and Disasters
This course will prepare administrators to effectively prepare for disasters and other emergencies in their communities. Topics addressed will include advanced disaster and emergency preparation; staff responsibilities and training; safety equipment and supplies; evacuations; disaster drills; and medical emergencies.

8. Building an Outstanding Activity Program
Administrators in RCFE and ARF facilities have a responsibility to provide an opportunity for each resident to maximize his or her personal potential for enjoyment and fulfillment. Successful activity programming begins with an assessment of individual needs and creation of a service or activity care plan. Activities are designed with a purpose to meet the individual and social needs of residents/clients through the use of a variety of program types. Specific suggestions for a variety of activities are presented including individual and group activities. Participants will prepare an appropriate activity, and experience activities through the eyes of the resident/client. Participants will learn resources available to assist in developing an outstanding activities program. Documenting program participation and individual progress is key to maintaining a successful activities program.

Source: Community Education, LLC (www.communityed.com)

FIGURE 7.2 *(Continued)*

Online Continuing Education

Online learning has become a popular and innovative way to provide continuing education to professionals. Sandi Flores, RN, and colleagues, in their work with Community Education, LLC, have created multiple model online continuing education courses for assisted living administrators and staff. Figure 7.3 demonstrates 20 model continuing education classes that provide administrators with innovative ways to utilize technology to enhance learning for themselves and assisted living staff (www.communityed.com).

1. Abuse, Neglect, and Exploitation Prevention
This course introduces the student to information regarding various aspects and types of abuse, neglect, and exploitation in residential settings for children, adults, and the elderly. Types of abuse, neglect, and exploitation are defined, described, and discussed within this course. Indicators of potential situations of abuse, neglect, and exploitation will be identified, and preventative methods demonstrated.

2. Common Infectious Conditions
This course will provide an overview of four common infectious conditions found in residential care and assisted living settings. The four conditions discussed are: methicillin-resistant staphylococcus aureus (MRSA), vancomycin-resistant enterococci (VRE), norovirus, and clostridium difficile. For each condition, the pathophysiology, the infectious process, modes of transmission, treatment, and prevention are discussed. Proper staff education, standard precautions, and isolation precautions are discussed as well.

3. Congestive Heart Failure
This program will provide an in-depth look at congestive heart failure, symptoms the patient exhibits and common treatments, risk, and lifestyle changes.

4. Constipation
This course introduces the student to current information related to the medical condition of constipation. An overview of the normal digestive system is discussed to better understand constipation. Such topics as causes, symptoms, and prevention of constipation are discussed. Examinations and tests to diagnose constipation and common treatments are presented. Learn the best practices for assisting individuals and residents who are experiencing constipation. Case studies will be utilized to apply the knowledge learned in this course to real-life situations.

5. Dementia Fundamentals
This course begins with an in-depth definition of dementia, its symptoms, specific types of dementia, and possible causes. This program will take participants through a dynamic process of care strategies from pre-admission through the progression of the disease including late stage complications. Also presented are unique behavior intervention techniques. Activities are analyzed with particular emphasis on quality of life issues. Research, new trends in care, pharmacological management of dementia, as well as self analysis of the quality of care carried out will also be discussed. Emphasis is placed on care provided in the residential care setting.

6. Depression and Suicide
This course will provide an overview of depression and suicide in the assisted living resident. Both the myths and facts surrounding depression and suicide among older adults will be discussed. The definition and symptoms of depression are presented. Ways to recognize if a resident is depressed will be addressed. Current statistics on depression among older adults is presented. The participant will learn how to identify a depressed resident, and ways to reduce the risk of depression among residents in the assisted living setting. The proper steps to take if a resident appears to be suicidal will also be discussed.

7. Digestive System
This program will provide an in-depth look at the anatomy of the digestive tract and many common disease processes affecting the elderly population. The pathophysiology of these disease processes are discussed in great detail, as well as potential complications and treatment. Assessment and care of the resident will be discussed as well.

FIGURE 7.3 Twenty model online courses for administrators and direct care staff.

8. Effective Communication Skills
We are all living in a technologically sophisticated world that continues to grow and change by the day. This course will identify the essential technology skills that all successful administrators should possess. A self-assessment is provided to assist administrators in identifying his/her technology skill strengths and weaknesses. Necessary skills are discussed and categorized into basic (must have), intermediate, and advanced skills. Threats of using email, including malware, are discussed with ways to protect personal computers from these threats. Learn common email and cell phone text messaging etiquette. An overview of text messaging uses, limitations, and jargon will get any administrator comfortable using this new technology. Resources for enhancing skills are provided.

9. Essential Technology Skills
We are all living in a technologically sophisticated world that continues to grow and change by the day. This course will identify the essential technology skills that all successful administrators should possess. A self-assessment is provided to assist administrators in identifying his/her technology skill strengths and weaknesses. Necessary skills are discussed and categorized into basic (must have), intermediate, and advanced skills. Threats of using email, including malware, are discussed with ways to protect personal computers from these threats. Learn common email and cell phone text messaging etiquette. An overview of text messaging uses, limitations, and jargon will get any administrator comfortable using this new technology. Resources for enhancing skills are provided.

10. HIV/AIDS for Care Providers
This course will provide the care provider relevant knowledge about HIV and AIDS. Demographic, geographic, and incident rate data is presented. To assist in their care of residents, care providers will obtain knowledge on the HIV/AIDS clinical signs, symptoms, modes of transmission, risk factors, prevention, and screening and diagnosis. Common HIV medical complications are presented. The participant will receive an overview of how the HIV virus duplicates, and the general classes of drugs that target each stage of HIV replication. Participants will gain an understanding of the psychosocial challenges of persons with HIV/AIDS and the importance of positive psychosocial support systems. Universal precautions and care facility considerations are presented to help care providers minimize accidental occupational exposure.

11. Lice, Scabies, and Bed Bugs
This program will provide an in-depth look at lice /scabies/bed bugs, defining infestations, transmission, myths, and common treatments, risk, and methods of elimination.

12. Seizure Alert
This program provides an in-depth look at seizures and epilepsy. Seizures are described in great detail as the presentation covers classification, causes, emergency procedures, treatment modalities, as well as current medical screening and diagnostic studies. This course will also include the history and incidence of epilepsy, risk factors, current treatment options, as well as discuss EEG and neuroimaging as they pertain to epilepsy.

13. Sexual Harassment
This course will provide the sexual harassment training for supervisors. The training will focus on federal and state laws, liability issues, harassment policies, employee rights, supervisor responsibilities, investigation procedures, and a number of other items necessary for the success of striving to provide a harassment-free workplace.

FIGURE 7.3 *(Continued)*

14. Staffing Skills for Administrators
The success of any assisted living or residential care community is dependent upon the skills of its administrative team. This course focuses on one of the key areas necessary to be a successful administrator: staffing. As many businesses know, a good company is only as good as its employees. This course will discuss one of the most challenging tasks to any administrator, which is to recruit, select, hire, train and motivate employees. Correct steps to provide performance corrections and terminations will also be discussed.

15. Substance Abuse and Treatment
This course will address the issues of substance misuse and abuse in residential care facilities. Participants will obtain insight on substance abuse risk factors and incidence. An overview of the human brain and ways in which abused drugs work in our brain is presented. Administrators and caregivers will learn the most common drugs of abuse, including their effects and risks. This course also presents the National Institute on Drug Abuse 13 Principles of Effective Drug Treatment. Various types of treatment programs and approaches to drug abuse treatment will also be addressed.

16. Tuberculosis
This program will provide an in-depth look at tuberculosis (TB) and the disease processes affecting today's population. The pathophysiology of this disease process is discussed in great detail as well as potential complications and treatment. Assessment and care of the resident will be discussed as well.

17. Progress Report on Alzheimer's Disease
This is an advanced course designed for administrators, nurses, and care providers desiring to better understand the in-depth issues related to Alzheimer's disease; causes, treatment, prevention, and care. The course summarizes the annual *Progress Report on Alzheimer's Disease* prepared by the National Institute on Aging. Focus is on current understandings as well as research projects currently underway.

18. Understanding MRSA
This program provides detailed information regarding methicillin-resistant staphylococcus aureus (MRSA) infections. Pathophysiology, the infectious process, modes of transmission, and prevention are discussed. Proper staff education, standard precautions, and isolation precautions are discussed as well.

19. UTI
Urinary Tract Infection (UTI): This program will provide participants with an in-depth look into urinary tract infections and its associated medical conditions. The signs and symptoms, appropriate interventions, treatment, and current research trends of UTI will all be discussed as well as complications, such as pyelonephritis. Focus is placed on prevention and treatment.

20. VRE
Vancomycin-Resistant Enterococcus (VRE): This course discusses vancomycin-resistant enterococcus (VRE) bacteria in great detail. Incidence of infection, pathophysiology, transmission, detection, and disease management will all be presented. Focus is placed on disease prevention with particular attention to the unique concerns of residents in long-term care facilities.

Source: Community Education, LLC (www.communityed.com)

FIGURE 7.3 *(Continued)*

CONCLUSIONS

This chapter has demonstrated the importance of continuing education for assisted living professionals, specifically administrators and direct care staff. Continuing education has been discussed in a manner to assist the reader in understanding the benefits of excellent continuing education programs, as well as the legal requirements which vary by state. Leaders in the continuing education field have shared their model programs, both with traditional classroom and online curriculum descriptions. Researchers and professionals continue to identify ways to improve the quality of care and quality of life of residents living in assisted living facilities. Continuing education is an important way to maintain and update the knowledge and skills necessary to run a successful assisted living community.

REFERENCES

Allegrante, J., Mooh, R., Auld, E., & Gebbie, M. (2001). Continuing education needs of currently employed public health education workforce. *American Journal of Public Health, 91*(8), 1230–1234.

Assisted Living Advantage. (2009). *On-line education.* Retrieved May 25, 2009, from http://www.aladvantage.com/states/online/online.htm

Community Education, LLC. (2009). *The leading provider of assisted living and residential care education.* Retrieved May 25, 2009, from http://www.communitycd.com/

Flores, C. (2005). Assessing the needs of RCFE administrators. In D. Yee-Melichar & A. Boyle (Eds.), *Aging in contemporary society: Translating research into practice* (pp. 17–25). Ann Arbor, MI: XanEdu Publications.

Hahk Training and Consulting. (2009). *Continuing education for license renewal.* Retrieved May 25, 2009, from http://hahktc.com/RCFE_ARF.html

Mollica, R., Sims-Kastelein, K., & O'Keeffe, J. (2008). *Residential care and assisted living compendium, 2007.* U.S. Department of Health and Human Services, Office of the Assistant Secretary for Planning and Evaluation, Office of Disability, Aging and Long-Term Care Policy and Research Triangle Institute. Retrieved June 21, 2008, http://aspe.hhs.gov/daltcp/reports/2007/07alcom.htm

Puetz, B. (1981). *Continuing education for nurses: A complete guide to effective programs.* Rockville, MD: Aspen Publications.

Todd, F. (Ed.). (1987). *Planning continuing professional development.* New York, NY: Croom Helm.

U.S. Department of Health and Human Services. (2000). *Healthy people 2010.* Washington, DC: Author.

CHAPTER **8**

Business, Management, and Marketing

With Contributing Author: Joseph F. Melichar

Learning Objectives

Upon the completion of Chapter 8, the reader will be able to:

- *Describe management theories, and how they can be implemented in assisted living facility (ALF) administration.*
- *Discuss how creating a management method and style is important to ALF operations.*
- *Implement a planning framework in order to provide a basis for efficient and effective ALF management and organizational structure.*
- *Understand business and operational plans, and how they can be used in the management and operation of an ALF.*
- *Understand the need for, and integration of, information and technology support systems.*
- *Understand the importance of marketing, and how it fits into the management and operation of an ALF.*

INTRODUCTION

An organization's managers seek the efficient use of resources to meet the end goals and objectives of the organization. For assisted living facilities (ALFs), the end objectives are related to the provision of residential services tied to the well-being of residents. Knowing the desired outcomes, the issue(s) faced by ALF managers is how to undertake management tasks, and then plan for success. Management has been defined as "both science and art" (Buttaro, 1994). There are numerous textbooks and articles addressing the topic of management for an ALF (Allen, 1999; Singh, 2010).

This chapter presents an overview on specific management methods that might be used in managing ALFs. The effective use of any management approach is dependent on the description of the organization and its business, operational, and marketing plans. These plans describe the selection and application of an effective management methodology and style. Irrespective of management style, there are constraints that must be met (e.g., budget, schedule, services, etc.); however, the planning system approach is a way of describing operations, expectations, and limitations to enable the execution of an effective ALF management.

This chapter contains information on: (1) management theories, (2) management method and style, (3) general constraints on management and operations, (4) organizing principles, (5) "system" as the basis for organization, management, and evaluation, (6) a framework to create a business and operation plan enabling evaluation of outcome, (7) evaluation and quality control, (8) business plan, (9) operational plan, (10) information and technology support services, and (11) marketing plan and approaches.

MANAGEMENT THEORIES

Managers control resource transformations into services and the implementation of those transformations. There are a large number of management methodologies with some common threads that include: participatory vs. non-participatory styles, quality control, and constant evolution of product quality. There also are recurrent themes through the different methodologies, and in some cases some of the "latest methodologies" almost appear like fads. It is best to remember the song lyric about everything old being new again (Allen & Sanger, 1979), and develop a management strategy from a mix of approaches. The following information outlines some of these main strategies.

Scientific Management

"Scientific Management" stems from the work of Taylor (1911), and was developed in a period that reflected "reductionism" as a principle. Taylor described a management approach that reduced management to controlling tasks with a high degree of division of labor. The focus is on producing well-defined tasks within the work profile making it is easier to train and assign workers to the task. The approach initially was focused on activities within a production process of physical objects, but has grown to be used more generally, and is imbedded in many subsequent methodologies. Its value to an ALF is the concept of looking at tasks and the division of labor and how these definitions affect the services provided within a broader and more facilitative management process.

Bureaucratic Method

The bureaucratic organizational form (March & Simon, 1957) was first described by the sociologist Weber (1947). It features clearly delimited functions by component elements with rigid boundaries, and well-defined tasks and lines of authority and reporting. A top-down chain of command is created with separation of an organization into functions and outputs. The categorization of function creates rigidity and limits decision-making within each organizational unit.

There is less room for individuality, adaptation, and ability to innovate than in most other forms of management, which spawned the concept of bureaucratic personality (Merton, 1940). People working in bureaucracies can become authoritative within their small portion of the organization and typically stay within the boundaries created for them. This form tends to be hierarchical, and the amount of authority and control grows as you move up the hierarchy.

There have been a series of analyses that suggest that bureaucratic form can be used without the rigidity and strong control lines (e.g., Alder & Borys, 1996). This view suggests that some of the strong points of this method can be used without accruing negative aspects. Organizational units can have delimited functions, a clear statement of boundaries, and enunciation of job descriptions. The use of team concepts and internal communications can avoid the rigidity of pure bureaucratic forms. An ALF can use this concept to help frame its organizational structure, define processes, lines of communication, and the expected lines of authority in different components.

Theory X and Theory Y

There was a growth of the role of the interpersonal and behavioral aspects of organization operation and management during the 20th century. It could be seen in Merton's (1940) (op.cit.) description of bureaucracy and escalated in the period of the 1960s (e.g., Hodge & Johnson, 1970). One major step in this growth was Theory X and Theory Y (McGregor, 1960) that stemmed from Maslow's (1943, 1954) "hierarchy of needs" (i.e., physiological need, safety needs, social needs, esteem needs, and self-actualization). The lowest level indicated a need for control that decreased across the hierarchy to self-actualization at the highest level. Theory X represents an approach that requires external direction and is reflective of a strong top-down authoritarian approach. Theory Y reflects an approach that seeks to develop each person's higher motivations and results in a participatory management style in which people are seen as assets.

Theory X seems to reflect most aspects of a rigid pure bureaucratic form. It assumes employees avoid work when possible, will not take responsibility, need reward systems to perform, and require a high degree of control. Theory Y presents the employee in an opposite manner. The employee becomes a source of support to the organization and is more participatory and can provide a degree of self management and creative support. The role of the manager changes from controlling and highly directive (X) to facilitative, sharing decision making, accepting input, and interaction with employees (Y) who are viewed as assets.

Theory Z

Theory Z (Ouchi, 1982) has often been thought of as a blend of Theory X and Y, yet having more in common with Theory Y. Theory Z was published over 20 years after McGregor's (1960) work (op.cit.) and after much of Deming's (1989) work proved successful in Japan. The theory underscores a "management style that focuses on strong company philosophy, a distinct corporate culture, long range staff development, and consensus decision making" (Ouchi, 1982).

There is a strong emphasis on: participatory management, shared decision-making, a strong organizational commitment, hiring the correct people, and giving them a focal role in their jobs. Ongoing training is important, and the managers and employees need to have a shared vision. As changes occur, all members of the organization adapt.

Deming Management Method

Deming's (1989, 1990, and 1993) management methodology is focused on quality of management and production outcomes, and grew from Deming's work in the mid-20th century. The framework for producing quality is the Deming cycle (Deming & Walton, 1989): *plan, do, check, and act*. A set of 14 points was defined by Deming and became the hallmark of the worldwide application of the Deming concepts. Deming's ideas were initially best received in Japan and many writings on the subject credit this approach as playing a large role in the revival of Japan's post-war economy.

Rienzo (1993) discusses Deming Management, and cited four interacting and interdependent basis for the approach: appreciation for systems, understanding of variation, appreciation and use of knowledge, and insights into human behavior and relationships. Deming's 14 Points (2010) are: *(1) create constancy of purpose for improvement of product and service, (2) adopt the new philosophy, (3) cease inspection, focus on evidence, and share information, (4) improve the quality of supply and resource and not focus solely on price, (5) improve constantly the system of production and service, (6) institute education and training (including concept of variation and statistics), (7) adopt and institute leadership and a culture of helping, (8) drive out fear and instill confidence, (9) break down barriers between staff areas, (10) eliminate slogans and targets for the work force, (11) eliminate numerical standard for the work force and management, (12) remove barriers and boundaries that rob people of pride of workmanship, (13) encourage education and self-improvement for everyone, and (14) take action to accomplish the transformation and ever-improving quality.*

Deming's work has spawned a number of adaptations of his framework. For example, Anderson (1994) synthesizes the steps into seven constructs: visionary leadership, internal and external cooperation, learning, process management, continuous improvement, employee fulfillment, and customer satisfaction. Rienzo (op.cit.) presented a method for applying the Deming Management Method to use in a planning framework for service organizations and processes, and is representative of a broad number of application approaches. Deming was well known as a statistician and wrote about use of statistical methods (1981/1982), and as pointed out by Grant and colleagues (1994), the methods developed by Deming evolved from statistical process control with connections to the scientific method. Deming's overall approach is not limited to statistical approaches and has focuses on long-term planning, and cooperation between all members of an enterprise (owners, managers, employees and customers).

Total Quality Management (TQM)

Total Quality Management (TQM) places quality and customer satisfaction as an organization's primary focus, and is also attributed to Deming (2010) (op.cit). The process was defined by the International Organization for Standardization (ISO) as: "TQM is a management approach for an organization, centered on quality, based on the participation of all its members, and aiming at long-term success through customer satisfaction, and benefits to all members of the organization and to society" (ISO 8402:1994).

TQM was first widely used in Japan and then spread internationally. In its use in Japan, it generally is attributed four distinct process steps: (1) continuous improvement, (2) a belief in the process working, (3) understanding how the product is used, and (4) the process should have an aesthetic property. An overview of TQM, its history, and associated methods can found by Pollack (2010; http://www.ischool.utexas.edu/~rpollock/tqm.html), and the UK Dept. of Industry (2010; http://www.businessballs.com/qualitymanagement.htm/).

The TQM step of "continuous improvement" termed "Kazien" (Imai, 1986; Japanese Human Relations Association, 1995; Kotlenikov, 2010) has evolved into a focus of some management styles. It is specifically focused on a team-based approach. In Japan, the concept is often imbedded in TQM and attributed to Deming (1989) and the Deming Cycle (namely; *plan, do, check, and act* in a continuous cycle). The focus is on maintaining a continuous improvement of management and the production process (or for an ALF service processes and outcomes).

Six Sigma

Six Sigma, developed by Motorola in the mid-1980s, is based on developing output quality by reducing defects in output products (De Feo & Barnard, 2004) and is an outgrowth of TQM. This management procedure evolved from many of the methods described herein, and uses the Deming Cycle in the form of: define, measure, analyze, improve, and control. The methodology is based on a continuous monitoring of processes and products for control and quality improvement (Juran, 1992).

Six Sigma relies on statistical methodologies based on standard deviations (sigma) from the mean of a normal distribution to achieve its goals. The methodology looks for deviations using a statistical analysis procedure aimed at process control and quality outcomes, and seeks to remediate the problems discovered. This method is usually applied by external consultants, tends to be costly, and is dependent on the ability to define end outcomes in forms adaptable to statistical analysis. The concepts of this approach are useful for an ALF, even if the statistical methodology is less of a fit. A review of its functioning at GE and other large companies is discussed by Morris (1996), and would be useful for ALF management to review.

Reengineering or Business Process Reengineering (BPR)

Reengineering or Business Process Reengineering (BPR) is a review and redesign of an organization and its processes (Hammer, 1990, 1993). According to Hammer & Champy (1993), reengineering is "the fundamental rethinking and radical redesign of the business processes to achieve dramatic improvements in critical, contemporary measures of performance . . . ." BPR is considered a means of a significant change in perspective or direction of the organization. Improvements can be sought in the output, production process, product quality, rapidity of production, and management of an enterprise. The focus is on the production or business processes that produce the organization's outcomes, and seem to bear some similarity to the reductionism approach suggested by Taylor (1911). The enthusiasm for the methodology seems to be waning, however (Davenport, 1995; Weicher et al., 1995), but the concept of periodically looking at the organization and its business and management strategies with a process focus has value for an ALF.

Planning, Programming, and Budgeting System (PPBS)

Planning, Programming, and Budgeting System (PPBS) is a methodology (Drew et al., 1967; Fisher, 1966) aimed at defining a project or organization, its plan, and looks to see if the resources are adequate to the task. It also looks to see if there are scheduling conflicts that would reduce the chances for timely success. If there is an inadequacy, the PPBS process is repeated until a balance is achieved. PPBS was developed in the Department of Defense in the early 1960s to better manage resources relative to desired outputs. Typically, the use was aimed at hardware development in large programs and most often used to develop a budgeting process.

One limitation for a service program is that the PPBS starting point did not sufficiently address contex or the desired service direction that is often the basis of human service programs (Melichar, 1972). One approach to remedying this deficiency is to begin with a description of environment, context, goals, and objectives. Secondly, it is desirable to link these elements to each part of the organization, service, and people receiving the service. The methodology suggested for this approach was NOBS (Melichar, 1972), which was a blend of PPBS and "the systems approach." Not only is it important to reach a balance between input resources and output products in an optimal manner, but it also must identify how the processes are used meet the organization's goals.

Management by Objective (MBO)

Management by objective (Odine, 1965; Drucker, 1981) is a process of relating outcomes to objectives. Managers hone processes until they produce outcomes defined by initiating objectives. This approach works best when imbedded with a PPBS type of system. One of the problems found by the author is that it is possible to achieve objectives without getting the outcomes desired. At least three potential sources of error occur: (1) the objectives can be badly written and not match the function or operation to which they are related, (2) the objectives may not add up to the goals and expected outcomes (please refer to the goal/objective hierarchy described later in this section), and (3) the measurement to determine the objective specified is in error. The concept is useful if these errors are avoided and is helpful in evaluation and quality control.

Zero Defects

Zero Defects is a methodology for developing quality control in the process of producing products (Crosby, 1982). The goal is to reduce the number of defective products and thereby decrease the cost of production, improve the quality of the end product, increase customer satisfaction, and reduce time spent on inspection and evaluation of the products. This approach has value within an ALF when used within a larger management framework and when the service outcomes are clearly defined.

Likert's Management Approach

Likert (1961, 1967) defined four types of management systems: *(1) exploitive authoritative system; managers decide direction and make decisions based on an organizational hierarchy; (2) benevolent-authoritative system; similar to the exploitive authoritative system except a reward system is provided within the hierarchy, (3) consultive system; there is up and down communication within the hierarchy, but decisions are still hierarchical, and (4) participative (group) system; directions and decisions are made across the organization hierarchy, and there is a shared responsibility for the specific direction and actions taken.*

MANAGEMENT METHOD AND STYLE

A management method can be a mix of multiple methods (see for example, Hall's [1963] discussion of bureaucracy as a continuum). The method selected should fit the organization as it is defined in the organization's business plan, and should have the support of upper managers.

A basis for conflict would exist if a participatory management style was selected and upper managers were focused on authoritative rigidity and control.

In contemporary management there is a strong focus on team-centered approaches, high degrees of communication, information flow, information support systems, and continuous improvement (plans, outcomes, management, and organization). An ALF needs to frame a management method that fits its goals, approach, and services.

Management Styles

Management often has been defined in terms of participatory vs. non-participatory styles. In a participatory style, all levels of the management can provide input to operations, and thereby produces a horizontal organization structure. A non-participatory style has a clearly defined supervisory-subordinate structure (e.g., the bureaucratic form) and a vertical framework.

Management styles can also be defined in terms of leadership. Lewin (1939) defined three types of leadership: authoritative, participative, and delegative. The styles also define how an organization will be formulated and managed. Implicit is the amount of control and delegation of responsibility. The definition is similar to that of Likert (1967) who identified four types of leadership: exploitive authoritative, benevolent authoritative, consultative, and participative.

The management methodology selected places limits upon the management styles selection. The style selected will have a large impact on: roles, reporting lines, organizational communication, operating tenor of the organization, task definition, and assigned responsibilities. The style defines who and how decisions will be made in the ALF, and in turn the character of the service process of delivery. The non-participatory and participatory styles of management are discussed in the following subsection. Lewin's delegative style is not included as it reduces the amount of control which seems appropriate for a service organization, except for highly specific services (e.g., medical).

Top-Down or Non-Participatory

The top-down or non-participatory management style is typically defined as Theory X (McGregor, 1960, 2002) and the bureaucratic form of management. Lines of authority are clearly delineated starting from the upper levels of management to the lower levels. There are clearly defined roles, delineated boundaries, and very strict lines of authority, control, and reporting. Any ideas, all control and decisions, flow from the top down. There are times where rigidity is important, for example in life-threatening situations when consensus management may be inappropriate.

Likert (op.cit.) also described a "benevolent authoritative" leadership style that had a reward system as its basis. This style still has a top-down control, and limits control and participation in decision-making by subordinates. This style does not provide very good communication to others about problems noted, as it lacks feedback, and isolates innovation from subordinates.

There are useful concepts in the bureaucratic form that can be used without absorbing the weaknesses. By loosening the rigidity of the form, the delineation of roles, lines of communication, definition of tasks and processes, creation of organizational units and structure, and lines of authority can be useful in consideration of how the ALF creates its management. For example, the definition of tasks does not mean there cannot be shared responsibility and decision-making.

Participatory

A participative management style is part of McGregor's (1960, 2002) Theory Y and also is described in TQM and Kaizen methods (op.cit). This management style uses a horizontal structure with weaker lines of authority and supervisory control. The management of the enterprise is more team focused with shared input and decision-making.

Team building has become part of the participatory management landscape. The use of a team includes a broader range of inputs and talents to management, planning, operation, decision-making, and quality control. There is shared responsibility across the team and within the organization. One example of this approach is the use of "Kaizen" (op.cit).

The team approach places a high value on knowledge and stresses the need of education for team members. The team approach still maintains lines of control, definition of roles, lines of authority, and information as well as flow. Constraints do exist on the team and its activities in the form of budgetary limitations for example. Team participation is aimed at consensus, but there are times to when a decision must be made and requires a determination of who will make it. As a service organization, services cannot become dysfunctional nor can a lack of a team decision negatively influence the residents.

Mixed Management Styles and Style Selection

A pure form of any management style is unlikely to exist. A better approach is to define a mixed management approach, based on all of the methods. In the planning framework suggested later in this chapter, there are references to almost all of the management methods defined earlier. For example, the overall structure of the planning system is a variation of the PPBS approach, and includes elements of the bureaucratic form, has a goal tree structure, is amenable to the use of MBO, and is consistent with TQM.

Rather than first selecting a specific management method, it would be more fruitful to decide how management will be used in the ALF. An ALF might consider what type of control structures it will use, and how decisions will be made within and across the organization. The approach also might include some areas of management in which the residents have input. An ALF has different focuses at different parts of the organization, and the mix of styles can vary by amount, focus, organizational level, or other organizational parameters. The selected management framework, mix of styles, and how they will be used should be made known across the ALF.

MANAGEMENT AND ORGANIZATIONAL STRUCTURE

The management method and style selected need to be integrated into the overall organization and its operation. The development of management and organization structures needs to include the following: (1) line staff relationships – who reports to whom and for what functions, (2) staffing of the organization, (3) organization chart, (4) a delineation of dispersal of decision making and authority as well as control, (5) feedback systems internal and external, (6) functions of the components of the organization with a clear delineation of responsibilities, and (7) definition of the information flow lines and how they are to be used.

It has been argued (Allen, 1999) that an ALF can be separated into an upper, middle, and lower level management structure with staff to carry out the directions of the managers. In a more horizontal organizational structure with a participatory style, these conceptual distinctions are less clear.

Constraints on Management and Operations

An ALF is managed under some fixed constraints, methodological limitations, and a large number of truisms:

1) The management approach must fit within the budgetary limitations of the ALF. Management should remain the means to achieve success and not be the end purpose.
2) The implementation of the management functions must fit the size of the organization. The discussions of the leadership roles often are by identification of key managers (e.g., executive, operating, financial, and compliance officers each with staff support). An ALF may not afford this executive staffing level, yet management must still fulfill the functions through existing staff sharing responsibility for the functions.
3) There is no universally accepted "best management approach." The best fit could vary with the ALF, its staff, and management team's personalities. In some cases a highly structured top-down organization is appropriate; in most situations it is the antithesis of a good approach.
4) The management approach and methodology should fit the needs and services of the ALF as opposed to selecting a management methodology, and then fitting the needs and services to the management methodology.
5) When examining both the overarching ALF organization and its specific components and activities, it is good to remember the often-stated truism "everything is connected to everything else" (generally paraphrasing John Muir, 1911). It is important not only to define the ALF's goals, activities, components, and functions, but also to describe how they are connected and reliant upon each other, and on the information requirements, flows, and exchanges needed to efficiently operate the ALF and its services. For a general review of management operations, see Lewis and Black (2003).

Organizing Principles

As many of the management methods share common elements, it seems best to facilitate this chapter's intended discussion upon creating an appropriate management style, methodology, and approach for an ALF by using the following organizing principles: (1) management is an ongoing and dynamic process, (2) adaptation and evolution are integral to developing the management process, the ALF organization, and the services it provides, (3) management and staff must focus on the quality of service outcomes and the well-being of residents, (4) feedback from across the organization into the management process is central to the improvement of outcome quality, management, operational service processes, and organizational development, (5) in order for feedback to occur there must be a set of organizational directions and an overarching plan, a set of operational plans, clarity of goals and objectives, a monitoring and measurement system, and clearly defined feedback and information flow lines, (6) communication within and across the organization is critical to successful management, and (7) information collection, flow, availability, control, and reporting are important to the communication process, oversight, and management. In simple terms, you cannot fix a problem of which you are unaware.

There is a broad collection of literature which defines the concept and creation of an organization, and stems from the seminal work of March and Simon (1957, 1993). An organization must be structured and have a stated purpose and direction. A review of the literature finds the term "system" used repeatedly. The "systems" concept (von Bertalanfy, 1968; Churchman, 1968) is the principles selected to plan and review an ALF's organization and its business and operational plans. Supportive and broadening views of the "systems concept" can be found in descriptions of "purposeful systems" (Acoff & Emory, 1972), "observing systems" (von Forester, 1981), and "inquiring systems" (Churchman, 1971).

System as the Basis for Organization, Management, and Evaluation

In the heuristic chosen, *system* is joined by *structure* and *process* (Melichar, 1972, 1972a) in a method for framing the organization, its services, operation, and projects. A systems representation of a management framework, business, and operational plans are models of the ALF and its operation. An evaluation framework is included and should ascertain how closely operations match the organization's plans and models.

A systems model of the organization includes all the organizational components as contributing subsystems that in turn can have subsystems. A hierarchy is created that includes relationships and connections within the system model that is representative of the organization's structure within its environment and context. Each component and its activities, tasks, and processes can be identified along with time lines and outcomes attached that form the service processes. The framework creates a basis for planning, evaluation, information flow, service provision, and management. The system diagrams make it possible to trace the flow of events, resources, and directives, as well as organizational connections, lines of authority, resource flows, and information flows. In using this single approach it is possible to outline: (1) a business model, (2) an operational plan and planning system, (3) an evaluation system, (4) resource management framework, (5) organization chart clearly defining jobs, responsibilities, staff, . . ., (6) service process models including definition of desired outcomes, (7) information systems, and (8) what the residents should expect, and definitions of their well-being.

The approach in framing the organization, its components, and activities acts as a foundation for the business plan and then the operational plan. The framework helps to address the full range of an ALF's organization and operation, and provides a way to tie the pieces together and form the basis for its management. This includes evaluation, a focus on quality, cost containment, and efficient use of resources. In the next section, a common planning framework for all aspects of an ALF is therefore presented.

Planning Framework

The following is a framework for planning, operation, and management of an ALF under the system type model (for an alternative, see Siegal & Bernstien, 1993). The framework (Melichar, 1972a) includes a direct link to the evaluation process and feedback loops which facilitate a constant improvement process leading to improved quality. Each part of the framework enables better use of management practices by indicating, "what is to be managed" and the ALF's structure with integration of all its parts and activities. The planning process is a means for improving management, operations, and service outcomes and is not an "end" outcome. The components of the planning framework are presented in Figure 8.1 and are briefly discussed below.

The *environment* sets the *context* and boundaries of the unit being described or planned. The definition for the business plan would differ from either the view of the overall operations or a unit of the organization. The ALF as an organization is responding to a *need* within the environment that also helps define its purpose. The lack of clear need limits the potential for the success of the ALF. The clearer the statement of need within the ALF environment, the more focused are the business and marketing plans, and their operations.

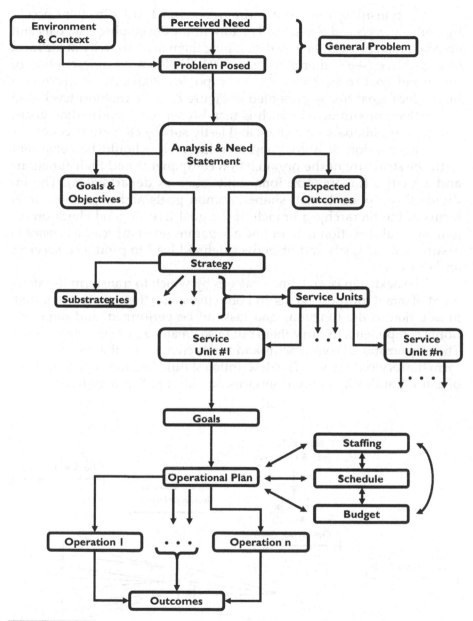

FIGURE 8.1   Planning format.

The transition from need and purpose to set ALF directions occurs by defining *goals and objectives*. The format for developing the goals and objectives can best be done by developing them in a hierarchy in the form of a goal tree (see Guiterez & Diaz, 2004, Section 4 for a description of the use of goal trees; Kavakli & Loucopoulos, 2004). An example of a hierarchical goal tree is presented in Figure 8.2. The topmost level is an overarching or supragoal which is then broken into contributing goals, followed by subgoals, objectives, and lastly subobjectives (if needed).

The creation of a goal/objective hierarchy should be consistent with the structure of the organization components and their functions and activities (or organizational units such as departments). The individual components will share common goals and objectives, or in terms of the hierarchy, a branch of the goal tree. A good check on organizational direction is to define a separate set of *expected outcomes* to assure that the goals and objectives defined lead to produced services and outcomes.

The next step is to define *strategies* by which to transform the statement of intent, purpose, goals and objectives, into the activities required, in addition to the functions and tasks to be performed, and organizational components to carry them out (also creates an organization chart). The organizational components and their activities are the processes that form the services created. The description should include: reporting, lines of control, authority, support services, and information requirements and

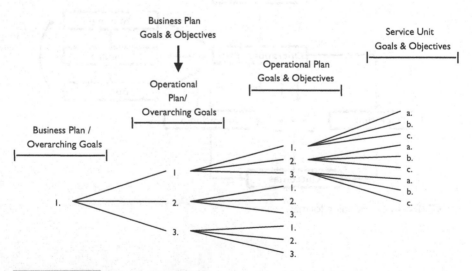

FIGURE 8.2 Goal tree hierarchy example.

control. Once the activities, components, and services are identified, then the needed *staffing* can be identified. The type and amount of staff needed to carry the service outcomes can be described.

A *schedule* should be defined for the various service and non-service activities, reports, operational milestones, decisions, and all other milestones. Based on the activities schedule, the *general resources* needed to operate them can be defined and may include: staff, facility, maintenance, cash flow, and income sources. The *budgeting* process balances the income needs, income sources, resource allocations, and the resource requirements for the planning unit being considered. The overall budget must insure that income and expense are at the least equal. The above definitions create the basis for an *evaluation system* (see Figure 8.3) that provides the measures of performance, outcomes, and client satisfaction, and establish the basis for quality control and effective management.

The multiplicity of variables and competing interests in an ALF require an *iterative* use of the planning framework. Using iterative planning will balance a budget, reduce conflicts between organizational elements, and produce better resource allocations to organizational components and services. Changes can be made in the ALF if future occurrences differ from those forecasted in planning the framework, or the evaluation and quality control program concerning services and resident well-being, and problems are indicated.

The planning framework provides a means of looking at the ALF or any component and its operation and management. The manner in which that framework is used and implemented is a decision made by the ALF governing body and management team. The decision could range from simply using the framework, informally reviewing the ALF, or drafting thorough written plans.

Evaluation Systems and Quality Control

Once business and organization plans are implemented and the organization is operational, a tendency can occur to let the operation simply continue and to only deal with problems that arise. The system model presented an alternate strategy using a continuous system of evaluating performance of both the total operation and its components. The purpose of this system is to insure that goals and objectives are being met, the overall facility and its components and services are effective, residents are receiving appropriate care, residents' well-being and outlook are positive, resources are adequate and effectively controlled, and all laws and regulations are met.

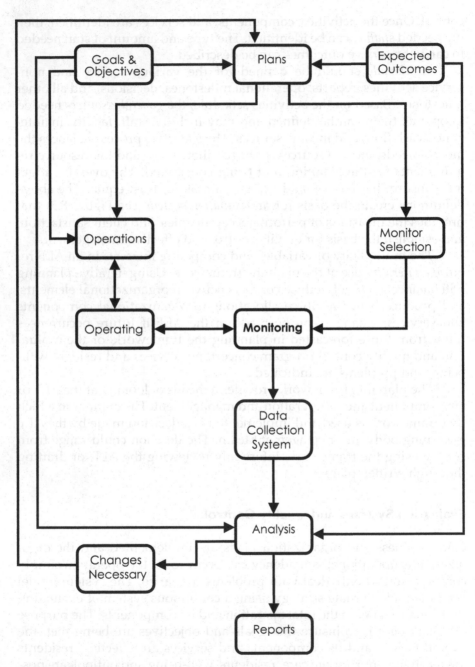

FIGURE 8.3 Evaluation process model.

Evaluation Strategies, Feedback Loops, and Quality Management

An evaluation process provides a clear picture of how the facility operates, and should provide feedback to aid in managing service and support processes, and identify problems. The development and maintenance of an evaluation system and quality management plan is dependent on monitoring defined parameters and their reporting to management. The feedback loops need to be developed in the operational plan along with the needed measures and procedures for transmitting evaluation results to management and the ALF operational units.

An effective information system will enable both capture and control of data, and can become the repository for feedback. One caveat of this system is that simply providing data and feedback does not assure action on that information. The overall evaluation design must include: the methodology, techniques, reports, and schedules needed to insure the data accrued are effectively used.

The evaluation system is integral to the information system. A profile of who needs what information, and when they need it, is an important part of the design. The design must also include methods to evaluate the evaluation and data systems. One of the goals, as earlier defined, was to create an adaptive and evolving system – it is this design that enables meeting this end.

For any evaluation or measure of effectiveness, it is important to define the target measures (e.g., goals, objective, intents, and types of information). Evaluation and management support information are based on having a meter to measure against. In simplistic terms, one cannot determine what "end" was accomplished if that "end" was never defined. Ad hoc afterthoughts are not overly effective information, the information requirements need to be designed as part of the facility design and management system. These requirements must include compliance requirements, resident protections mechanisms, and support an ALF's focus on the quality of its operations and services. A TQM type methodology that focuses on the production of quality in a continuous manner, by looking at process outcomes and customer satisfaction, requires an appropriate evaluation and information support system.

Evaluation and the Change Process

Upon completion of an evaluation, an organization must decide how to utilize the information gathered to better its operation and assure quality. An ALF has been presented as a multi-tiered organization; one with multiple component activities, supports, and services. The evaluation data must be weighed to determine whether there is a need to change the overall structure of the organization, alter the system model, or make changes in components, processes or services. A decision is also required as to whether or not to make small corrections on a continuous basis (typical of TQM approaches), or more abrupt changes found in the BPR methodology. Whatever decision is made, any change must: (1) focus on service processes and their outcomes, (2) have an adaptive process for the organization, (3) a basis for improvement, (4) provide ways to adapt to changing conditions or new knowledge, and (5) have a means to correct failure to meet goals and objectives, provision of less than optimal service, or improve its cost basis.

THE BUSINESS PLAN

An ALF operates under a business plan model (Osterwalder et al., 2004; Ing, 2009) that also serves as an ongoing overarching or strategic plan for the organization. The operational plan is separate, but would use the business plan directions to guide the operation of the facility and function as a mechanism to transform input resources into resident centered outcomes. The two plans serve the organization differently, and although they share a common interface, they must be kept separate.

The business plan should address exactly what is expected from the business and its creation as described in Figure 8.4. The expectations should address: (1) fiscal resources such as expected income and cash flow requirements, (2) the expectation of added resources from external agencies and community sources, (3) the services expected from the board of directors, (4) the expected mix of residential types and expected occupancy rates, (5) reporting of progress of the organization toward expectations by management, (6) the services to residents, their well-being, and the quality expected to be provided, (7) management performance, and (8) potential staff availability and the community demographic profile.

The business plan focuses on the viability of the organization, the oversight of the ALF's operation, and is used to review the effectiveness of its operation. Typically, the business plan is focused at issues addressed by investors, owners, and/or board of directors. This section reviews some of the main aspects of the business plan, but due to space limitations, it is not put into the planning system framework as earlier described.

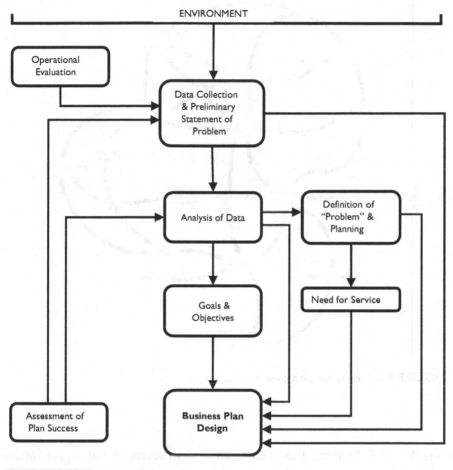

FIGURE 8.4 Business plan development.

Business Plan Perspectives

An organization is a system of interacting parts (as described earlier, and is summarized in Figure 8.5). This system (ALF) can be viewed from many different aspects, and may appear different to various viewers (operators, providers, residents, families of residents, staff, managers, and external agencies), each with a unique perspective and desired set of outcomes

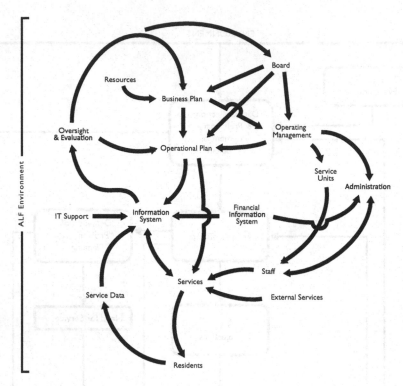

FIGURE 8.5 Business plan overview schematic.

from the ALF. In total, they create an overall sense of the organization and its operation, and yet they all are a part of it. The organization's management must take these perspectives into account while maintaining or producing a steady organizational framework, ongoing operations, the input resources needed to underwrite the operations, marketing and acquiring residents, and the desired outcomes from the business model.

The identification of organizational and management approaches, along with organization components begins with the business model. The business model addresses how the overall organization is formulated, the desired operational strategy, and the financial model needed to maintain operations. The business plan presents what the facility intends to produce, its resource utilization approach, and a timeline for major outcomes. From that framework, the business plan can develop, monitor, and maintain a plan of operation to actualize its goals.

The business plan should show organizational components and the interrelation of those components that is needed to make each part of the organization a performing entity within the overall ALF system. Each operation is integrated with the other operations to provide the residential care services. Management is the control element of these processes, and occurs relative to the entire organization or to any of its components. Each component must fit into the overall system that is the facility, and thereby the management of each component must synergistically fit within the overall ALF management.

Business Plan Issues

The first step in creating a business plan is to develop and/or maintain a viable business model. A business model evolves from the following questions: What is the organization to be? What are its goals? How will it maintain itself economically? How will it be operated? A business plan should at a minimum answer these questions in a clearly written statement that becomes the organization's framework for its existence and operation. The business plan should also be viewed as a strategic plan that at a minimum will include: (1) the context and environment for the organization including competing services, (2) the purpose and goals of the organization and the services it will provide, (3) the resources required and how they will be used, including cash flow requirements, estimate income and expenses, and source of income, (4) who is/will be served including a target population profile, (5) the time frame of the business plan and its components, (6) business strategies, (7) facility operation, and (8) an understanding of the consumer and their expectations.

Furthermore, the real estate market in the area should be surveyed. One reason is that the ALF either owns a real property or is leasing a real property. The business plan needs to address how the real property is treated as an asset and cost item, which includes its cost basis, assets, and liabilities. Competing services that may affect income streams also should be identified, and include the number of clients served, cost profile, type of client served, residential unit mix, and a general organizational structure. This information along with knowledge about the population targeted also should help identify an advantageous residential unit mix and becomes an internal resource for the facility's planning, financing, and marketing.

The data should determine if it is advantageous to target populations different from the competing services, focus on private clients vs. public support, low vs. high-income groups, or consider focusing upon underserved populations. Marketing of the facility should be addressed. Even if an effective facility is created, there is little social or economic value if the facility is not populated with residents. The issue is approached under the term "marketing" at the end of this chapter.

The community in which the facility exists helps to define some of the parameters in planning. It enables planning to take advantage of community resources or lack thereof. Will the residents be drawn only from the community? Does the community accept and encourage this type of facility? What is the pool of workers for the staffing needs? Is there adequate housing in the community for the staff? What is the cost-of-living in the service area? Links to other organizations in the community (including a parent company if a chain or franchise) should be identified including potential partners and services available to the ALF and its residents.

The above framework is useful as both a start-up guide and prospectus, but should be updated as the facility evolves. It should provide a basis for assessing how a facility is doing for both management and its oversight board. The framework also provides a set of parameters in planning the operation and services of the facility, and is an important element in maintaining the ALF's focus over time.

Once operational, a facility must look at how it is performing from the multiplicity of perspectives described in the business plan. Is it meeting the goals and objectives as outlined in the business plan, in addition to the processes of the operational activities? Are resources being used effectively and are costs being controlled? Can the facility and its services be improved? Are the needs of residents, resident's families and staff being met? Is the operation meeting all regulatory requirements? The business plan should provide methods for continuously looking at these questions systematically, and how to best make changes based on the assessment of performance as was earlier addressed.

Business Plan Directions

The ALF exists for a specific reason, and should be defined as part of the business plan (or overall strategy) in a clear statement of purpose, goals, and expectations to substantiate the "why" of the organization. The ALF's core ideology should be clear and part of the basis for determining the direction set by the board. The business plan should include residents' perspectives and the ALF's expectations for maintaining well-being and satisfaction of residents.

The definition of expectations should include how the organization will adapt to change (economic, cultural, knowledge, capital, and technological). If the organization is not in a static environment, it should have an adaptive potential built into its strategic plan. Lack of adaptive potential means the organization at some point will become uncompetitive and unresponsive to the needs that it addresses.

A clear set of financial goals and objectives (including time frames) to rate accomplishments should be identified. This identification should form the basis for the overall financial operation of the ALF and represent the requirements and outcomes expected by owners, investor's, and the board. The financial plan's goals and objectives should be identified, and includes the operational, financial, and management strategies.

A set of goals and objectives for the board of directors needs to be defined. This is a statement of intent, and should frame the expectations of the board, criteria for board membership, and expected performance guidelines. The role of the board with respect to the business plan, how the board will evaluate the achievement of the business plan, and how the board itself will be evaluated should be included in the set of goals and objectives.

The business plan should address exactly what is expected from the business. The expectations should address: (1) financial issues such as income and cash flow requirements, (2) the expectation of added resources from external sources, (3) the services expected from the board of directors, (4) the expected mix of residential types and the expected occupancy rates, (5) reporting of progress of the organization toward expectations by management, (6) the services to residents, their well-being, and the quality expected to be provided, and (7) the internal management performance.

Implementation Strategy

The business plan should address the framework and methods needed to implement the business plan. This strategy is focused on the creation and maintenance of the ALF, and not the operational level strategies. The basis for the marketing of the ALF should be identified. The method for transitioning the business plan into the operational and marketing plans should be addressed.

The strategy should address the physical plant and its continuing role in the business, in addition to how the insurance aspects will be addressed. The mix of housing types within the ALF operation and the business model need to be addressed as well. The framework for the needed financial arrangements should be addressed. The way the ALF will relate to other services in the area. A strategy for developing a management framework for the operation of the ALF should be defined.

Activities and Services to be Provided

The result of the preceding descriptions should enable the description of the organizational framework including the main components and the activities needed to maintain the viable operation of the ALF and any constraints or limitations faced. The structure of the board should be identified along with its operational guidelines; the roles to be ascribed to the board. A similar description should be provided for the operational units and any activities needed to meet the ALF goals, objectives, expectation, and strategies. The differentiation of lines, flow of resources, information, services, and authority should be identified, which in turn will create the basis for identifying activities within the operational plan and its execution. A framework for the ALF's information system should be addressed along with the technological framework for the physical plant, services offered, management and administrative needs, and technologies to be offered to residents.

Resources: Available Income and Input-Output Expectation

The operation of the facility was described as the transformation of input resources into outputs. The business plan should outline the expectations of the output creation to the input resources. The determination of input-output transformation is based on the sources of the input flow of resources and monies, and the determination of output is defined by the operational plans across the organization. The budget process is about matching these inputs and outputs.

The business plan should define the expected and existing resources of the facility. Resources include the facility, equipment, staff, community resources, and income. The resources also should include the cash flow and monies needed to supplement income flow and lags in payment. Specific definitions of access to cash, via loans or other sources, need to be explicitly defined. The definition of resources should be extended to include existing and expected sources of income.

Organizations acting as resources to the ALF include those related to services in the community or those that might exist within the ALF. Additionally, these resources may be external if the facility is a franchise or chain. Some of the most basic external services are the health care and social services systems. Links to educational facilities and other training sources should be identified as these programs are needed to maintain licensure in many different disciplines, as well as providing the ALF with interns and graduates.

The business plan also should identify general categories of expenses; facility costs, administrative costs, management costs, overhead ratio, operational cost profile, and the ability to carry out the operation(s) during periods when expenses exceed income. The adjustment of income and expenditure on a scheduled basis should be a part of the business plan. The budget also should review the value of the real property of the ALF and provide a periodic financial report.

The budgeting process has to be iterative. Part of the input resource flow is the income stream from the residents. The sources of income per resident must be defined, as well as the expected total population. The definition of the output or services provided is the basis of the cost estimates and the monies that must be accrued. The time lines for all financial parameters, fiscal reports, and general performance reports should be included.

Evaluation and Quality Control

The business plan should define how the organization as a whole deals with the concept of quality and evaluation of quality, customer satisfaction, operational performance, cost-effectiveness, and management performance. The board and those in top management positions need to identify how they want to be informed of quality and performance matters.

The business plan evaluation process will lead to necessary revisions to maintain effective operation of the facility. Performance assessments and analysis of operations must provide a feedback loop to the board and upper management. If target goals are not being met (financial, operational, service, etc.), then the business plan needs to be reviewed and appropriate changes made. In turn, the operational plan and the actual operation must be adjusted. These revisions could alter the business model or any of the various operations undertaken within that model. Cost-benefit and cost-effectiveness can be included in the evaluation.

Implementation Design

The business plan should also address its implementation to form operational units and processes. There need to be links between the strategic business and operation plan, and activity. Defining how the broad targets and directions are transformed into the specificities of an operational plan and process is important. The goal of the implementation design is to provide a basis for the operational plan and service operation.

OPERATIONAL PLAN AND PLANNING SYSTEM

The business plan focuses on overall strategies, while the operational plan and planning system focus on the organization and operations that make the facility function (see Figure 8.6). The operational plan takes direction from the business plan, but transforms the broad strategy into an organizational structure with an organization chart, goals and objectives, management, administration, financial and bookkeeping activities, functioning service units, output processes and services, and operational control mechanisms. The control mechanisms also aid in determining effectiveness measures for any component, component activity, and service, as well as their use of resources.

Managers must maintain control, effectiveness, and focus within the organization. Some control points are resource utilization and the budget, service program control, monitoring process, quality controls, and resident inputs. Inherent to management is providing leadership for the ALF and supporting leadership within the components of the organization.

The Environment and Context

The external environment, context, and general constraints can be drawn from the business plan. On the operational level, it is the physical plant, support services, board directives, internal support, and community inputs, services, and resources that form the operational environment. These elements are the resources management can draw upon informing the constraints on operations, ancillary service availability, and the ALF's overall environment. The environment will vary between ALFs, communities, and even the neighborhoods in the same community.

The strengths and weakness of the ALF should be identified along with its neighborhood and the safety of that area. Local community resources available to residents (e.g., banks, library, markets, post office, restaurants, stores, etc.) should be identified along with the availability of transportation, health care, and recreational services. The restriction of local weather on residents should be reviewed, along with methods for adjusting services offered for either good or bad weather according to season.

Goals, Objectives, and Expectations

Goals and objectives should be set for overall management and for individual services; they should remain consistent with the business plan. A goal tree should be used to enable increasing specificity of goals for

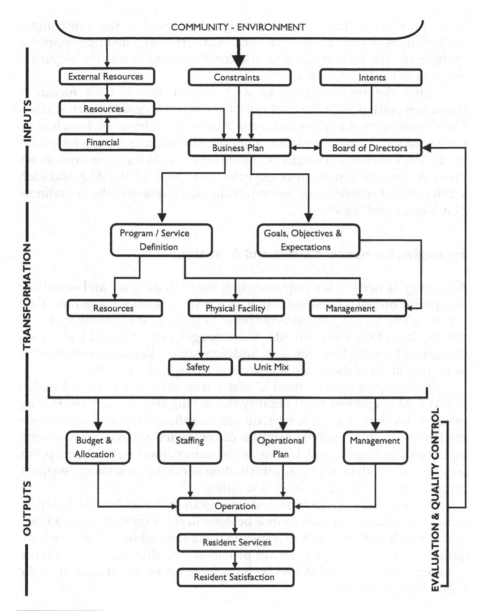

FIGURE 8.6 Operation plan overview schematic.

service operations. Each branch of the goal tree should reflect one component of the ALF (e.g., maintenance or food services). The upper portions of the goal structure should provide common links across the organization and to the business plan.

After defining subgoals in each branch, an objective hierarchy should be crafted with the final objectives being specific to each service. The definition of objectives includes: "who will do, by what, by when, as measured by" helping to define a specific direction and basis for evaluation. The lower level objectives should combine to form the ones above them. A separate statement of expected outcomes for the ALF and each service would enable an assessment of the effectiveness of the operational plan's goals and objectives.

Strategies, Component Units, and Activities

A strategy is needed for implementing the various goals and objectives for specific organizational units (e.g., reception or food services) and their services. The strategy should comprise all parts of the organization and the services offered to residents. The management for the ALF and each component should be defined, in addition to the planning, coordination, and integration of them into one service and operating system.

The support services needed may not be able to be provided within the ALF. Management must identify the lacking support services that *are* needed, and how they will be acquired and then integrated into the organization. Some possible examples of contracted services are: accounting, bookkeeping, payroll, billing, maintenance, food services, reception, specialized resident services, information services, technology support, nursing service, transportation, and safety.

Each of the organization services needs to be addressed independently. As addressing each cannot be done in the limited space available, two examples of the types of issues that must be addressed for each organization component/service are provided. The first example is administration, and information and technology services are discussed in the following subsection.

Administration Example

Administration is a separate function from management. Management seeks to provide the best use of resources in a facilitative manner. Administration is the combination of support services needed to maintain the organization and its operation. Administrative services generally do not provide direct client services with the possible exception of support in the completion of forms needed to maintain residents' status at the facility. Administration is an arm of management to maintain the control and flow of resources, interaction with government and insurance agencies, banking services, and internal control of personnel and budgeting issues.

Like management, there are a multiplicity of definitions of administration and its functions. What is important to the ALF is how it defines administration, administrative functions, the support it provides, its integration into the organization, and management's expectation for input from the administrative unit.

Maintaining control of the flow of monies into and through the organization is needed. Accounting practices need to be identified from simple bookkeeping to annual statements. The inflow and outflow of resources must be logged and ascribed to the correct functions/departments, control of the function/department expenditures must be maintained, and is it necessary to develop methods to also maintain payroll, billing, and control of receivables. There also must be a strategy for defining banking and borrowing relationships as defined in the business plan. The accounting function can be met internally or externally, but is necessary to use resources expeditiously and produce good cost-benefit and cost-effectiveness.

Personnel services also are part of the administrative function. The services must be provided, but it is done as part of the management design. The other administrative support services also must be identified. For example, a personnel department provides personnel support services (e.g., taxes and insurance), provides employ support, provides grievance procedures, and remains current with human resources requirements.

Schedule, Staffing, Resources, and Budget

The schedule for each activity identified should be defined. This definition assures that processes/activities are completed in a timely manner. The schedules for different functions can have a large variation (e.g., schedules for daily, weekly, monthly, and annual time horizons).

A staffing profile needs to be created for all the components and activities within the ALF. The staffing profile needs to identify the education, skills, and experience required for each staff position. Job descriptions should be produced from the staffing profile, as well as the resources for finding appropriate staff, and the methods needed to locate them. Interviewing methods should also be identified, and a salary profile for the staff types must be set.

The budget and resources needed to operate the ALF, by component and activity, should be defined and matched to the activities defined, including staffing, and the schedule. The balancing of activity and resources should be an ongoing process. The ALF needs to provide guidelines to the components and activities of the resources allocated to them, and create a feedback loop for those expenditures that need to be identified.

It is important to define how the information from the units will flow back to management and administration. Control systems need to be identified, and support systems for the ALF's activities need to be provided. The link to management, administration, in addition to record and reporting systems are important to define and maintain.

Evaluation and Quality Control

An evaluation system for the entire ALF and each of its components and activities, should be designed from the goals and objectives. The operational plan needs to define how to measure the progress towards the objectives and performance quality established. Measures of some performance such as maintenance can be made using hard measures, but measures of resident well-being and satisfaction will be harder to define. In both instances, quality of the organization's output is dependent upon these monitors, and how the data retrieved is reported and used. These feedback loops are the basis for ongoing planning and quality control.

INFORMATION AND TECHNOLOGY SUPPORT SERVICES

The basic technical nature of our society is such that any ALF will house multiple technological systems. These systems provide support to the ALF's administrative, management, financial, and direct care services. The physical facility also includes a range of technologies that include heating and air-conditioning, safety, and security. Patient services include both support systems for the provision of care, but also for the use of residents' recreation and communication. The facilities are likely to have a wireless network, patient data online, medication control systems, and many other support services.

The management team needs to be aware of technological advances and new methodologies. The goal is to increase and improve service levels, and to utilize technologies that help to control costs. The Internet has also become a resource for management, staff, and residents.

As with every benefit, there are associated costs. The facility is responsible for locating, evaluating, securing, and maintaining the system, in addition to training users. The ALF must have an IT department or equivalent services. The technical support staff becomes an increasing cost, while the technologies themselves become less expensive per unit function.

Information Systems

Organizations run on information. Systems are needed to accrue this information, manage it, and make it available in appropriate reports and queries. The sustainment of various organization functions is dependent on the information system chosen. Equally important is that the information system be integrated into the operational and management system. Cost savings come from synergy and meeting the needs of the entire staff. The system design must look at how the various organization processes use the information, and how the information gathered is put back into the system.

The information management system should be created as part of the overall facility design. The management and operational plans must include the information system as an integral part. The design process includes identifying: (1) the supported processes within the organization, (2) how the information will be used by various staff, departments, and management, (3) the cost of information in terms of monetary costs and staff time costs (designing a system that increases staff demands over gains is not desirable), (4) the information needs of the evaluation, compliance, and quality control system implemented by the facility, (5) the security needed at different levels of the organization, (6) who will share what information (e.g., administration may only need a portion of patient information, and direct services will not access personal and payroll records), and (7) who has overall responsibility for the information and information system.

Records Systems

One function of an information system is to maintain an organization's records. Part of an ALF's design is to determine what records are required to be maintained, and what additional information will be required by the organization to operate effectively. Information collection, control, management, and storage all have costs. The concept of "necessary and sufficient" should be a controlling concept, but must be applied to all parts of an organization. What is necessary for the service process may be soporiferous for administration and vice versa.

Once a data system has be designed, built, and implemented, perhaps the most costly aspect of its operation is the collection of data. A careful review is needed to determine how the data will be gathered on a continuing basis, and also what technologies can be used to reduce the costs in both monies and staff time. The definition of when and how data is collected may also determine its utility and uses.

The selection of information gathered has to be developed by department, section, function, or task. It must also fit within the processes undertaken by each component/service both in terms of their operational and functional needs, and how the recording of the information will fit into their day-to-day operations. These definitions also determine the parameters of the information system: input processes, data availability, reporting, interactive data, and patient support services. Some elements may have common uses; for example, provision of medications and their control provide support to service staff, protection of patients from wrong medications, inventory control, and fiscal reporting.

Resident Records System

The management system must identify what records about each resident are needed, and how the data will be recorded and accessed. There should be implemented a reliable set of standards concerning the amount and type of personal information, medical information, medication history, services provided, location, schedules, and support service assigned to each resident. Any compliance data (HIPAA) required must also be integrated. This records system is typically integrated into the overall information system of the facility with privacy and security safeguards.

The more technology is used, the more the facility is responsible for providing adequate support staff that is knowledgeable about "computing." As the ALF's resident records, medication lists, and schedules become computerized, the amount of time that the computer system can be down decreases without it influencing ALF operations. The need for available and knowledgeable staff increases in order to gain the rapid response in maintaining the information technology. The availability of computer support staff makes responses to problems timelier and better, but at the cost of providing the support.

Technical and Technology Support

The main support requirement will be in the information technology and computing areas. The various technologies utilized will be to improve systems, and will require upgrades and staff support of these systems. The facility itself will have a series of technological systems in addition to the information systems. These systems also are increasingly computer based, more reliable, and often easier to repair, but still require maintenance, error recovery, and updates. The management plan must include the manner in which these systems will be maintained and what support is needed. For example, is the facility large enough to have technical staff or should it find support through an independent consulting agent?

Critical systems need to be identified, including a definition of acceptable downtimes for each. Data back-up and recovery should be defined for each system including the individuals responsible for addressing any problems. The facility should expect that its residents will want and need computer and Internet access. The residents should have access to each facilitates communication with family, information gathering, and entertainment. The amount and range of services need to be defined by the facility as part of its management plan, in addition to how much technological support will be provided to residents.

MARKETING APPROACHES

Successful operation of an ALF is dependent upon maintaining an inflow of resources which is related to the admission of new residents. The flow of income is resident based unless the facility is a non-profit, in which they might also receive donations and/or grants. A base level of income is needed to meet necessary expenses and overhead, which is equated to a base level of occupancy. A marketing program must focus on attaining and then exceeding this base occupancy level to ensure the facility can remain in existence.

Marketing Strategies

A first step in developing a market strategy is to define the marketing targets. A strategy then needs to be formed to undertake the actual marketing. An implementation plan is needed, which will be enacted by the staff. The last step is to define an evaluation strategy to determine the effectiveness of the marketing strategy. For overviews of ALF marketing, information is contained in Dixon et al. (2001) and Allen (1999).

The business plan should provide a community profile, types of services to be offered, competitors and their characteristics, the market segment targeted, and a clear delineation of the ALF from a nursing home (Dixon et al., 2001). The potential means for reaching the target population is part of the marketing strategy along with the community links for the ALF (especially if co-marketing is desired).

The marketing plan needs to identify the types of living arrangements available in the facility, including the cost of each option. Based on the cost structure and housing types available, the marketing plan and marketing strategy can be focused at an appropriate segment of the population. The mix of living arrangements will have been identified in the business plan as well as the physical structure of the facility.

Marketing Message

The marketing plan should have a clearly identified message – "this is who we are, these are the services we provide, these should be your expectations of our facility." The potential client can better evaluate the ALF if all the parameters of living at the facility are known. Potential assistance in presenting the facility should be identified; working with community organizations may help to create these links.

The marketing effort needs to provide advertising through media or mailings, links to community and health care organizations, tours of the facility, brochures, an on-line presence (e.g., a website), E-marketing (Straus & Frost, 2008), E-marketing effectiveness (Ranchhold et al., 2001), and virtual tours and/or DVDs/CDs about the ALF and its services. Developing a specific marketing team is essential because team members will know about the preceding efforts in relation to current goals and future focus of the overall marketing plan. In addition, staff responsibilities for each part of the marketing plan should be identified.

Ultimately, marketing should locate potential residents, provide the message of ALF existence, provide information to people interested in the ALF, follow-up information to interested parties, and then an onsite tour capability. A specific team of people should be identified in order to ensure the implementation of all aspects of the marketing strategy. Roles should be defined and appropriate training provided.

Marketing Team and Activities

The onsite and interactive aspects regarding inquiries about the facility, requests for more information, or visitation, need to be identified. Reception will be the initial face of the ALF for either telephone inquiries or people arriving. The role needs to be clearly identified, and appropriate training given. The responsibility for responses to the inquiries needs to be identified. A similar responsibility needs to be offered to postal mail or email inquiries.

The marketing team should include assignments for provisions of onsite tours. The ability to answer both potential resident and family concerns needs to be considered. The team should have a clear understanding (and training if necessary) regarding the process of conducting tours and explaining the resources available within the ALF as part of the overall presentation of the facility to a potential resident. Each member of the team should understand the types of units offered, the size of each unit, and what is physically included (the services provided by the ALF) and all associated costs. The team should also be able to answer any questions about services available within the community: such as health care, recreation, cultural resources, transportation, and any unique aspects of the community. This discussion should also include the way in which residents can access these external services.

All presentations should address safety issues either within the facility, within the residence units, and in the community. The safety features of the facility should be presented, and the team must be able to answer questions. Safety should address both resident based issues such as falls or health emergencies, as well as external threats to the facility. The team should also be prepared to address concerns about the safety of resident belongings.

The team should also present the services available within the facility. The food services (if offered) should have a clear description along with sample menus. Shopping facilities for food and other necessities need to be identified for potential residents, along with how they might access those services. Other services offered should be detailed (e.g., broadband, resident nursing, exercise facilities and programs, and visitor areas).

Assessment of Marketing Effectiveness

The ALF should have a program for evaluating its marketing activity (Churchill, Jr., 1978). Is it meeting the goals of the business plan? Are the methods being used cost-effective? How do the methods being used compare with those of competitors? How will the information from the evaluation be used to improve marketing, and what parts of the evaluation should be provided to other parts of the organization.

CONCLUSIONS

This chapter has provided the reader with information on how management is an ongoing process with built-in quality control and resident satisfaction measures. An ALF should have business, operational, and marketing plans against which it manages. A planning system is useful in developing the plans and should include the systematic aspects of the ALF as well as an evaluation and quality control method. Management methods and styles need to be selected from the broad range of existing methods. Information systems and technology are important components of an ALF. Marketing must be matched to the business and operational plans, as well as to the specific target populations they define.

REFERENCES

Ackoff, R., & Emery, F. (1972). *On purposeful systems*. Seaside, CA: Intersystem Publications.

Allen, J. (1999). *Assisted living administration: The knowledge base*. New York: Springer Publications.

Allen, P., & Sanger, C. (1979). "Every Thing Old Is New Again." Song Lyric, *All That Jazz soundtrack*.

Anderson, J., Rungtusanatham, M., & Schroeder, R. (1994). A theory of quality management underlying the Deming Management Method. *Academy of Management Review, 19*(3), 472–509.

Buttaro, P. (1994). *Basic management for assisted living and residential care centers*. Aberdeen, SD: HCF Educational Service Publishers.

Center for the Advancement of Study of Educational Administration. (1968). *Toward a source of organization*.

Champys, J. (1995). *Reengineering management*. Retrieved from http://en.wikipedia.org/wiki/HarperCollins

Churchill, Jr., G. A. (1979). A paradigm for developing better measures of marketing constructs. *Journal of Marketing Research, 16*(1), 39–53.

Churchman, C. W. (1968). *The systems approach*. New York: Delacorte Press.

Churchman, C. W. (1971). *The design of inquiring systems: Basic concepts of systems and organization*. New York: Basic Books.

Crosby, P. (1982). *Zero defects subjective vs. objective, step 7 of Philip Crosby's 14 step quality improvement process*, Winter Park Public Library. Retrieved from http://www.wppl.org/wphistory/PhilipCrosby/grant.htm

Davenport, T. (1995). *The fad that forgot people*. Fast Company.

Davenport, T. (1995, January). Will participative makeovers of business process succeed where reengineering failed? *Planning Review*.

DeFeo, J., & Barnard, W. (2004). *Juran's six sigma breakthrough and beyond*. New York: McGraw-Hill.

De la Vera Gonzalez, J., & Sanchez Diaz, J. (2004). *Business process-driven requirements engineering: A goal based approach.* Retrieved from http://citeseerx.ist.psu.edu/viewdoc/download?doi=10.1.1.92.4477&rep=rep1&type=pdf

Deming, W. E. (1975). On some statistical aids toward economic production. *Interfaces, 5*(4), 1–15.

Deming, W. E. (1981–1982). Improvement of quality and productivity through action by management. *National Productivity Review, 1*(1), 12–22.

Deming, W. E. (1986). *Out of the crisis.* MIT Center for Advanced Engineering Study.

Deming, W. E., & Walton, M. (1989). *The Deming management method.* Dodd, Mead & Co.

Deming, W. E. (1990). A system of profound knowledge. *Actionline,* 20–24.

Deming, W. E. (1993). *The new economics for industry, government, education.* MIT MA: Center for Advanced Engineering Study Cambridge.

Deming, W. E. (2010). *Deming's 14 Point plan for TQM.* Retrieved from http://www.1000advices.com/guru/quality_tqm_14points_deming.html

Dixon, G., Parshall, P., Pratt, D., Salinger, J., & Young, D. (2001). In Namazi and Chafetz (Eds.), *Assisted living: Current issues in facility management and resident care* (Chap. 4). Westwood, CT: Greenwood Publishing.

Drew, E. B., et. al. (1967). PPBS: Its scope and limits. *The Public Interest, 8,* 3–48.

Drucker, P. (1981). What results should you expect? A user guide to MBO. *Public Administration Review, 36*(1).

Drucker, P. (1981). Management by objectives: As developed by Peter Drucker assisted by Harold Smedly. *The Academy of Management Review, 6*(3).

Drury, H. (1915). *Scientific management: A history and criticism.* New York: Columbia University.

English, J., & Morely, H. (1968). *Cost-effectiveness: The economics of engineered systems.* New York: John Wiley.

Erez, M. (1977). Feedback: A necessary condition for the goal setting relationship. *Journal of Applied Psychology, 62,* 624–627.

Grant, R., Shani, R., & Krisman, R. (1994). TQMS challenge to management theory and practice. *Sloan Management Review, 35*(2).

Hall, R. (1963). The concept of bureaucracy: an empirical assessment. *The American Journal of Sociology, 69*(1), 32–40.

Hammer, M. (1990). Reengineering work: Don't animate, obliterate. *Harvard Business Review,* 104–112.

Hammer, M., & Champy, J. (1993). *Reengineering the corporation: A manifesto for business revolution.* New York: Harper Business.

Hodge, B., & Johnson, H. (1970). *Management and organization behavior: Multidimensional approach.* New York: John Wiley.

Ignizio, J. (1994). *Goal programming and extension.* MA: Lexington Books.

Imai, K. (1986). *Kaizen, The Kaizen: the key to Japan's competitive success.* New York: McGraw Hill/Irwin.

Ing, D. (2009). Value creating business models. Message posted to coevolving.com ISO 8402:1994, Geneva, Switzerland: International Organization for Standardization, *International Organization for Standardization (2000) Quality Systems - Model for Quality Assurance in Design, Development, Production, Installation and Servicing.*

International Standard ISO 9001:2000(E), Geneva, Switzerland. Retrieved from http://en.wikpedia.org/wiki/International_Organiztion_for_Standardization

Japanese Human Relations Association. (1995). *The improvement engine: The Kaizen Teian approach*. Portland, OR: Productivity Press.

Juran, J. M. (1992). *Juran on quality*. New York: Free Press.

Kavakli, E., & Loucopoulos, P. (2004). Goal modeling in requirements engineering: Analysis and critique of current methods. In J. Krogstie, T. Halpin, & K. Siau (Eds.), *Information modeling methods and methodologies*. London: Idea Group.

Kotelnikov, V. (2010). *Kaizen and total quality management*. Retrieved from http://www.1000ventures.com/business_guide/mgmt_kaizen_tqc_main.html

Lewin, K., Lippit, R., & White, R. (1939). Patterns of aggressive behavior in experimentally created social climates. *Journal of Social Psychology, 10*, 271–301.

Lewis, M., & Black. N. (Eds.). (2003). *Operational management: Critical perspectives on business and management*. New York: Routledge.

Likert, R. (1967). *The human organization: Its management and value*. New York: McGraw-Hill.

Likert, R. (1961). *New patterns of management*. New York: McGraw-Hill.

Locke, E., Shaw, K., & Brawley, L. (1981). Goal setting and task performance 1969-1980. *Psychological Bulletin, 90*, 125–152.

March, J., & Simon, H. (1958). *Organizations*. New York: John Wiley.

March, J., & Simon, H. (1993). *Organizations* (2nd ed.). Cambridge, MA: Blackwell Pub.

Maslow, A. (1943), A theory of human motivation. *Psychological Review, 50*(4), 370–396. Retrieved from http://psychclassics.youru.ca/maslow/motivation/htm

Maslow, A. (1954). *Motivation and personality*. New York: Harper & Row.

Maslow, A. (1965). *Eupsychian management: A journal*. Homewood, IL: Irwin-Dorsey.

Maslow, A. (1970). *Motivation and personality*. New York: Harper & Row.

McGregor, D. (1960). *The human side of the enterprise*. New York: McGraw-Hill, Inc.

McGregor, D. (2002). Theory X and Theory Y. *Workforce, 81*(1).

Melichar, J. F. (1972). *NOBS: New or better systems*. San Mateo: URS Corp.

Melichar, J. F. (1972a). *An evaluation system structure*. San Mateo: URS Corp.

Merton, R. (1940). Bureaucratic structure and personality. *Social Forces, 8*(4), 560–568

Morris, B. (1996). *New rule: Look in not out*. Retrieved from http://money.cnn.com/2006/07/10/magazines/fortune/rule4.fortune/index.htm

Muir, J. (1911). *My first summer in the Sierra*. Boston: Houghton Mifflin.

Namazi, K., & Chafetz, P. (Eds.). (2001). *Assisted living: Current issues in facility management and resident care*. Westwood, CT: Greenwood Publishing.

Odine, G. S. (1965). *Management by objective*. New York: Pilman Publishing Corporation.

Osterwalder, A., Parent, C., & Pigneur, V. (2004). *Setting up ontology of business models*.

Ouchi, W. G. (1982). *Theory Z*. New York: Avon Books.

Pollack, R. (2010). Retrieved from http://www.ischool.utexas.edu/~rpollock/tqm.html

Ranchhod, A., Zou, F., & Tinson, J. (2001). Factors influencing marketing effectiveness on the web. *Information Resources Management Journal, 14*(1).

Rand Corporation. (1966). *The world of program budgeting. P-3361*. Santa Monica, CA: Fisher, G.H.

Reengineering Reviewed. (1994). Retrieved from *The Economist Wiki:* http://en/wikipedia.org/The_Economist

Renzio,T. (1993). Planning Deming management for service organizations. *Business Horizons, 36*(3).

Siegal, E., Ford, B., & Bernstein, J. (1993). *The Ernst & Young business plan guide.* New York: John Wiley.

Singer, D. A. (2010). *Effective management of long-term care facilities* (2nd ed.). Ontario, Canada: Jones and Bartlett.

Strauss, J., & Frost, R. (2008). *E-Marketing.* Upper Saddle River, NJ: Prentice Hall. Retrieved from http://www.ibiblio.org/eldritch/fwt/ti.html

Taylor, F. (1911). *The principles of scientific management.* Retrieved from http://www.ibiblio.org/eldritch/fwt/ti/html

UK Dept. of Industry. (2010). Retrieved from http://www.businessballs.com/qualitymanagement.htm/

Walton, M. (1986). *The Deming management method.* New York: Putnam Publishing.

Weber, M. (1947). *The theory of social and economic organizations*: New York: Oxford University Press.

Weicher, M., Chu, W. W., Lin, W. C., Le, V., & Yu, D. (1995). *Business process reengineering: Analysis and recommendations.* Retrieved from http://www.netlib.com/bpr1.htm

Von Bertalanfy, L. (1968). *General system theory: Foundations, development, applications* (rev. ed.). New York: George Brazllier.

Von Forester, H. (1981). *Observing systems.* Seaside, CA: Intersystem Publishers.

Financial Management in Assisted Living Facilities

With Contributing Author: Raymond Yee

Learning Objectives

Upon the completion of Chapter 9, the reader will be able to:

- *Describe accounting systems (cash basis and accrual basis) and accounting records (accrued expenses, accrued income, revenue, deductions from revenue, expense accounting).*

- *Discuss the organization of an accounting system (chart of accounts, documentary evidence of financial transactions, a journal and general ledger).*

- *Define common accounting job titles and positions that exist in assisted living facilities (ALFs).*

- *Describe financial reports (balance sheet, cash flow statement, profit and loss statement).*

- *Discuss financial standard operating procedures for cash, accounts payable, resident accounts receivables, and credit and collections.*

- *Understand the need for account records such as payroll records, time and earnings records, federal payroll taxes, payroll journal, employee personnel file.*

- *Describe budget preparation in relation to operating, plant and equipment (capital), and cash.*

- *Discuss ratio analysis (current ratio and quick ratio) as an indication of future solvency problems.*

- *Understand risk management including commercial insurance, liability insurance, property insurance, consequential loss insurance, and theft insurance.*

INTRODUCTION

This chapter is intended to present a summary of information on financial management in assisted living facilities (ALFs) covering the following topics: accounting systems, organization, financial reporting, department titles and staff, the use of accounting and financial software, standard accounting procedures, accounts records, budget preparation, financial ratio analysis, risk management and common accounting terms and definitions. The information contained will help administrators and operators of ALFs to learn about basic financial concepts and accounting terminology.

This chapter will also relate the functions of accounting and accounting systems to ALF management. Two functions of management previously considered were planning and controlling. One of the purposes of the planning function is to make very basic decisions concerning the types of service to be provided by the ALF. In addition to management objectives, ALFs must also be concerned with fiscal objectives in order to have adequate funds to carry out the purposes and goals of the facility. Fiscal objectives should take into consideration income and expenditures within the various organizational units or departments will be expressed in monetary or statistical terms to allow coordination of operations in the various departments.

ACCOUNTING SYSTEMS

To have effective management functions relative to the planning and controlling of an ALF, a strong organizational structure must be established for fiscal operations. There must be some sort of information and statistical data relating to each department or aspect of the business. Accounting is the system which accumulates data of quantitative nature relating to the activities taking place in the facility. Senior management and the financial administrator must be able to utilize this information to make key and sound managerial decisions. Accounting is also the interpretation of the results of the data, involving not only accumulation, but the correct interpretation and then effective communication within the organization. Accumulation means the mechanical process of actually recording financial transactions. Interpretation responds to the analysis of the information (key financial ratios and trends) in order to assist senior management in making correct financial decisions of the ALF. Lastly, communication corresponds with the reporting of this information, and presenting the data in a manner to help senior management understand and then make decisive financial decisions.

The accounting system should accurately reflect detailed aspects of the assisted living industry. Sophisticated methods of accounting are not required. The system however should be able to allow for basic cost accounting so that senior management will be aware of all expenses and revenues relating to each department. The accounting system should also be able to collect data such as the number of admissions, readmissions, resident transfers (upgrades/downgrades), and discharges in order to help senior management perform their strategic planning.

Accounting is a discipline that is based on basic and evident concepts which should be understood by the financial manager. Some of these basic concepts are:

(a) The ALF is considered a legal entity that is capable of buying, selling and carrying additional business activities;

(b) The ALF is capable of continuity of activity; it has both a life of its own and a business life divided into parts. These parts are timed measurements to determine the amount of dollars earned and the expenditures in each piece;

(c) The facts ascertained by the accounting process must be capable of being objectively documented. That is, an accounts payable invoice should be supported by the proper documentation that includes a purchase order (P.O.), vendor invoice, receiving report, and a paper check issued in payment of the bill;

(d) The accounting system must be consistent year to year. Consistency means that standardization and uniformity of accounting policies and procedures are used in the accounting process every year;

(e) Full disclosure relating to accounting procedures is essential. That is, all pertinent and important financial information used to generate each accounting report must be reported by the ALF;

(f) Historical cost is the acting term for the evaluation of assets and the recording of most expenses. The term "cost" signifies that the amount of cash or cash equivalent given in exchange for property or services;

(g) Any acquisition of donated property does not involve cost; this property should be recorded at fair market value (FMV) when it is obtained. Failure to do so will result in the underreporting of assets, revenues and expenses.

In accounting there are two basic systems: cash basis and accrual basis.

Cash Basis

In cash basis accounting system, revenues are recognized when the cash is actually received by the ALF. All expense and asset items are NOT recorded until the cash is actually disbursed. The operating statement, or the profit and loss statement, that results from cash basis accounting methodology is the summary of cash receipts and disbursements or a recording of cash flow. Items such as accrued income, accrued expenses, depreciation, expense accounting, revenues and deductions are NOT included.

Accrual Basis

In accrual basis accounting system, the primary accounting method used by ALFs (especially large ALFs and those facilities that are part of a nationwide chain), the information that is provided can be developed into more meaningful data, giving senior management a more detailed and expanded picture of the overall obligations and prospects of the ALF. The accrual system of accounting provides recognition to all revenues in the time period they are actually earned, and to all expenses when they are actually incurred. The cash flow has very little to do with recording these types of transactions as they are reflected when they take place irrespective to the flow of cash between the ALF, its residents, and vendors.

Furthermore, the typical ALF accounting records should include the following six items: accrued income, accrued expenses, revenue, deductions from revenue, expense accounting, and depreciation.

(a) **Accrued expenses**
Accrued expenses are those incurred by the ALF, but not yet paid in cash.
(b) **Accrued income**
Accrued income is income that already earned by the ALF, but the cash has not yet received in-house.
(c) **Revenue**
Revenue is the income received at the ALF's established rates, or charges for all services rendered to the resident whether or not these amounts have not been paid to the ALF by the resident or third party payee (e.g., State Medicaid, long-term care insurance carrier). The purpose of revenue accounting is to keep precise records of gross revenue earned. The revenue is allocated to the appropriate departments within the ALF, which establishes a meaningful comparison as to earning potential of the various departments in the facility. Those

departments with earnings potential (e.g., physical therapy, home aide, cafeteria, et al.) may also be compared in terms of expense in order to determine which ones are making a profit.

(d) Deductions from revenue

At times, the ALF may receive less than its full charge for goods and/ or services rendered to its residents. It is essential to note that the comparisons between potential revenue and revenue losses due to partial resident payments at less than full charges, be recorded in the accounting system. These revenue losses or deductions are of three basic types as follows:

* Contractual allowances

A contractual allowance is the uncollectable difference between the full established charges and what is actually paid by state Medicaid or negotiated contractual rate by a long-term care insurer and the ALF. For example, the ALF posted charges for per-diem resident rate are $400, and the long-term care insurer negotiated payment rate is $300 per day. The $100 per day difference is considered to be the contractual allowance and thus deducted from resident revenue. The same methodology also exists for state Medicaid payment rates.

* Deductions for charity care

All charity care provided to a resident by the ALF is deducted from resident revenue. The charitable care should be first recognized by the ALF as established set rates. It should be noted that a charitable care deductions cannot be taken after a service had been billed to a resident.

* Bad debt provision

These are estimated amounts in "Accounts Receivable" which cannot be collected by the ALF from the resident, and therefore are considered credit losses. The Bad Debt provision is NOT the same as Deductions for Charitable Care. If there had been any collection effort by the ALF to obtain the monies owed by a resident and/or long-term care insurer and that effort is not successful, there would then be a reduction of resident revenues by utilizing the Bad Debt Provision to offset the difference.

(e) Expense accounting

Expense accounting is used to collect on an accrual basis. It is a meaningful record of the operating expenses that relates to the ALF and/or individual facility department.

(f) Depreciation

All ALF assets, whether they are purchased or donated, must be included in the facility's balance sheet. All assets (except land) depreciate, or lose value over time through use, wear and tear, or technological obsolescence. The assets would eventually need to be replaced and is considered an operating expense that reflects the actual cost to replace it. If the asset were recognized and the depreciation expense not taken into consideration, the assisted living facility's real cost of operations would be significantly understated. Therefore, depreciation must be recorded as an operating expense. There are five depreciation methodologies that are recognized and allowed by the United States Internal Revenue Service (IRS) as follows:

1) Line depreciation
The straight line depreciation method is the easiest to use and record, in addition to being the easiest to understand. It basically provides for equal periodic charges to expenses over the estimated life of the asset. For example, an ALF purchases physical therapy equipment for $5,000 to service its residents. This exercise apparatus has an estimated life span of 10 years. Therefore, for 10 continuous years, $500 would be the depreciation value each year.

2) Units of production method
This depreciation method is based on asset usage. That is, the more an asset is utilized, the faster it depreciates. The asset life is expressed in terms of hours, miles, or number of operations. For example, in order to conserve energy and save monies, an ALF purchases CFL light bulbs for its resident's quarters and common use areas. Each CFL light bulb costs $5.00, and has a life span of 5,000 hours. Therefore, each CFL light bulb would depreciate at a rate of .001 cents per hour.

3) Declining balance method
The declining balance method is illustrated by a declining periodic depreciation charge over the estimated life of the asset. A common method is to double the straight line depreciation rate and then apply the resulting rate to the cost of the asset. For example, the ALF bought a sonogram machine to use in the facility's health clinic. The state-of-the art diagnostic equipment cost $20,000, and you would double the straight 10% line depreciation rate, therefore depreciating 20% of the $20,000 which provides a $4,000 first year depreciation expense. At the end of the second year, the depreciation formula would be $20,000 subtracted by $4,000, and equal $16,000 times 20%, equal to $3,200, which is amount depreciated. Furthermore, the original formula is applied each year thereafter until the $20,000 (the original amount) is exhausted.

4) Sum of the years digit method
This depreciation method can be best portrayed as a steady decreasing periodic depreciation charge over the life of the asset so that a progressively smaller fraction is used each year to the original first year

of the asset. For example, an ALF licenses an advanced drug tracking software for $15,000 in order to track resident medication dosages for its pharmacy department. The software developer guarantees that the application will have an estimated useful life span of 5 years. Therefore, the drug software is depreciated where the denominator is 5 + 4 + 3 + 2 + 1 or 15. For the first year, the numerator is 5, for the second year it is 4 and so on as illustrated in Table 9.1.

5) Accelerated depreciation

Accelerated depreciation such as the prior declining balance and the sum of the years digits methods, allow for a higher depreciation charge in the early part of an asset's useful life, especially during the first year as it then gradually declines therefore. The Accelerated Depreciation method is preferred by the ALF along with most other institutions and companies in other industries because of the increased depreciation expense in the early years that help to reduce taxable earnings. Furthermore, under IRC Section 179 deductions (or First-year expensing), the IRS would allow an ALF a full deduction for investments in depreciable business equipment during the year the property is placed in service. The expensing limit for First-Year Expensing Deduction was $108,000 in 2006, and was adjusted for inflation in 2007 through 2009. In 2010, the IRC Section 179 deduction limit fell back to a maximum of $25,000 per year.

TABLE 9.1   Depreciation – Sum of the Years Digit Method

Year	Asset Cost	Depreciation Rate	Depreciation Amt.
1	$15,000	5/15	$5,000
2	$15,000	4/15	$4,000
3	$15,000	3/15	$3,000
4	$15,000	2/15	$2,000
5	$15,000	1/15	$1,000
Total:			$15,000

ORGANIZATION

The accounting system itself contains the following items: chart of accounts, documentary evidence of financial transactions, a journal, and general ledger.

The ALF's Finance Department must establish a Chart of Accounts before any financial transactions can be recorded. The Chart of Accounts is basically the manner in which the financial information is recorded and classified. It helps to systematize data of a financial nature, as well as assist in meeting the reporting requirements of the U.S. Internal Revenue Service, state Medicaid, and other government regulatory agencies. A sample Chart of Accounts is depicted in Table 9.2.

Furthermore, to illustrate a more detailed chart of accounts, a chart of accounts for the Riverdale Premier Assisted Living Corporation is depicted in Table 9.3. Note how detailed cash, accounts receivables, salaries, etc. are expanded and recorded compared to prior sample Chart of Accounts.

TABLE 9.2 Sample Chart of Accounts
Assets (items of value owned by the ALF)
101- Cash (money in banks and investments such as U.S. Treasuries that are very liquid)
102- Accounts Receivables (monies owed to Facility by residents for past services provided such as rent and physical therapy)
103- Inventory (stock such as the cost of unused supplies like food stuff, cleaning materials, and CFL light bulbs)
104- Investments (money market funds, CDs, and depreciation fund)
105- Land (the cost of land)
Liabilities (items of debts owed by the ALF)
201- Accounts Payable (the amount of monies owed to creditors for supplies and services)
202- Salaries (the amount of monies and wages owed to full and part-time employees that have not been paid)
203- Interest Payable (the amount of monies owed to financial institution on the loan principal)
204- Employee Benefits Payable
205- Taxes Payable – (can be separated into federal, state, and municipal)
Capital (items that are the equity of the owners of the ALF. It is the amount of the owners' investments. For a publicly traded company, it would be the corporate ownership rather than a proprietary ownership in private investor hands)
301- Owner's Capital
302- Owner's Withdrawals
303- Revenue and Expense Summaries
Revenues (items that are income for ALF)
401- Resident Daily Room Charges
402- Resident Cafeteria Charges
403- Resident Physical Therapy
404- Resident Nursing Care Charges
405- Gift Shop Revenues
Expenses (items that are expenditures for ALF)
501- Facility Salaries
502- Consultation fees (e.g., outside Auditor)
503- Employee Health Insurance
504- Facility Telephone/Internet
505- Employee Travel

TABLE 9.3	Riverdale Premier Assisted Living Corporation – Chart of Accounts		
Assets		**Liabilities**	

Assets		Liabilities	
Current Assets		*Current Liabilities*	
1101-	Cash- Petty	2102-	Accounts Payable- supplies
1103-	Cash- Payroll Account	2104-	Notes Payable- short-term
1106-	Cash- Operating fund	2107-	Mortgage Payable- short-term
1112-	Investments- Money Market Fund	2109-	Debts Payable- current
1114-	Investments- CDs (less than one year)	2111-	Employee Benefits Payable
1117-	Investments- Depreciation Fund	2113-	Employee Health Insurance Payable
1122-	Accounts Receivable- Medicare Part B	2115-	Salaries Payable
1123-	Accounts Receivable- Medicaid/DSS	2201-	Taxes
1124-	Accounts Receivable- Resident Self Pay	2204-	Taxes Payable- New York State
1126-	Accounts Receivable- Other Payers (e.g., Commercial, VA, Workers' Compensation)	2205-	Taxes Payable- New York City
1163-	Unexpired liability insurance	2207-	Taxes Payable- Federal
		2221-	Interest Payable
Noncurrent Assets			
1302-	Land	*Noncurrent Liabilities*	
1305-	Land Improvements	2303-	Notes Payable- long-term
1402-	Building- Primary	2313-	Mortgage Payable- long-term
1414-	Building- Secondary	2323-	Bonds Payable
1426-	Building- Garage/storage	2401-	Pensions Payable
1430-	Building Improvements		
1502-	Furniture- Primary	*Capital*	
1504-	Furniture- Secondary	3001-	Shareholders' Equity
1512-	Equipment- Primary	3101-	Net Income (loss)
1514-	Equipment- Secondary		
1516-	Equipment- Office	*Revenue (Health Care)*	
1518-	Equipment– Kitchen	4001-	Medicare Part B
1519-	Equipment– Laundry	4003-	Medical Department of Social Services

(Continued)

TABLE 9.3	Riverdale Premier Assisted Living Corporation – Chart of Accounts (*Continued*)		
Assets		**Liabilities**	

	Assets		Liabilities
1521-	Transportation	4005-	Other Payers (e.g., Commercial, VA, Workers' Compensation)
1524-	Equipment– Land Maintenance		
		Ancillary	
Contra Assets, Accumulated Depreciation		4212-	Physical Therapy
1602-	Accum. Depr. – Primary Building	4214-	Occupational Therapy
1604-	Accum. Depr. – Secondary Building	4216-	Social Services/Activities
1606-	Accum. Depr. – Garage/Storage	4218-	Speech Therapy (contract)
1630-	Accum. Depr. – Building Improvements		
1642-	Accum. Depr. – Furniture Maintenance	*Uncompensated Care*	
1644-	Accum. Depr. – Furniture (Secondary Building)	4311-	Contractual Allowance– Medicare Part B
1651-	Accum. Depr. – Equipment (Primary Building)	4313-	Contractual Allowance– Medicaid 1651
1654-	Accum. Depr. – Equipment (Secondary Building)	4315-	Contractual Allowance– Other Payers (e.g., Commercial, VA, Workers' Compensation)
1666-	Accum. Depr. – Office Equipment	4332-	Donated Charitable Care
1668-	Accum. Depr. – Kitchen Equipment	4341-	Bad Debts
		4315-	Resident Refunds
1669-	Accum. Depr. – Laundry		
1671-	Accum Depr. – Transportation		
1674-	Accum. Depr. – Land Improvements		
1680-	Accum. Depr. – Building Improvements		

Expenses	
Administration	
5001-	Salaries- Management
5002-	Salaries- Clerical
5003-	Consultation Fees
5006-	Health Insurance
5011-	Payroll Tax
5013-	Taxes- Income

(Continued)

TABLE 9.3	Riverdale Premier Assisted Living Corporation – Chart of Accounts (*Continued*)	
Assets		**Liabilities**
5015-	Taxes- Property	
5022-	Insurance- Liability	
5026-	Retirement Fund	
5032-	Supplies	
5034-	Telephone/Cellular/Internet	
5035-	Travel	
5037-	Postage/Mailings	
5039-	Licenses and Professional Dues	
5042-	Repairs	
Plant Operation		
5101-	Salaries	
5106-	Health Insurance	
5111-	Payroll Tax	
5122-	Utility- Electricity	
5124-	Utility- Gas	
5126-	Utility- Water	
5128-	Utility- Sewage	
5132-	Supplies	
Health Care Workers		
5201-	Salaries- Nurses	
5202-	Salaries- Health Aides	
5206-	Health Insurance	
5211-	Pharmacy	
5224-	Laboratory	
5237-	Uniforms	
5242-	Repairs	
Dietary		
5301-	Salary- Management, Food Services	
5302-	Salary- Kitchen Staff	
5306-	Health Insurance	
Assets		**Liabilities**
5311-	Payroll Tax	
5332-	Supplies	
5342-	Repairs	

(*Continued*)

TABLE 9.3	Riverdale Premier Assisted Living Corporation – Chart of Accounts (*Continued*)	
	Assets	**Liabilities**

Laundry
- 5401- Salaries
- 5406- Health Insurance
- 5411- Payroll Tax
- 5432- Supplies
- 5442- Repairs
- 5461- Contract Services

Housekeeping
- 5501- Salaries
- 5506- Health Insurance
- 5511- Payroll Tax
- 5532- Supplies
- 5542- Repairs

Rehabilitation (Physical Therapy)
- 5601- Salaries (or Contract)
- 5606- Health Insurance
- 5611- Payroll Tax
- 5632- Supplies
- 5642- Repairs

Occupational Therapy
- 5661- Salaries (or Contract)
- 5666- Health Insurance
- 5671- Payroll Tax
- 5682- Supplies
- 5692- Repairs

Social Service/Admissions
- 5701- Salaries (or Contract)
- 5706- Health Insurance
- 5711- Payroll Tax
- 5732- Supplies
- 5742- Repairs

Activities
- 5801- Salaries – Beautician
- 5802- Salaries – Arts & Crafts
- 5806- Health Insurance

(Continued)

TABLE 9.3	Riverdale Premier Assisted Living Corporation – Chart of Accounts (*Continued*)	
Assets		**Liabilities**
5811-	Payroll Tax	
5832-	Supplies – Beauty	
5833-	Supplies – Arts & Crafts	
5835-	Transportation	
5837-	Special Events	
5842-	Repairs	
Capital Expenses		
5904-	Interest – Mortgage	
5907-	Interest – Long-term debt	
5914-	Debt Service – Mortgage	
5917-	Debt Service – Long-term debt	
5934-	Depreciation – Plant	
5936-	Depreciation – Equipment	

Documentary Evidence for Internal and Independent Auditors

Whenever the assisted living facility dispenses monies for various transactions, it is an important requirement in the accounting cycle that these disbursements be recorded by various pieces of documentation. For example, the items that would record the issuance of a bank check for an item bought by the facility would be the store register receipt of the item, purchase order, vendor invoice, credit card statement, or other evidence that this transaction had occurred. The reliability and accuracy of the facility's accounting systems is based upon the extent of the necessary documented evidence for the various transactions that occurred. The typical accounting cycle is described below:

(1) First, the transaction is recorded in the billings journal on a daily or chronological basis;

(2) Second, from the billings journal, there is a posting to the General Ledger;

(3) Next, from the General Ledger, an electronic accounting spreadsheet (e.g., Microsoft Excel and/or Great Plains software, IBM Lotus 1-2-3) is produced;

(4) Lastly, from the spreadsheet, various financial reports (e.g., profit & loss statement, balance sheet, income statement) are generated.

Billings Journal

The billings journal is a chronological record of increases and decreases affecting transactions. Adjusted and closing entries are made at the end of each month. These entries do not reflect the account balances which are required to be documented as part of the various financial statements for the facility at the close of each month. The financial data in the billings journal must be transferred to a book called the "General Ledger."

General Ledger

A general ledger is kept for each facility account in the chart of accounts. At the close of each month (i.e., "closing the books"), the financial data recorded in the billings journal is transferred to each of the accounts in the general ledger. This accounting procedure is called "posting."

Electronic Accounting Spreadsheet

After all financial transactions for the month have been journalized and posted, and after the balances have been determined for each general ledger account, an electronic accounting spreadsheet is prepared. The accounting spreadsheet is the work sheet of which the facility accountants compile important financial statements such as the profit and loss statement, the income statement, and the balance sheet.

DEPARTMENT TITLES AND STAFF

The following are a list of common accounting job titles and positions that one would encounter within the accounting department of an assisted living facility. The larger the size of the ALF, the more departmental titles and accounting personnel are required.

Accountant

By analyzing revenues, costs, financial liabilities, and assets, accountants are able to calculate future cash flows fairly accurately. Financial reports such as balance sheets or profit & loss statements must be maintained and reported to administrators. The majority of an accountant's day is spent completing or analyzing paperwork, but communication among departments is also necessary.

Accounting Manager/Supervisor

Accounting professionals must often calculate, input, and verify data on a regular basis. These managers and supervisors oversee all of these basic functions in addition to maintaining all financial records. These positions may require a great deal of time spent researching or reviewing the work of others.

Assistant Controller

Controllers assist in leading the daily activities of an accounting organization. They are responsible for preparing, evaluating, and presenting budgets and reports directly to management. Their duties range from establishing, to implementing company practices and procedures, and extensive knowledge of accounting principles is mandatory.

Auditor

Auditors are responsible for carefully analyzing reports, statements, and accounting software of an internal or external facility to ensure accurate calculations. They must have a thorough knowledge of all laws and regulations relating to accounting practices, because their job is to detect and report any discrepancies within a company's financial records. If an error has occurred, it is their duty to trace it back to the source, and make recommendations to ensure more accurate accounting in the future.

Bookkeeper

Familiarity with standard accounting procedures is required for a bookkeeper position, due to the fact that they are responsible for recording a company's business transactions. Bookkeepers are responsible for maintaining records within given ledgers or computer programs. They must keep accurate records and balance all reports and ledgers on a monthly basis.

Clerk

Associates planning on working towards higher level positions often start as accounting clerks. Duties are often redundant, but allow candidates to learn the processes of an accounting office or department. Daily activities generally include ledger maintenance and the preparation of basic financial reports.

Controller

Developing and implementing efficient policies, procedures, and practices is the main priority of a controller. They must oversee all aspects of the accounting department, such as budget or report maintenance and preparation. Once they are positive data has been compiled properly, they are responsible for presenting the data to management.

Chief Financial Officer

Immense creativity and independence is necessary for a CFO career because they are held accountable for organizing and directing the assisted living facility's overall financial policies. Insurance, tax, treasury, accounting, budgeting, and many other aspects are included in this grouping. An in-depth education of accounting practices and higher education will be needed for these professionals. A CPA and/or MBA degree in Accounting or Managerial Finance would be helpful.

Director

Accounting, payroll, and cost accounting functions are direct responsibilities of the accounting director. They are responsible for a number of tasks and applications, therefore extensive education and experience is generally mandatory. They must have the capability to lead others within the department as well as work within deadlines.

Financial Analyst

Reconciling and forecasting the internal accounts are a large part of an analyst's career. They spend an immense amount of time compiling data, ensuring accuracy, analyzing information, and creating reports. They monitor all documents and report any trends to management.

Office Administrator

The development of policies and procedures of all office activities is the primary responsibility of the office administrator. They supervise all associates and proceedings on a daily basis. Duties, including filing, typing, faxing, mailing, and dictating, are often delegated to clerks or administrative assistants. They must maintain order among all records.

Office Manager

These careers often require extensive experience and good judgment. Office managers are expected to direct the general duties of multiple business office operations. They must be capable of directing and coordinating others within their department.

Payroll Administrator

Although this position focuses mainly on payroll functions, a keen understanding of all accounting practices is necessary to adequately fulfill this role. Typical duties include compiling accurate records of timesheets within a software system, computing earnings, and withholding mandatory amounts such as taxes or benefits. Accuracy and attention to detail are traits a payroll administrator must possess.

Payroll Specialist

Payroll specialists are often in charge of compiling timecards within a computer system, or inputting data from hard copies of timesheets or production records. They have the ability to balance payroll when completed and ensure proper the State, Federal, and local tax payments are made. Since pay is generally issued at a specific time, these professionals must be able to complete all work within a given deadline.

Principal

As the highest authority in the accounting department, principals assume numerous duties. They oversee all accounting functions from preparing reports and entering data, to collaborating with other departments, and organizing special projects. Principals are commonly responsible for performing audits of departments, monitoring department workloads, and creating and monitoring databases. They handle any communication necessary among fellow administrators and management.

Specialist

Common duties for accounting specialists revolve around the direction and planning of financial statements, cost control systems, and ledger accounts. Basic accounting skills are mandatory for these positions, and immense organization is integral. They watch over all aspects of basic accounting tasks.

Staff Assistant

Duties are often varied for these occupations. Staff assistants may handle duties from basic administrative tasks such as filing or organizing data to running reports. They take on more responsibility as experience is gained, but these are generally entry-level positions. An understanding of accounting principles is generally required.

Tax Specialist

It is often easier to maintain detailed tax information year round rather than attempting to organize wide-ranging information within a short period of time. As a result, many organizations employ tax specialists year round. Their duties are not only limited to preparing tax returns.

USE OF ACCOUNTING AND FINANCIAL SOFTWARE

Today, assisted living communities require state-of-the-art technologies and innovative processes to operate efficiently and cost effectively. ALFs must have systems and processes in place that help them financially operate the facility with timely and accurate tracking of revenues and expenses information. The processing of invoices must be paid on time, collecting monies owed to them by residents should be done on a regular basis, and paying their employees accurately, as well as reporting critical financial and utilization data to federal and state government agencies, is important. Thus, in order to successfully operate an assisted living facility, the fiscal administrator must automate the financial function with computer technologies and accounting software.

Accounting software is application software that records and processes accounting transactions within functional modules such as accounts payable, accounts receivable, payroll, and trial general ledger balance. It functions as an accounting information system. It may be developed "in-house" by the assisted living facility, or it may be purchased from an outside software developer. It may also be a combination of a third-party application software package with homegrown modifications. Overall, accounting software varies greatly in its complexity and cost.

The accounting software market has been undergoing considerable consolidation since the mid 1990s with many vendors ceasing to exist or being bought out by larger companies.

Typical accounting software that is used in assisted living facilities is composed of various modules, different sections dealing with particular areas of accounting. Among the most common modules are:

Core Modules

- Accounts receivable—where the facility enters money received from residents/patients
- Accounts payable—where the facility enters its bills and pays money it owes vendors
- General ledger—the facility's "books" that are used to generate its monthly, quarterly, and annual financial statements
- Billing—where the facility produces bills/invoices to residents and outside vendors
- Stock/Inventory—where the facility keeps control of its inventory/supplies/parts
- Purchase Order—where the facility orders its inventory/supplies/parts
- Sales Order—where the facility records resident sales for the patient census

Noncore Modules

- Debt Collection—where the facility tracks attempts to collect overdue resident bills (sometimes part of accounts receivable)
- Electronic payment processing
- Expense—where facility employee business-related expenses are entered
- Inquiries—where the facility looks up information on screen without any edits or additions to resident and/or vendor records
- Payroll—where the facility tracks employee salaries, wages, and related taxes
- Reports—where the facility prints out management, financial, and utilization census data
- Purchase Requisition—where requests for purchase orders are made, approved, and tracked by the facility

In many cases, implementation (i.e., the installation and configuration of the accounting system at the facility) is a bigger consideration than the actual software chosen when considering the total cost of ownership for the assisted living facility. Most mid-market and larger accounting software applications are sold exclusively through resellers, developers, and consultants. Those vendors generally pass on a licensing fee to the software vendor and then charge the facility for installation, customization, and support services. Facility clients can normally count on paying roughly 50-200% of the price of the software in implementation and consulting fees.

Small-sized assisted living facilities typically use inexpensive accounting software that is limited in function, but allows most general business accounting functions to be performed. The modules used are accounts payable type accounting transactions, managing budgets, and simple account reconciliation. Many of the low-end accounting software products are characterized by being "single-entry" products, as opposed to double-entry systems seen in many businesses. Some products have considerable functionality, but are not considered GAAP or IFRS/FASB compliant. Some low-end systems do not have adequate security or audit trails.

The most complex and expensive business accounting software used by a larger assisted living facility (ALF) chain are frequently part of an extensive suite of software often known as Enterprise resource planning or ERP software. These applications typically have a very long implementation period, often greater than six months. In many cases, these applications are simply a set of functions which require significant integration, configuration, and customization to even begin to resemble an accounting system. The advantage of a high-end solution is that these systems are designed to support individual facility specific processes as they are highly customizable and can be tailored to exact business requirements. This usually comes at a significant cost in terms of money and implementation time.

Crane (2007) describes the importance of accounting software in assisted living facilities and states that:

> . . . Yardi Senior Housing Management software, from Yardi Systems in Santa Barbara, CA, is a Web-based program that does it all–from running financial reports to managing residents' care schedules. For those services, there are substantial start-up costs and annual license fees. Initial costs, including implementation and training, might start at $30,000 for smaller operators; annual fees are in the neighborhood of $4,000 per community and include hosting through Yardi servers, plus product updates and some telephone support.

FINANCIAL REPORTING

There are three major financial reports that all businesses produce: the balance sheet, the cash flow statement, and the profit and loss statement. Listed below are descriptions of these reports and other tables an ALF generates.

The Balance Sheet

The balance sheet is used to depict the entire financial operation of the facility in terms of its assets, liabilities and capital (stockholder's equity) at a given period in time. It is usually prepared and reported monthly, quarterly, and annually. The items in the balance sheet are: (1) assets that include current assets, long-term investments (such as stocks, bonds, etc.), and fixed assets (property, equipment and assets having a value to the facility over a long period of time); (2) liabilities that include both current liabilities and long-term liabilities (debts that are due in one year or more) such as mortgages, capital equipment loans, and corporate debt (long-term bonds). Capital or stockholder's equity is the amount of monies provided by the owner(s) of the business. This can come from the sale of company stock, retained funds (earned for the owner[s] but is left in the business) and equity funds (considered as a long-term and/or permanent investment by the owner[s]). The net worth of the facility can be calculated as the total assets minus total liabilities equal the owner's equity. Therefore, the total liabilities plus the owner's equity must represent the total assets of the facility.

The balance sheet is the essential financial statement that reports the main types of assets owned by the assisted living facility (ALF). Assets are only half of the picture; the ALF also borrows money. At the date of preparing the balance sheet, the facility owes money to its financial lenders who will be paid sometime in the future. Also, most ALFs purchase many things on credit and owe money to their vendors, which will be paid in the future. Amounts owed to lenders and suppliers are called *liabilities*. A balance sheet reports the main types of liabilities of the facility and separates those due in the short-term and those due in the longer-term.

At times, an assisted living facility might have its total liabilities greater than its total assets. This would occur if the ALF has been losing money. In the vast majority of cases, a facility has more total assets than total liabilities. That is true because: (1) its owners have invested money in the business, which is not a liability of the business; and

(2) the business has earned profit over the years and some of the profit has been retained in the business (profit increases assets). The sum of invested capital from owners and retained profit is called *owners' equity*. The excess of total assets over total liabilities is traceable to owners' equity. A balance sheet reports the make-up of the owners' equity of a business.

You generally see the balance sheet in the following layout:

Assets

Assets are the economic resources of the business. Examples are cash on deposit, long-term investments, equipment, and buildings.

Liabilities

Liabilities arise from borrowing money and buying things on credit from banks and investment firms.

Owners' Equity

Owners' Equity arises from two sources: money invested by the owners, and profit earned and retained by the assisted living facility.

One reason the balance sheet is called by this name is that the two sides balance, or are equal in total amounts:

Total Recorded Amount of Assets = Total Recorded Amount of Liabilities + Total Recorded Amount of Owners' Equity

Owner's equity is sometimes referred to as *net worth*. You compute net worth as follows:

Assets – Liabilities = Net Worth

Net worth is not a particularly good term because it implies that the assisted living facility is worth the amount recorded in its owners' equity accounts. Though the term may suggest that the business could be sold for this amount, nothing is further from the truth.

An example of a typical balance sheet is shown in Table 9.4 for Riverdale Premier Assisted Living Corporation:

TABLE 9.4	Riverdale Premier Assisted Living Corporation-Balance Sheet	
	July 31, 20XX	July 31, 20XX
Assets		
Current Assets		
Cash	$182,100	$8,502
Accounts Receivable (less bad debts of $27,096)	160,551	184,191
Securities	675,825	31.500
Inventory	186,018	164,640
Prepaid Insurance	7,200	10,800
Total Current Assets	1,211,694	399,211
Noncurrent Assets		
Equipment	5,949,000	5,943,600
Plant	17,301,012	17,301,012
Less Accumulated Depreciation	8,316,576	7,086,900
Plant and Equipment	14,933,436	16,157,712
Property	7,950,000	7,950,000
Total Fixed Assets	22,883,436	24,107,712
Total Assets	**24,095,130**	**24,507,345**
Liabilities		
Current Liabilities		
Accounts Payable	8,556	73,818
Notes Payable	100,875	1,065,813
Benefits Payable	74,529	2,114,751
Current portion of long-term debt		
Mortgage	692,040	576,699
Long-term debt	225,000	225,000
Total Current Liabilities	1,101,000	3,832,494
Noncurrent Liabilities		
Mortgage Payable	10,380,606	11,072,649
Debts Payable	2,025,000	2,250,000
Total Noncurrent Liabilities	12,405,606	13,322,649
Total Liabilities	**13,506,606**	**17,155,143**

(Continued)

TABLE 9.4	Riverdale Premier Assisted Living Corporation-Balance Sheet (*Continued*)		
Assets		July 31, 20XX	July 31, 20XX
Net Worth			
Retained Earnings			
Year to date		106,875	82,521
Total		1,112,868	1,005,993
Shareholder's Equity		9,368,781	6,263691
Total Net Worth		10,588,524	7,352,205
Total Liabilities and Capital		24,095,130	24,507,345

The Cash Flow Statement

The cash flow statement for an assisted living facility presents a summary of the sources and uses of cash during a financial period. Successful financial administrators have to manage both profit and cash flow. Assisted living facilities are a two-headed dragon in this respect. Even with a successful profit-making approach, ignoring cash flow can bring ruin upon an ALF. Still, some financial managers become preoccupied with making profit and overlook cash flow, thus causing vendor bills, and then causing employee payroll to be paid late. For financial reporting, cash flows are divided into three basic categories:

Basic Format of the Cash Flow Statement

(1) **Cash flow** from the profit-making activities, or *operating activities*, for the period. (*Note*: *Operating* means the profit-making transactions of the ALF.)
(2) **Cash inflows and outflows** from *investing activities* for the period.
(3) **Cash inflows and outflows** from the *financing activities* for the period. You determine the bottom-line net increase (or decrease) in cash during the period by adding the three types of cash flows shown in the preceding list.

Section one of the cash flow statement explains why net cash flow from sales revenue and expenses – the business's profit-making operating activities – is more or less than the amount of profit reported in the profit and loss account. The actual cash inflow from revenues and outflow for expenses run on a different timetable than the sales revenue and expenses. The sales revenues and expenses are recorded for determining profit. Imagine two different airplanes going to the same destination: the second plane (the cash flow aircraft) runs on a later schedule than the first plane (the recording of sales revenue and expenses in the accounts of the business).

Section two of the cash flow statement records the major long-term investments made by the business during the year, such as constructing a new assisted living building or replacing machinery and equipment. If the business sold any of its long-term assets, it reports the cash inflows from these divestments in this section of the cash flow statement.

Section three records the financing activities of the business during the period, which concerns borrowing new money from lenders and raising new capital investment in the business from its owners. Cash outflows to pay off debt are reported in this section, as well as cash distributions from profit paid to the owners of the business.

The cash flow statement reports the net increase or net decrease in cash during the year (or other time period), caused by the three types of cash flows. This increase or decrease in cash during the year is never referred to as the *bottom line*. This important term is strictly limited to the last line of the profit and loss account, which reflects net income: the final profit after all expenses are deducted.

An illustration of a sample Cash Flow Statement for Riverdale Premier Assisted Living Corporation is shown in Table 9.5.

The Profit and Loss Statement (a.k.a. "The Income Statement")

The purpose of the profit & loss (P&L) statement is to portray the results of the financial operations in the terms of the amount of revenues the facility has earned. This includes current assets (assets consumed in less than one year) such as cash, short-term investments (interest and dividends), patient accounts receivables, inventory, and the amount of expenses the facility has incurred which includes current liabilities (obligations to be paid in one year or less), such as accounts payables for vendors, wages/ salaries & taxes (e.g., FICA, Medicare) payable for employees in the given year. The P&L statement is sometimes known either as the "income statement" or the "statement of income and expenses," and is usually prepared monthly. The time periods reported by the P&L is monthly, quarterly, and annually. Furthermore, the statement of expenses should be departmentalized, thus enabling senior management to determine

TABLE 9.5   Riverdale Premier Assisted Living Corporation – Cash Flow Statement

	Week 1	Week 2	Week 3	Week 4
Beginning Cash Balance	$330,000	$300,000	$294,000	$246,000
Cash Inflow				
Commercial	570,000	510,000	540,000	660,000
Medicaid/DSS	345,000	345,000	345,000	345,000
Medicare Part B				35,000
Self Pay	195,000	150,000	165,000	195,000
VA				20,000
Workers' Compensation				5,000
Short-term investments	300,000		300,000	
Short-term loans			150,000	
Miscellaneous (Gift Shop, Beauty Salon, etc.)	90,000	75,000	60,000	90,000
TOTAL	1,500,000	1,080,000	1,560,000	1,350,000
Cash Outflow				
Payroll	1,050,000		1,095,000	
Accounts Payable	600,000	540,000	675,000	540,000
Delayed Payments	(210,000)	210,000	(198,000)	198,000
Interest Payable				50,000
Taxes	45,000			
Plant in Progress Payments				30,000
Purchase short-term investments		300,000		300,000
Pay short-term loans				100,000
Miscellaneous	36,000	45,000	36,000	48,000
TOTAL	1,530,000	1,086,000	1,608,000	1,266,000
Ending Cash Balance	300,000	294,000	246,000	330,000

the actual income and expense of each department for proper analysis of efficiency (utilization of resources), profits (either a profit center or loss center), etc. It should be noted that the percentage of resident occupancy figure is significant because it helps senior management determine how many residents are required for the assisted living facility to operate profitably or "in the black." As an industry benchmark, assisted living facilities break even financially at about 70% to 75% resident occupancy and achieve financial stabilization (attain long-term economic viability) at approximately 93% occupancy. The profit and loss account is the all-important financial statement that summarizes the profit-making activities (or operations) of a business over a period of time. In very broad outline, the statement is reported like this:

Sales Revenue

Sales revenue is the sales of products and services to customers.

Less Expenses

Less expenses include a wide variety of costs paid by the business, including the cost of products sold to customers, wages and benefits paid to employees, occupancy costs, administrative costs, and income tax.

Equals Net Income

Equals Net Income (which is referred to as the *bottom line* and means final profit after all expenses are deducted from sales revenue), the profit and loss account gets the most attention from business managers and investors – not that they ignore the other two prior key financial statements. The very abbreviated versions of profit and loss accounts that you see in the financial presses, such as in *The Wall Street Journal and The Financial Times*, report only the top line (sales revenue) and the bottom line (net profit). In actual practice, the profit and loss account is more involved than the basic format shown here. Table 9.6 contains the Income Statement for the Riverdale Premier Assisted Living Corporation.

Other Financial Reports

In addition to the Balance Sheet, the Cash Flow Statement and the Profit and Loss Statement, a well-managed assisted living facility would also use additional financial reports concerning supplies and expenses. Several of these reports that the fiscal administrator need to successfully

TABLE 9.6	Riverdale Premier Assisted Living Coporation – Income Statement	
Revenues	July 20, 2010	Year to Date (YTD)
Operating Revenues		
Health Care	$1,072,809	$6,623,442
Total Health Care	$1,072,809	$6,623,442
Ancillary		
Physical Therapy	29,922	185,517
Occupational Therapy	29,670	178,020
Social Services	8,598	50,727
Total Ancillary	68,190	414,264
Gross Operating Revenues	1,140,999	7,037,706
Less Deductions	136,920	844,524
Net Operating Revenues	1,004,079	6,193,182
Nonoperating Revenues		
Miscellaneous		
Meals	1,290	7,482
Concession	4,074	26,073
Beauty Shop	2,370	14,457
Total Miscellaneous	7,734	48,012
Interest	7,920	45,936
Nonoperating Revenues	15,654	93,948
Total Revenues	1,019,733	6,287,130
Expenses		
Operating Expenses		
Salaries		
Health Care Personnel	405,576	2,499,453
Dietary	46,746	280,476
Administration	28,653	163,323
Laundry	10,227	61,362
Maintenance	15,861	96,435
Physical Therapy	28,956	182,424
Occupational Therapy	10,350	62,205
Social Services- Admissions	6,438	39,915

(Continued)

TABLE 9.6	Riverdale Premier Assisted Living Coporation – Income Statement *(Continued)*	
Revenues	July 20, 2010	Year to Date (YTD)
Total Salaries	552,807	3,385,593
Supplies	94,179	569,784
Activity	6,195	37,170
Capital Equipment	600	4,800
Utilities	26,292	157,752
Telephone/Cellular/Internet	489	3,129
Insurance	12,000	72,054
Taxes (Real Estate)	9,939	59,634
Capital Costs		
Interest	83,448	500,688
Mortgage Payment	72,087	432,522
Depreciation	118,881	713,286
Total Capital Costs	274,416	1,646,496
Total Expenses	1,017,234	6,180,255
Net Income (loss)	2,499	109,875
Income Tax	1,125	48,093
Profit after Taxes	1,374	58,782

manage and grow the facility's operations are: a daily report of cash receipts and disbursements, a resident accounts receivables report and an accounts payable report.

Cash Report

The cash report (Table 9.7) provides the fiscal administrator a working knowledge of the amount of cash on hand. It is usually generated monthly and at the end of the month.

Resident Accounts Receivable Report

The resident accounts receivable report (Table 9.8) checks the assisted living facility's fiscal operations from the income perspective. It includes only income from residents (cash) and third party payers (state Medicaid,

TABLE 9.7	Cash Report
Cash on Hand (3/31/2010)	$125,000.00
Plus Cash Receipts	+5,000.00
Total Cash	130,000.00
Less Cash Disbursements	−10,000.00
Cash on Hand (4/30/2010)	$120,000.00

TABLE 9.8	Resident Accounts Receivable Report
Resident A/R (1/31/2010)	$2,000,000.00
Plus Resident Charges	+500.000.00
Total A/R Outstanding Balance	2,500,000.00
Less Resident Payments	−800,000.00
Resident A/R (2/28/2010)	$1,700,000.00

commercial long-term insurance). Furthermore, it indicates the effectiveness of the facility's collection procedures, billings, and efforts to maintain positive cash flow. It is also generated monthly, at the end of the month.

Vendor Accounts Payable Report

The vendor accounts payable report (Table 9.9) also assists the fiscal administrator in keeping track of operating expenses (e.g., outstanding debts to vendors) in line with monthly cash flow. The operating expenses that are included in this report are only those payable within one year (short-term liabilities). Moreover items that include employee salaries and benefits, mortgages, and loan interest payments are not included.

TABLE 9.9	Vendor Accounts Payable Report
Facility A/P (1/31/2010)	$500,000.00
Plus Facility Purchases	+75,000.00
Total A/P Outstanding Balance	575,000.00
Less Facility Payments	−125,000.00
Facility A/P (2/28/2010)	$450,000.00

ACCOUNTING PROCEDURES

In order to operate successfully and profitably, an assisted living facility must have tight departmental management controls in place. Four of the most essential financial standard operating procedures are for: cash, accounts payable, resident accounts receivables, and credit and collections.

Cash Handling Procedure

The significance of cash in any kind of business is important because it is evident that this is a method of financing the business operations. Cash transactions occur more than any other kind of transaction in an assisted living facility. In addition, cash is the asset that is most susceptible to theft, fraud, and misappropriation. As part of financial management, it is important to have some type of internal control for cash receipts. Listed below is a standard operating procedure (SOP) list as an internal control for the ALF's cash receipts:

(1) Incoming mail is opened by someone who does not have access to the accounting records and is not responsible for bank deposits;
(2) Whoever opened the mail prepares a remittance list of all cash items received. One copy of the remittance slip is given to the person actually making the bank deposits;
(3) All personnel who are handling cash are bonded (insurance – see Risk Management section);
(4) A cash receipts slip is prepared for all cash received by the assisted living facility; one copy of this is provided to the person paying the cash with a duplicate copy to the accountants. All cash receipts are recorded in the appropriate accounting records at the earliest time practicable. Separate staff personnel that do not handle cash or record cash transactions prepare the bank reconciliation. Cash receipts must be deposited in the bank daily. Immediately upon receipt of checks, endorsement is made by indicating on the back of the check "For Deposit Only to the Account of XYZ Assisted Living Facility"; and,
(5) Using copies of the cash receipts slips, the accountant then records all cash receipts in a cash receipts journal on a daily basis. Finally, the cash receipts are also posted to the resident's ledger.

Handling Accounts Payable Accounts

An accounts payable account is a creditor of the assisted living facility. A standard operating procedure for handling this type of account is:

(1) Start a file folder for each vendor/supplier/service contractor with which the assisted living facility does business.
(2) A purchase order (P.O.) number is issued or a purchase order written for all facility purchases.
(3) Have a central storeroom where all shipped vendor goods are received.
(4) When supplies, equipment, or goods are received at the central storeroom, a receiving slip must accompany the items. Ensure that the number of cartons that is received corresponds to the items on the receiving slip. Document any item(s) that are backordered.
(5) The receiving slip after being checked by the storeroom (materials management) manager is then sent to the bookkeeper in the accounting department.
(6) When the assisted living facility receives the invoice from the vendor, the accountant or the accounts payable clerk: (a) reviews the invoice to determine that the purchase order is signed by the person authorized to order the item, (b) then against the purchase order to determine if the unit price and any extensions are correct, and (c) finally against the receiving slip to determine if all ordered goods were received.

The last step is that the above information is given to the individual responsible for authorizing payment (typically either the Chief Financial Officer or Controller). All approved hardcopy invoices are lastly filed away in accounts payable folders by alphabetical order of vendor names.

Handling Resident Accounts Receivable

This is the most important accounting procedure for the assisted living facility, since the survival of the assisted living center depends on adequate cash flow from resident revenues. Therefore, the standard operating procedure to establish correct residential rates and to properly record resident revenue plays an essential role in the operation of the facility. The bulk of all revenues received by the assisted living facility come from resident revenues for room and board, routine preventive medical and housekeeping services, special rehabilitation, and private duty nursing services. The typical procedure for handling resident accounts receivable is:

(1) Review and establish the proper rental rate structure for each residential unit, routine services and special services at least on an annual basis.

(2) At the time of resident acceptance into the assisted living facility, set up a ledger card in the name for each resident, noting important data such as resident name, unit number, source of payment (i.e., private pay, commercial long-term care insurance, state-funded Medicaid) and any pertinent routine and special service charges.

(3) At the end of each week and/or month, prepare a resident accounts receivable journal for each resident income. This would act as a check and balance on the ledger.

(4) Gather all charge slips for any special services for each resident that are not included in the monthly rent. Keep a special service revenue journal to act as a check and balance. Residential charge receipts should also be summarized and reviewed on a daily basis.

(5) At the end of each month, the totals in these resident A/R journals should be posted to the general ledger and the resident's ledger card. Invoices for residential rent and board, routine services, and special services are prepared and submitted to the responsible financial parties.

Handling Credits and Collections

The accumulation of residential accounts receivable that are not collected can cause a major concern and financial crisis for an assisted living facility. It might cause a severe cash flow problem that would require the facility to borrow funds at a high interest rate from a financial institution. For this particular reason, an effective credit and collection procedure must be implemented. A recommended procedure would be:

(1) Financial information as to the source of payment should be obtained from the resident upon acceptance to the assisted living facility. If third party payers are to pay for the resident's room & board and routine services, verify that these benefits are actually covered as soon as possible.

(2) Determine if the resident is eligible for state Medicaid or other governmental assistance (Medicare might pay for certain special services).

(3) Explain to the resident the types of services and their respective charges for them at the time of his/her/their acceptance. Have them sign off on a written letter of agreement to these services and charges.

(4) Furthermore, explain the assisted living facility's billing and collection policies. Have them sign off on their acceptance to a written document detailing this.

(5) Prepare an accounts receivable aging schedule for each resident. If a resident account is over a month old, send the resident or third party payer a notice of the past due account.

(6) Further stringent and harsher collection efforts must be made if a resident account is more than 60 days past due. Instead of a gentle collection notice, a more personalized collection letter by senior management may be sent to remind the resident of their past due bill. In this situation, a great deal of tact and diplomacy must also be made by senior management in collecting past due accounts. The assisted living facility must determine, as a matter of corporate policy, whether to utilize an outside collection agency or an attorney to collect unpaid resident bills.

ACCOUNT RECORDS

The assisted living facility must maintain under federal and state laws and regulations specific account records for internal management controls and outside governmental regulatory audits. The most important accounts deal with human resources and staffing since employees are the major cost items to the assisted living facility. The five essential account records are:

Payroll Records

Employee salaries/wages and benefits represent 50% to 60% of an assisted living facility's operating expenses. Therefore, adequate, accurate, and up-to-date payroll records are critical.

Time and Earnings (T&E) Records

A method of precise time keeping should be utilized for hourly and salaried full-time employees. In the past, a manual time clock and punch cards located at a central location were used to record employee hours worked. These days, electronic hand scanners at various locations are used at the assisted living facility to clock in employees as they arrive for work and clock out when they finish their work. Some assisted living facilities pay their lower salaried nonmanagement employees bi-weekly or weekly. Senior management and higher paid employees are usually paid monthly. The rationale in paying higher-level employees once per month is to conserve cash for the facility. For lower salaried employees, where a bi-weekly pay period is used, the following procedure is typically utilized:

(1) At the first day of the pay period, the employee's name and date of pay period is recorded on the employee T&E Record.
(2) The T&E Record is then given to the employee's supervisor.
(3) At the end of each day (sometimes at the end of each week) the employee or supervisor enters the number of hours the employee worked in each department.
(4) At the end of the pay period, the T&E record is returned to the accountant who calculates the employee hours worked, gross pay, and deductions.

Federal Payroll Taxes

Federal law requires that the employer make income tax withholdings from the employee's salaries and wages each pay period and remit these withholdings to the Internal Revenue Service. Most states and certain municipals also require employers to withhold income taxes. The federal, state, and city withholding rates are determined from tax tables furnished by federal and state governments. Employers must also withhold F.I.C.A. (Social Security— 6.2%) and Medicare (1.45%) taxes from employee wages. For both deductions, the amounts that are withheld are a percentage of the wages up to a certain amount. The employer must also match this amount paid by the employee to the Internal Revenue Service. Please note that President Barack Obama has proposed to eliminate the cap on F.I.C.A. and Medicare taxes for high wage earners to pay for health insurance reform.

Payroll Journal

The employee time and earnings record serves as a basis for entries into the payroll journal. Two separate accounts are maintained as follows: "Cash in Bank – General Checking" and "Cash in Bank – Payroll Checking." Accounts payable and wages/ salaries should not be paid out of the same account as listed above.

Once the total net payroll for the time period is determined from the payroll journal, a single check for the total net payroll is written out of the general account and place into the payroll checking account. When the payroll check clears at the bank, the payroll checking account should have a minimal balance. As an internal control, there should be different colored bank checks and different checking accounts (or have payroll and general checking from different banks) for the payroll checking and general checking accounts. Nowadays, most assisted living facilities payroll is handled electronically and the payment is automatically deposited into the employee's bank at each pay period.

Employee Personnel File

An individual hardcopy folder and/or electronic file (scanned documents) should be maintained for each employee. The employee file should contain all personnel data such as resume, reference checks, physical exam, drug testing results, salary increases, promotions, employee awards and reprimands, and payroll information (earnings records, W-2 form, citizenship verification, copy of social security card, etc.). Some older assisted living facilities post from manual cards to employee's individual earnings records. Others prepare payroll checks in duplicate and file the duplicate copy to the employee's personnel folder.

BUDGET PREPARATION AND EXECUTION

The survival of any business is in direct correlation to its financial solvency. One of the most important tools for sound financial management is the budget, a planning and management control device. The budget is defined as the projection of financial data for a specific period of time, that period of time typically measured as one year. A budget should not be completely restrictive and static. That is, after one or more administrative reviews of the budget throughout the year, it may be necessary to make several adjustments of the revenues and expenses, either upward or downward.

In managerial accounting, there are three basic kinds of budgets: operating, plant and equipment, and cash. Businesses that maintain all three are said to have comprehensive budgets.

The Operating Budget

The operating budget is a financial projection or forecast for 12 months of revenues, including the deductions from revenues and expenses. If the assisted living facility's budget encompasses the 12 months from January 1, 2010 to December 31, 2010, the budget would be for the calendar year. Otherwise, the assisted living facility's budget would be projected for the fiscal year (e.g., July 1, 2009 to June 30, 2010). In establishing the revenue budget, it is necessary to carefully review the monetary and statistical data concerning the income by each department in the assisted living facility. Trends in the data should be considered carefully, established, analyzed, and then forecasted for the upcoming year. It may be necessary to review anticipated changes in the internal operations of the assisted living facility which consists of the following items:

(a) Changes in the number of units (e.g., residents, employees).
(b) New services to be added (e.g., physical therapy, on-site pharmacy).
(c) New or amended corporate by-laws to be placed in effect.
(d) New or amended federal and/or state & local government regulations that are imposed on the assisted living facility.
(e) A realistic projection of resident days (the more days the more resident revenue for the assisted living facility).
(f) A projection of the volume of service in each department for the entire budget period (assist in forecasting departmental revenues such resident revenues, gift shop income, PT/OT special services and their contribution to overall company profitability).

To view revenues realistically, it is also necessary to budget deductions from resident revenue. The following budgetary steps will assist to project these deductions:

(a) Relate the past facility's experiences to the total budgeted resident service revenue.
(b) Take into consideration the above changes in relationship to applicable government laws or new resident acceptances that relate to fiscal matters.
(c) Develop a percentage of deductions to gross revenue that is classified by each type of deduction.

It is also important to establish a budget regarding expenses. Each year, senior management and each departmental administrator should sit down and discuss and review in detail the projected budget figures for expenses in their departments to remove unnecessary costs and/or over ordered cost items. The participation by departmental heads in this level of detailed fiscal planning would encourage acceptance of responsibility by each middle-level manager and help provide them with the sufficient information, and current up-to-date knowledge as to what is expected of his/her department. Steps in the budgeting expense process are:

(a) The use of a master human resources staffing plan that contains the proper titles of all employee positions in the assisted living facility.
(b) Prepare salary projections for 12-month time period for each department.
(c) Determine supplies for each department.

Plant and Equipment Budget (Capital Budget)

The following is a financial projection for 12 months of construction for new buildings costs, obtaining additional properties (e.g., adjacent land) and new or replacement equipment. The procedure for establishing a plant and equipment budget is as follows:

(a) Each departmental administrator should submit proposals to senior management for anticipated purchases of equipment in his/her department.
(b) The proposal should indicate what equipment is needed, why the equipment is needed, how many pieces are needed, the cost for each piece, any vendor discounts if applicable, and how the obtainment of the equipment would help either to generate additional revenues or minimize risks/liabilities.

Cash Budget

This reflects the projection of the cash balance at the beginning and end of each month. It forces senior management and even the company's Board of Directors to pay particular attention to the flow of cash in a given month. For example, the cash budget would help senior management anticipate the possible shortage of cash in the 6th and 7th months of a 12-month budget time period. The assisted living facility can then make plans to either borrow monies from a bank loan to supplement this cash shortfall, or make adjustments such as raising resident rates and/or ancillary fees, cutting expenses, postponing capital equipment purchases, new building capital construction or delayed repairs. Most cash receipts for the assisted living facility would come from the following sources:

Resident's Accounts Receivable

A review of residents' accounts receivable would provide senior management with a guide to the budgeting of cash receipts from residents or third party payers. For example, if past experience indicates that 85% of the current billings are collected in the month billed, 10% the following month, 4.9% the subsequent month and 0.1% sent to collections, senior management would have a good idea of the monthly cash flow to pay expenses.

Interest (Money Market Funds, CDs) and Dividends (Bonds, Stocks)

If the assisted living facility has excess cash for investment purposes, estimated income from these investments can then be based on information regarding the rate of interest, the probable yield of the investments and a determination of which month, quarter, or year end the dividends and interests are paid out. In addition, there may be potential capital gains from stock equities for the assisted living facility, but this cannot be predicted.

Bank Loans

Bank loans are budgeted for periods when the cash flow is low. If the assisted living facility needs to borrow monies from a bank, a cash budget would help. It is quite often that banks require the prospective borrower to submit a cash flow report as part of the loan application. This is to help the bank determine if the borrower can repay the loan within the time period specified Lastly, in setting up a cash budget, it is also important to project cash disbursements from employee payroll, tax payments, and other ongoing expenses (e.g., insurance payments, maintenance contracts, equipment rentals, etc.).

FINANCIAL RATIO ANALYSIS

Liquidity ratios help indicate an assisted living facility's ability to meet its short-term obligations and help financial analysts assess this aspect of a company's performance from the results of a financial model or financial statements.

There are two common liquidity ratios that a financial modeler is likely to encounter:

Current Ratio

Current assets are those assets that will be realized as cash within the next 12 months. Current liabilities are debts that are due for payment within the next 12 months. The current ratio gives an indication of whether the ALF will be able to pay its debts in the short term (i.e., the next 12 months). Clearly, this ratio should be as high as possible. A prudent ratio is 2:1

Current ratio = Current assets/Current liabilities

Quick Ratio

The quick ratio, or acid test, focuses on whether the assisted living facility could pay its debts in the very short-term (i.e., tomorrow, or next week). As company stock cannot always be sold quickly it is removed from the calculation of current assets. Again, this ratio should be as high as possible, and a prudent ratio is 1:1

Quick ratio = (Current assets less inventory)/Current liabilities

Both the current ratio and quick ratio give an indication of future solvency problems (i.e., whether the assisted living facility will be unable to pay its debts).

Performance Ratios in Financial Modeling

There are four common types of financial ratios that a good financial analyst will use to assess the performance of a business or project in building or interpreting the results of a financial model. These four performance ratios are by no means exhaustive, but provide a good indication on the most important ratios of which to be aware.

Return on Assets (ROA)

This ratio provides an indication of how effectively a business is utilizing its investments in assets:

ROA = Net income/Average assets

Operating Margin

A good high-level indicator of profitability and profit potential or "wiggle room" (robustness to competitive and external factors that may reduce profitability in the short-run):

Operating margin = EBIT/Sales

Asset Turnover

This ratio provides a further indication of the effectiveness of capital/asset utilization and relative "capital intensity" of a business:

$$\text{Asset turnover} = \text{Sales}/\text{Average assets}$$

Return on Equity (ROE)

This is also known as the return on average common equity or return on net worth, and measures the rate of return on the ownership interest (shareholders' equity) of the common stock owners. ROE measures a firm's efficiency at generating profits from every dollar of net assets, and shows how well a company uses investment dollars to generate earnings growth.

Working Capital Ratios in Financial Modeling

Working capital ratios demonstrate a company's efficiency at managing its resources, with particular reference to cash flow, and allows a good financial analyst to quickly and efficiently assess this aspect of the company's performance in a financial modeling project. Some typical working capital ratios that a financial analyst will come across include:

Days Inventory

This tells us the amount of time on average each unit of stock is in the shop/warehouse before being sold. Clearly, the shorter this length of time, the better.

$$\text{Days inventory} = (\text{Average inventory}/\text{Cost of goods sold}) \times 365 \text{ days}$$

Debtor Days

Days sales in receivables or debt collection period tells us the amount of time on average each debtor takes to settle their debt to the business. For the facility, clearly, the shorter this length of time, the better. A very large debtor collection period might indicate that the business may be unable to collect its debts.

$$\text{Debtor days} = (\text{Average accounts receivable}/\text{Sales}) \times 365 \text{ days}$$

Creditor Days

This refers to the days accounts payable or credit period, and tells us how long on average the business takes to pay its creditors. The longer the length of this time, the better. However, a very large credit period may indicate that the business does not have the cash to pay its debts.

Creditor days = (Average accounts payable/Cost of sales) × 365 days)

Solvency Ratios in Financial Modeling

Solvency ratios indicate the risk inherent in the assisted living facility as a result of its debt. A good financial analyst will use solvency ratios to keep tabs of the forecasts made in a financial modeling exercise on debt accumulation to ensure that they are realistic and prudent. A good financial analyst will also use solvency ratios to assess the debt profile of a company from its financial statements, and analyze whether the company needs to undergo debt restructuring exercises (such as mortgage refinancing, debt consolidation, etc). There are two common solvency ratios that a financial analyst is likely to come across when building a financial model.

Leverage Ratios

The leverage ratio, or gearing level, effectively measures the fixed debt payment commitment. Too high a gearing level can imply a high risk upon the cash flow of a public assisted living facility and its ability to pay dividends to shareholders.

Leverage = Debt/[Capital employed (i.e., equity + debt)]

Interest Cover

Measures the ability of an assisted living facility to pay interest out of profits. Most banks would expect the cover to exceed 1.5 times.

Interest cover = Profit before interest and tax/Loan interest expense

Limitations of Financial Ratios in Financial Modeling

While financial ratio analysis can provide us with important insight into a company's performance, a good financial analyst will be aware that there are some important limitations which should be noted when using financial ratios as an analytical tool in financial modeling. Limitations include:

- Ratio analysis is a retrospective, not prospective examination.
- Ratio analysis is based on accounting, not economic data.
- Ratios don't capture significant off-balance sheet items.

- Basic ratios can be manipulated through acceptable alterations of accounting policies (e.g., LIFO/FIFO).
- Financial statement accounts reflect historical cost, not necessarily current economic value.
- Cash flow measures have been proven to be more closely correlated with stock price movement that income based measures.

Table 9.10 illustrates how traditional accounting based profitability financial ratios often yield ambiguous results.

TABLE 9.10   Limitations of Financial Ratios in Financial Modeling

Issues	ROA	ROE	ROI	Profit Margin
Do not incorporate opportunity cost or risk	x	x	x	x
Often mislead managers to slash assets rather than invest	x	x	x	
Ignore cost of capital investments required to generate earnings		x		x
Difficult to compare with other opportunities when used in isolation	x	x	x	x
May be affected by financing decisions (e.g., tax implications of interest on debt, dividend policy)		x	x	

Notes: ROA = Return on Assets; ROE = Return on Equity; ROI = Return on Investments (Owner's Capital–Shareholder's Equity; Profit Margin–Operating Margin).

RISK MANAGEMENT

Some of the potential hazards in an assisted living facility relate to its employees. These hazards include injuries and illnesses suffered from helping residents, slipping and falling on wet floors while on the job, and having contact with residents with communicable diseases (e.g., tuberculosis, hepatitis). The federal government mandates that the assisted living facility (ALF) carry Workman's Compensation liability coverage and adhere to the applicable rules and regulations of the Occupational Standards of health and Safety Act. A second area of possible liability is with the residents, their guests and others (suppliers, repair & service personnel) who come onto the facility's grounds in order to legally conduct business.

In addition to required commercial building insurance, it is also important that the ALF have an operational safety plan (major disaster, fire, and earthquake), safety committee and periodic evacuation practice drills. Any facility accident and incident reports must be reviewed by senior management along with the safety committee on a regular basis to determine the causes, as well as to implement any remedial safety corrections. Furthermore, employee safety orientation and in-service training programs also must be schedule for all staff members to emphasize safety precautions regarding residents, guests, and outside visitors.

Commercial Insurance

The major risks that assisted living facilities typically face can be broken down into two categories:

(a) Those liabilities risks where the insured may be liable to others because of his/her own actions, or those of his/her staff members and invited guests and/or suppliers, outside contractors and business service agents; and,

(b) Those liabilities involving property loss risks where the insured may suffer loss or injury to property as a result of his/her own actions or the actions of others.

Liability Insurance

Most liability insurances are divided into two separate categories: bodily injury and property damage. The assisted living facility itself is also exposed to lawsuits for its own negligence and negligence of others. The most common liability insurance policy provides coverage only for amounts that the insured becomes legally obligated to pay that results from accidents and does not provide coverage for incidents that are not considered accidents (such as illness that is caused by repeated exposure to unsanitary conditions – hepatitis and tuberculosis). Other incidents for which the insured is legally obligated to pay that are not covered in a basic insurance policy, include: liabilities for which the insured is not obligated under negligence law until fault is proven and liabilities where the insured voluntarily admits fault. Expanded insurance coverage can be obtained on basic policies for an additional premium, and by substituting such words as "occurrence" for "caused by accident."

That is, Comprehensive General Liability and add-on insurance riders that would provide broader coverage can be obtained by the assisted-living facility to minimize its insurance risk. The assisted living facility should be aware of the following basic liability insurances available in the marketplace.

Owners and Corporate Board of Directors Liability Coverage

The basic policy insures against claims that result from ownership and operation of the facility. This is usually a scheduled policy in as much as it designates specific properties and risks assured against suit. The Comprehensive General Liability offers similar coverage via added optional insurance riders.

Workman's Compensation

All businesses are required by Federal/State law to cover any employees who may be injured while working on the job.

Professional Liability

Also often known as malpractice insurance, where the insured is covered under the areas of malpractice, error, negligence in rendering, or failure to render proper medical, nursing and other professional treatment (e.g., resident OT/PT therapies, resident drug regiment), this insurance does not cover the liability of employees working in the assisted living facility unless it is provided in a schedule within the insurance policy. In addition to paying insurance claimants, commercial liability insurance also provides a number of valuable services and benefits as follows:

Defense of Law Actions

The insurance company would defend in the insured's name all lawsuits or actions brought against the assisted living facility employees even if determined to be false or groundless. This insurance policy would pay all costs that include the investigation of the claim, in addition to procuring supporting witnesses and legal counsel. Furthermore, it also pays for bonds that may be required in appeal of any lawsuit, including bonds to release attachments.

Medical Payments Coverage

This is a rider that can be added to the liability policy for an additional premium. This rider would cover all reasonable medical, surgical, and funeral expenses incurred within 1 year of an accident to each person who sustains bodily injury, sickness, or disease caused by a workplace accident regardless of whether the insured is legally liable. Normally, without this rider, the insured or employees of the insured are not covered for these medical payments.

Property Insurance

The assisted living facility must also consider insurance against direct loss to its tangible properties (e.g., the assisted living facility's buildings, equipment, supplies). These insurances and coverage include:

Fire Insurance

Fire Insurance covers direct loss by fire and lighting. It also covers certain types of property damage (either insured separately or uninsured) caused by heavy smoke resulting from the fire. Smoke damage caused by defective heating devices is typically not covered by a basic Fire Insurance policy.

Extended Property Riders

Extended insurance coverage for other perils can be added to your basic Fire Insurance policy for additional premiums. The additional endorsements would insure against windstorm and hail (damage to the interior of a building and/or its contents resulting from water, rain, snow or dust is covered but the actual building must be damaged itself by the force of wind and hail as well), heating oil/natural gas explosions (excludes steam boiler usually), riot or civil disobedience (includes direct loss due to theft, looting, etc.), and aircraft crash (includes objects falling from airplane/helicopter or actual strike by airplane/helicopter).

Additional Extended Property Coverage Endorsement

The extended coverage must be written for the same amount as the basic fire policy, whereby not increasing the face amount of the insurance policy. These endorsements merely extend the coverage to include additional perils such as building collapse, explosion of steam or hot water boiler, vehicles owned or operated by the insured, falling trees, insect and rodent damage to building, equipment or supplies, glass breakage, vandalism and water damage, ice, snow, and freezing to facility property and equipment.

Other Property Insurance Coverage

Additional endorsements to the basic fire insurance policy or separate coverage that the assisted living facility might consider are earthquake insurance (especially in earthquake prone areas in California, Washington, and Oregon), federal flood insurance (especially located in cities close to major rivers in the mid-west like the Mississippi and Missouri Rivers), automobile insurance (that includes all risks of damage and collision of vehicles owned by the ALF), war and military conflicts, and steam boiler and machinery insurance (two types: narrow form that limits coverage to damage caused by explosion, cracking, bulging, etc. to the boiler alone, and broad form that covers all damage caused by explosion, etc. to the boiler and surrounding properties).

Consequential Loss Insurance

A successful assisted living facility must also consider the possibility of an indirect loss following destruction preventing the use of all of or certain parts of its facilities(s). Three examples of consequential loss insurance are as follows:

(a) Building Interruption Insurance

This provides a source of recovery for loss of resident income because of a reduction of business due to destruction or breakdown of the assisted living facility or part thereof.

(b) Extra Expense Insurance

This insurance covers the costs of operations associated with emergencies.

(c) Accounts Receivable Insurance

This insurance protects assisted living facility against physical destruction of the resident accounts receivable records. To determine the amount of coverage, beforehand, the insurer would perform an analysis of prior patterns of resident accounts receivable of the facility.

Theft Insurance

The assisted living facility should also review the need for theft insurance to protect itself. There are two broad categories of theft insurances as follows:

Burglary and Theft Insurance

Five various policies are: (1) *Open Stock Burglary policy* (insures against the loss by burglary of merchandise, furniture, fixtures, equipment and damage to the premises because of the burglar by all but the facility's employees or agents. It does not cover the loss of cash, securities, records, accounts); (2) *Mercantile Safe Burglary Policy* (covers loss of cash, securities, other property and damages that results from the burglary of the safe); (3) *Money and Securities Broad Form Policy* (comprehensive coverage for most mercantile risks that provides coverage for all risk for cash and securities); (4) *3D Policy* (protects the ALF against comprehensive employee dishonesty, records disappearance, and employee destruction of property and equipment); and (5) *Blanket Crime Policy* (similar to 3D policy, but provides a single fixed amount for all coverage – not open ended). There are also *Fidelity Bonds* that the assisted living facility can purchase which covers an employer against the loss of any kind of property (cash, securities, raw materials or merchandise, and equipment) that results from dishonest acts by its employees. Such bonds insure only the named individuals (usually senior management); others may cover all employees at the assisted living facility.

Multiple Peril Coverage

This type of coverage is sometimes called package policies, and combined into one policy from many different insurance policies. The advantage of the Multiple Peril Coverage is broader coverage, elimination of overlapping coverage and claims, and a lower cost. Some policies cover all risks while others only insure specified perils.

MOST COMMON ACCOUNTING TERMS AND DEFINITIONS

Accounting, financial analysis, and financial modeling are integrated disciplines of which any good financial analyst will be familiar. In particular, it important that a sound knowledge of fundamental accounting principles and accounting terms is had to ensure a common basis and language for understanding, interpreting, and analyzing financial statements and financial model results. Appendix A provides a useful list of the most common accounting terms that an assisted living accountant/analyst/ financial administrator may encounter.

CONCLUSIONS

This chapter has provided the reader with a comprehensive summary of information on financial management in assisted living facilities (ALFs). It is clear that knowledge about accounting systems, organization, financial reporting, department titles and staff, the use of accounting and financial software, standard accounting procedures, accounts records, budget preparation, financial ratio analysis, risk management and common accounting terms and definitions will help administrators and operators with efficient and effective management. In addition to management objectives, ALFs must also be concerned with fiscal objectives in order to have adequate funds to carry out the purposes and goals of the facility and meeting the needs of the residents.

REFERENCES

Brealey, R. A., & Myers, S. C. (1988). *Principles of corporate finance* (3rd ed.). New York, NY: McGraw-Hill Book Company.

Brigham, E. F., & Gapenski, L. C. (1987). *Intermediate financial management* (2nd ed.). Chicago, IL: The Dryden Press.

Crane, M. (2007). *How to run a senior living home: technology.* Forbes.com. Retrieved from http://www.forbes.com/2007/02/28/yardi-assisted-living-ent-manage-cx_mc_0228assisttech.html

Davidson, S., Stickney, C. P., & Weil, R. L. (1985). *Financial accounting – an introduction to concepts, methods, and uses* (4th ed.). Chicago, IL: The Dryden Press.

Weston, J. F., & Brigham, E. F. (1982). *Essentials of managerial finance* (6th ed.). Chicago, IL: The Dryden Press.

10

Legal Concepts and Issues in Assisted Living Facilities

With Contributing Author: Anthony Chicotel

LEARNING OBJECTIVES

Upon the completion of Chapter 10, the reader will be able to:

- *Comprehend liability in relation to the administration of assisted living facilities.*
- *Describe tort law in relation to personal injury lawsuits; negligence; corporate negligence; respondeat superior; governing body; elder abuse; and liability limits.*
- *Discuss the important elements of, and need for, contracts and admission agreements in assisted living facilities.*
- *Understand the procedures for evictions and state-ordered relocations; appeals process; and readmission following a hospital stay.*
- *Comprehend elder law in relation to estate planning including wills and trusts.*
- *Describe advance planning in relation to elder law with attention to financial and health care management.*
- *Discuss surrogate decision-making including powers of attorney, conservatorships, guardianships, and other forms of surrogacy.*

INTRODUCTION

Most assisted living owners and operators probably have a negative perception of legal issues. The law is often associated with burdensome regulations and costly lawsuits. However, the law can and should be an ally of assisted living providers. Laws and regulations that help establish an expected standard of care for residents can serve as helpful guides to owners and operators. Other laws clarify the relationship between facilities and their residents, ensuring that both parties understand their roles with respect to one another. Finally, the law enables residents to plan for their incapacity, particularly with regard to their health care and finances, which accommodates and directs their care and reduces a provider's burdens.

TORT LAW

Tort Law and Personal Injury Lawsuits

Tort law is the law governing people's relationships with one another as general members of a civil society. A "tort" is committed any time a person or a business violates a basic expectation of a civil relationship. Examples of torts include battery, slander, and medical malpractice. Tort law is different from contract or criminal law. Contract law governs relationships between the participating parties only. Criminal law is similar to tort law in that it governs individual conduct within society, but violations are addressed by society as a whole, operating as a prosecuting agency, instead of by the victim. The key elements to tort law are: 1) a civil wrong against a person or property 2) prosecuted by the victim or their representative. Many torts are addressed by courts as "personal injury" lawsuits.

Common Law, Statutes, and Regulations

The law comes from many different sources which can create confusion even for seasoned lawyers. When most people think of laws, they think of statutes. Statutes are laws passed by a legislative body and codified in writing for all citizens to read and follow. Statutes come from federal, state, and local governments and usually vary considerably.

Another form of law is regulations. Regulations are similar to statutes in that they are written and created at the federal, state, and local levels. However, regulations are not passed by legislatures but by government agencies operating within the executive branch of the government. Agencies that address assisted living are often called departments of health or departments of human services. Regulations do not have the same force as statutes, so if they conflict in any way, the statute prevails.

One last form of law is the common law. Common law comes from judges, often dating back hundreds of years to fill voids caused by a lack of statutes and regulations. Common law developed as courts considered cases and rendered decisions based on principles of general fairness. As more and more cases were decided, the law was refined and became more and more stable. The common law is particularly prominent in tort law involving negligence. While some tort law derives from statutes and regulations, it is predominantly grounded in common law.

P*ractice Tip*
Law comes from all three branches of the government. Statutes come from the legislature, regulations from the executive branch, and common law from the judicial branch.

Remedies

An important part of tort law is the remedies available to victims. There are many remedies available but they generally fall within one of two categories: monetary and equitable relief.

Monetary remedies are focused on compensation and making a victim whole. The money that is awarded to the victim is intended to return the victim to the position they were in prior to the commission of the tort. The computation of money damages begins with measuring the loss to the victim. For example, if the victim suffered a theft of $100, the perpetrator would be liable for $100. The victim is entitled to all reasonably foreseeable financial damages, including lost wages, medical expenses, and the replacement value of damaged property. These damages are often called "compensatories" as their purpose is to compensate victims for the harm they suffered.

Another form of monetary remedies is known as general damages, and is more difficult to precisely quantify. General damages cover an array of issues such as pain and suffering, loss of consortium, and loss of enjoyment. As these types of damages are not easily ascertainable, they are often controversial because they can lead to huge money awards based on mixed evidentiary support.

P*ractice Tip*
Elderly and disabled residents of assisted living facilities are often limited in recovering monetary damages because they often have very low incomes and do not suffer much in lost wages. In addition, they have shorter life expectancies which restrict the amount of compensable future damages.

Equitable relief is based on common law but is often supported by statutes as well. There are two main forms of equitable relief: injunctions and specific performance. Injunctions are court orders that typically prohibit a party from engaging in a particular action. Restraining orders are one well-known type of injunction. Specific performance is a court order requiring a party to complete its promises made in a contract. Orders for specific performance are rare.

Negligence

Negligence is perhaps the most significant tort for assisted living facilities. The key to negligence is neglect: a failure to live up to the applicable standard of care. Negligence does not require a failure to act; positive actions can constitute negligence. The key to determining negligence is whether the action or inaction at issue violated the suitable range of reasonably expected action or inaction. Over the past couple hundred years, common law has established four elements of a negligence claim:

1) The allegedly negligent party must have a duty of exercising due care to the victim;
2) There must have been a breach of the standard of care;
3) The breach must have caused actual harm to the victim; and
4) The harm must be measurable in damages.

Duty of Care

The most important element of negligence for assisted living facilities is the duty of care. By law, all assisted living facilities have important duties of care for their residents and even their visitors and family members. The critical issue is defining the standard of care that facilities owe their residents. The applicable standard generally comes from two legal sources: state laws and professional standards. State laws vary, but a close examination yields generally applicable standards nationwide.

Practice Tip

The laws regarding assisted living facilities are almost entirely state laws. There are virtually no federal laws. The only noteworthy mention of assisted-living facilities in federal law relates to the receipt of Supplemental Security Income ("SSI") by residents (42 U.S. Code § 1382). The law allows states to reduce SSI payments to assisted living facilities that do not meet quality of care standards. The statute has had no meaningful impact on care as SSI reductions would actually discourage providers from serving SSI recipients (Carlson, 1999). The paucity of federal law reveals a national policy to leave assisted living matters to the state control.

Required Services

The first applicable standard of care expressed by state laws is required services. Required services are those mandated by state law to be provided in any facility that engages in assisted living services. The services consistently required, regardless of the state, are shelter, food, supervision, and assistance with activities of daily living. Room and board are staples of assisted living but the most salient feature is the provision of living assistance. Most states delineate the types of living assistance to be provided. Vermont, for example, requires certain facilities to assist with "meals, dressing, movement, bathing, grooming, or other personal needs" (33 VT Statutes Annotated § 7102[1] [A]). North Carolina requires facilities to provide transportation for residents to "necessary resources and activities" (10A NC Admin. Code R. 13F.0906). Most state laws simply mandate facilities to provide oversight and assistance with the residents' personal care needs.

Care Plans

A second applicable standard for assisted living facilities in many state laws is the formulation and revision of resident care plans. Alabama requires a care plan that documents each resident's personal care needs and required services, updated whenever the resident's needs change, and reviewed by a physician at least annually (AL Admin. Code § 420-5-4-.05 [3][d]). Care plans in Indiana and South Carolina must be updated at least semi-annually and after any change of condition (410 IN Admin. Code § 16.2-5-2[a]; SC Code Regs. § 61-84-703[A]). Regardless of state law requirements, professional standards of care seem to mandate a fair amount of care planning for residents. The elements of good care planning include a careful assessment of resident needs, a plan for addressing those needs, and continuous revision.

While good care planning is definitely helpful to quality resident care, some providers may be wary of written documents that could ultimately be used against them in a lawsuit. If care planning is documented but not effectively implemented, it could serve as evidence of the care that was needed, but not provided. In that way, care planning becomes a liability. However, the advisable approach to care planning is not to abandon it, but to ensure that it is performed carefully and that implementation is routinely scrutinized. Most state laws and professional care standards require a fair amount of care planning and it cannot be shirked. Care planning should be viewed as an active, fluid process involving both assessment and implementation.

Staffing Levels

Another prominent care standard involves minimum staffing levels in assisted living facilities. New Mexico is a typical state, requiring at least one staff person be on duty at all times in facilities with 15 or fewer residents (7 NM Admin. Code § 8.2.18[A]). For facilities with more residents, the staffing requirements increase. Florida uses a weekly standard of total staffing hours closely correlated to the number of residents (58 FL Admin. Code Ann. R. 58A-5.019[4][a][1]). Other states, like Alabama, do not require a specific number of staff members but refer to "sufficient staff" necessary to provide "adequate care" to the residents (AL Admin. Code § 420-5-4-.04[1]). Regardless of whether the state sets a minimum number of staff or staffing hours, facilities should always carefully monitor staffing levels and the care needs of the residents. Attorneys who litigate cases against assisted living facilities will often target staffing levels whether or not staffing was an initially an issue. If an attorney can demonstrate that the staffing was inadequate to satisfy the care needs of the residents, compliance with state prescribed staffing levels will not immunize the facility from legal action.

Medication Management

Medication management is a universal issue for assisted living facilities; hence, the handling of medication is addressed by every state. Most states rely on an assumption that residents retain the mental capacity to give consent to the administration of medications, and the physical ability to take medications on their own. These states authorize facility employees to store and distribute medications to the hands of residents but usually prohibit actually placing the medication in the mouths of residents. The result is a fairly confusing process for medication administration where the law is inadequately matched to reality. Massachusetts provides for "self-administered medication management," limiting facility staff members to:

> "reminding residents to take medication, opening containers for residents, opening prepackaged medication for residents, reading the medication label to residents, observing residents while they take medication, checking the self-administered dosage against the label of the container, and reassuring residents that they have obtained and are taking the dosage as prescribed" (MA General Laws Ann. 19D §§ 1, 2[iv]).

Illinois and Ohio allow staff members to place medications into containers and then place the containers into the mouths of residents with physical impairments provided they are mentally alert (77 IL Admin. Code § 330.1520[c][2]; OH Revised Code Ann. § 3721.011[B][2][c]). Similarly, Alaska law allows staff to guide medication in a resident's hand to the resident's mouth (AK Stat. Ann. § 47.33.020[c][7]). With laws that allow such leniency in the "self-administration" of medication, drawing a clear line between permissible and prohibited medication management is challenging.

A few states have addressed the problematic distinction between self and assisted administration of medication by allowing nurses to designate or train staff members in medication issues (TX Health & Safety Code Ann. § 247.026[g]; 6 CO Code of Regs. § 1011-1, chapter XXIV). In these instances, staff members may operate in a nursing capacity, provided the legal requirements are satisfied.

The issue of medication management, like that of care planning, poses a potentially significant legal dilemma for assisted living facilities. In most states, where medication assistance is limited to helping with resident "self-administration," staff members must avoid conduct that is not expressly permitted. Residents with mental or physical incapacity therefore must have some ability to recognize medications and take them on their own. Facilities face liability concerns whenever a medication mistake is made, particularly when residents are overdosed. If a resident is incapable of self-administration as defined within their state, the facility better be able to explain how the resident nonetheless continued to receive medication. In states where nursing duties can be delegated, facilities have to ensure that all staff designations and training requirements are completely satisfied. If facilities employ nurses, they should carefully supervise the nursing performance, as the appropriate care standard may be higher than a customary assisted living standard.

Resident Falls

Risks of resident falls present another interesting dilemma to assisted living facilities that is often found when dealing with the legal issues of elderly people, or people with disabilities. On one side of the dilemma is resident autonomy, allowing residents to make their own decisions regarding risk and benefits, and choosing when and how they would like to walk or ambulate. On the other side of the dilemma is resident safety, which suggests that facility staff have a duty to prevent residents from falling. Falls, after all, can be a catastrophic event for residents, often leading to severe injuries and permanent declines in functioning or death.

Therefore, falls often lead to personal injury lawsuits against assisted living facilities. However, the only way to truly prevent falls is to restrain the resident. State laws usually prohibit restraining residents but do not set any care standards for preventing falls.

Common law standards do impose a duty to prevent falls on assisted living facilities. Resident care plans should assess a resident's fall risk and the staff should implement appropriate measures to limit that risk as much as possible, including assistance to and from the bathroom, consensual use of modest restraints such as wheelchair lap belts, and even facilitating the acquisition of ambulatory aids such as walkers, wheelchairs, or mobility carts. Facilities should carefully document its resident fall care plans and be sure to note residents' acceptance or refusal of recommended fall prevention techniques. In addition to resident-centered approaches, facilities should also be cognizant of simple environmental issues such as carpeting, grab bars, lighting, and spill cleanup. The law does not require that falls be prevented; it rather expects reasonable measures will be undertaken to minimize them at all times.

Aside from preventing falls, facilities should be sure to have a detailed post-fall procedure that, at a minimum, assesses the resident for a physician visit, documents the incident, and triggers additional care plan revision. Seemingly insignificant falls can cause significant latent injuries and even falls resulting in no injury at all can be evidence that more falls may be imminent. Post-fall procedures will be scrutinized by attorneys whenever a fall leads to significant injury.

Resident Wandering and Supervision

Preventing resident wandering is much like preventing falls in that it sometimes pits resident autonomy against resident safety, and state laws provide very little direction and cannot be relied upon as setting a specific standard of care. Again, as with falls, staff should be vigilant regarding resident wandering and care plan accordingly. The law requires that facilities allow residents to move freely about their environment and prevents the use of physical restraints barring an emergency medical situation. However, facilities are also expected to provide significant supervision to residents, particularly those with dementia, by ensuring they do not leave the facility unless they are supervised or have a safety plan in place. Facilities must be careful to balance the rights of residents to be free from restraints with the expectation that they will be supervised and safe. In terms of legal liability, residents who wander and suffer injury are likely more problematic than overuse of restraints. Nonetheless, liability can be incurred whenever a facility fails to properly balance the two competing interests.

Conclusion on Duty of Care

The standard of care means different things for assisted living facilities in different states. While certain national standards are discernible, state laws that specifically set forth minimal care standards are exceptionally important to facility owners and providers. Even in instances where there is no state statutory or regulatory guidance, facilities should be aware of common law standards set forth in case law, and understand that appreciably specific standards can exist outside of what is stated in state code books. The requisite standard of care is of paramount importance in assisted living and tort law liability.

Breach of Duty

Once the appropriate standard of care has been identified, the next step in assessing a facility's liability for negligence is determining whether or not the standard was breached. A breach is simply a failure to satisfy the duty of reasonable care. An old-time U.S. Appellate Court Judge, Learned Hand, devised a simple method for determining whether a breach of reasonable care had occurred by comparing the cost of an untaken precaution versus the expected benefit such precaution would have had. If the cost outweighs the potential benefit, there is no breach. Few states use the Learned Hand "formula" for determining breach of duty, but the efficiency of actions taken or not, does play a role in evaluating whether a breach has occurred. Providers should carefully document efforts made and costs considered whenever a resident's care needs are being evaluated.

Causation

The third element of a negligence claim is causation. The alleged injuries of the victim must have been caused, at least in part, by the breach of the duty of care that occurred. The perpetrator or the tort is only liable if the tort was the primary reason for the victim's damages. Causation is usually broken down into two elements: 1) factual causation and 2) legal causation.

Factual causation is concerned with whether the action or nonaction at issue caused the victim's damages. One rule of thumb for establishing factual causation is to use a "but-for" test: would the victim's damages have occurred but for the perpetrator's action or nonaction? If the answer is no, then factual causation likely exists.

Legal causation, also known as proximate causation, is concerned with the chain of events between the perpetrator's actions or nonactions and the damages at issue. The perpetrator is held liable for all of the reasonably expected consequences of negligence. If a subsequent act causes additional damages, the chain of causation is broken and the initial negligent actor is not liable for those additional damages.

Related to the causation issue in a negligence claim are the defenses of contributory and comparative negligence. Contributory negligence is a doctrine by which an alleged tortfeasor (a person who has committed, or allegedly committed, a tort) can avoid any liability for damages if the victim's own conduct contributed in any way to the causation of the damages. Contributory negligence is used in a handful of states, including Alabama, Maryland, North Carolina, and Virginia, as well as Washington, DC. Most states instead use a related concept of comparative negligence. Under comparative negligence, the alleged tortfeasor's liability is limited to the proportion to which their conduct caused the damages. If the tortfeasor's negligence was 75% responsible for the damages suffered, their liability is limited to 75%. Contributory and comparative negligence can be powerful tools in a lawsuit. Assisted living owners and providers should therefore have an even greater incentive to carefully document all instances where a resident's risk of injury was assessed and communicated to the resident or their legal decision maker.

Damages

The fourth and final element of a negligence claim is quantifying the damages. Damages are the amount of money the tortfeasor will owe for the negligence. Damages were briefly discussed in the review of remedies above. Compensatory damages are the money needed to make the victim "whole," including lost wages, medical expenses, replacement property, and pain and suffering. In addition to compensatories, many states allow for punitive damages, money that is not meant to compensate the victim, but rather to punish the tortfeasor to send a clear public message that such behavior will not be tolerated. Punitive damages are usually not available unless the tortfeasor has acted recklessly or intentionally; thus, negligence does not usually generate punitive damages. Some states, like California, allow for damages to be multiplied in cases where the victim is an elder or adult with disabilities to provide further protection to such populations.

Corporate Negligence

Corporate negligence is a relatively recent concept, holding corporate health care providers liable for negligence that occurs from a flawed system as opposed to a single identifiable incident. While corporate negligence is most often associated with hospitals, its principles can easily be extended to assisted living facilities. Corporate negligence assigns health care systems a duty to oversee the general quality of their care as provided by individual members whether they are "staff" or not. The system manager, in this case the facility owner or operator, is to remain alert for patterns of incompetent behavior and to address those issues in a timely manner. For assisted living facilities, corporate negligence may impose additional duties to carefully supervise staff members, and terminate those who provide inadequate care, as well as to constantly review its overall delivery of care and identify and address problem areas.

Governing Body

Assisted living facility owners must also be cognizant of potential personal liability for personal injury claims of residents. Owners or corporate directors may be liable under various legal theories including "piercing the corporate veil" and "governing body." If alleged resident injuries are the result of particularly egregious conduct that was known or should have been known by any reasonably diligent owner or director, they may be personally liable. As with corporate negligence, the issue is oversight of the entire care system at issue, especially the quality and performance of the direct care staff members. In health care settings, this oversight must be particularly focused as life or death outcomes may be at stake. The law presumes that owners and corporate directors are immune from liability and piercing corporate veils and governing body liability are rarely realized; however, corporate providers should be careful to exercise diligent oversight and must take action whenever they are informed of significant problems within an assisted living facility.

Respondeat Superior

Respondeat superior is a Latin term that means "let the master answer." For legal purposes, the doctrine of *respondeat superior* is used to hold employers liable for the actions of their employees. The liability in such situations is often called "vicarious" liability because the actual wrongdoing is performed by one person (the employee) but may be answered by another (the employer). Generally *respondeat superior* does not exist unless the employee was acting within the scope of employment at the time the alleged wrongful conduct occurred. If an employee that is not "on the clock" takes a resident to the movies and the resident chokes on some popcorn, the employer facility would not generally be liable. However, the resident or his family may allege the facility had inadequate policies regarding staff member outings with residents, or that the resident did not have capacity to decide about outings at all. The facility may be also be liable if it knew that this staff member was engaging in risky activities with residents after hours. Facilities can reduce their liability by having detailed policies governing the actions of its employees regarding all aspects of a resident's care. Some states have "strict liability" provisions whereby certain actions create liability for employers even if employees were acting outside of the scope of their employment.

Elder Abuse

Most states treat elders and disabled adults together as protected classes in abuse prevention statutes. For simplicity's sake, this chapter will use the term "elder abuse" to cover both elder and disabled adult abuse. Elder abuse is a special tort in some states, while in others it is merely a method of enhancing the penalties for conduct that is some other form of tort. For assisted living facilities, there are two concerns regarding elder abuse liability: one, perpetrating elder abuse, and two, failure to report elder abuse.

Elder abuse occurs in assisted living facilities. Often, the perpetrator is a staff member of the facility itself. Abuse can be overt and obvious, including the hitting or emotional harming of residents, but it also covers instances of neglect, where the facility's inaction is the problem. Assisted living providers are at particular risk of elder abuse tort actions because they have legally assumed the responsibility of caring for the elder; thus, any failure to provide reasonably expected care could be treated as both negligence and elder abuse. Most elder abuse statutes require that the neglect be significant, including reckless or intentional conduct, and more than simple negligence. Facility owners and operators can be liable for elder abuse perpetrated by their employees.

The second issue regarding elder abuse in assisted living facilities is compliance with mandatory reporting requirements. Every state has statutes that require certain professionals that are expected to regularly assist elders and disabled adults to report any suspected incidents of abuse or neglect to a state agency for investigation. The list of "mandated reporters" varies from state to state but usually includes law enforcement officers, nurses, and social workers. Assisted living facility staff members and administrators are often named mandated reporters (e.g., VA Code Ann. 63.2-1606[A][1]). States may issue civil fines to mandated reporters for failing to report suspected elder abuse, but failure to report could also subject the facility to tort litigation, particularly if proper reporting would have prevented potential harm from occurring.

Limiting Liability

MICRA caps. Many states have instituted laws to limit the liability of health care providers in personal injury lawsuits to counter what they perceived as the deleterious effects of excessive money judgments against them. California was the first state to address this issue when it passed the Medical Injury Compensation Reform Act ("MICRA") in 1975. MICRA placed a $250,000 limit on awards for noneconomic damages, the main target of which was pain and suffering. Many states have followed California's lead, including Florida, Maryland, Massachusetts, Michigan, Oregon, and Wisconsin, by also limiting the recovery of noneconomic damages in cases of medical malpractice. The application of MICRA caps for assisted living facilities depends on whether or not they are considered health care providers in their particular state.

Tort Reform

Tort reform is the name given to efforts that aim to reduce both the number of personal injury lawsuits filed, and the awards given to victorious claimants. Well-publicized cases of million dollar judgments for seemingly insignificant torts, such as the McDonald's coffee burning case (where a woman was awarded nearly three million dollars by a jury), have precipitated various movements for tort reform in states and in the federal government.

As previously discussed, one of the primary methods of tort reform is capping noneconomic damages. The Texas legislature recently passed a law, HB 4 (2003), imposing a $250,000 noneconomic damages cap that expressly includes actions against assisted living facilities. Several times in recent years, Congress has considered imposing damages caps nationwide, although without success. Another type of tort reform targets punitive damages, which can often far exceed the actual damages suffered by the victim. Several state courts and even the U.S. Supreme Court have weighed in on punitive damages, finding that the amount of punitive must bear some relation to the actual damages, often expressed as a ratio. For example, an award of punitive damages that is more than 10 times that of the actual damages may be considered unconstitutional. Other efforts have focused on limiting class action lawsuits and attorneys fees. One proposal, yet to be adopted in any state, is to create a "loser pays" system in which the loser of a lawsuit has to pay the attorney fees and court costs of the winning side. Such a proposal would likely dramatically reduce the number of lawsuits because the plaintiff would risk significant costs if the lawsuit ultimately fails.

Licensing Reports' Admissibility

Another issue concerning legal liability is the admissibility of reports generated by state licensing agencies during their investigations of complaints or during annual inspections. The reports, if admitted in court, could be influential with judges and juries as a definitive opinion on whether a facility was incompliance with state standards of care. The admissibility of these reports varies from state to state but the possibility should remind providers to be especially responsive to visits from licensing. Licensing reports not only publicly reflect on a facility's performance, they also serve as ammunition for savvy plaintiffs' lawyers.

CONTRACTS

The General Law of Contracts

For assisted living providers, contract law may be nearly as important as state laws that establish basic care standards. The contract between providers and residents establishes many of the rules that will govern their relationship. The contract, usually known as the admission agreement, is critically important.

Elements of a Valid Contract

Although there are differences among states regarding contract law, most share consistency in identifying the basic elements of a contract. The four most important elements of a valid contract are:

– Offer and acceptance;
– Consideration;
– Capacity;
– Writing.

The first element of a valid contract is offer and acceptance. An offer must be made by one party that is accepted, in full, by the other. An offer and acceptance do not need to be formal steps, one right after the other; rather they must simply reflect a "meeting of the minds." Both parties to the contract must have a mutual understanding of what is being agreed, and intend to be bound by it. A counter-offer made in response to an offer is not the same as acceptance and does not create a contract unless the counter-offer itself is accepted.

Practice Tip
The law regarding offer and acceptance should encourage assisted living facilities to scrutinize their marketing materials used to promote the sale of their services. Marketing materials are often considered by courts in lawsuits to convey promises that go beyond the legal standard of care. Marketing materials often describe services to be provided, creating expectations and becoming part of the offer that is implicitly extended to prospective residents.

The second element of a valid contract in many states is consideration. Consideration is a term for the exchange of something of value. In other words, a valid contract requires that each side give something up in the agreement. The value of the consideration can be minimal (i.e., one penny). Consideration can be particularly important for assisted living facilities, where relatives or other third parties often sign the admission agreement as financial guarantors. If consideration is required for a valid contract, third party agreements to undertake financial responsibility for the resident may be unenforceable. Third parties can claim that they did not receive anything of value in a resident admission agreement and thus have no obligation to pay for services provided to another person. Facilities should check with a local attorney if it uses a third party financial responsibility clause in its admission agreements.

The third element of a valid contract is capacity of the signing parties. This is a key issue in assisted living facilities where residents often have questionable capacity to make their own decisions. If a proposed agreement is signed by a person without capacity, it is unenforceable. Providers should demand that a legally authorized surrogate, along with the resident, sign an admission agreement if the resident has questionable capacity. Signing issues will be discussed further below.

The fourth element of a valid contract is that is be committed to writing. The law does not require that all contracts be in writing but all states have a "statute of frauds" that requires some types of agreements be in writing. Usually, contracts with duration of more than 1 year and those involving a fair amount of money ($500 or more in many states) must be in writing. Other states require that all leases involving residential use of property be in writing. Regardless of whether a written agreement is required or not, good practice dictates that providers reduce their agreements with residents to writing. Facilities should also ensure that all residents have a written agreement *prior to* move-in, because once a resident has moved in, they potentially receive the protection of landlord-tenant laws and might have a residency claim without having signed anything.

Unconscionability

Sometimes, a contract that meets all of the above elements is nonetheless legally unenforceable because it is considered unconscionable. Unconscionability is a concept of fairness whereby a contract that is manifestly unfair to one of the parties can be declared void by a court of law. Unconscionability has two elements that must be satisfied to void a contract: an absence of meaningful choice by one of the parties, and contract terms that are unreasonably favorable to the other party. The absence of meaningful choice is always a potential problem when both sides of a contract are perceived to have drastically unequal bargaining positions. The formation of a contract is supposed to be an interactive process. The more one side dictates the terms; the more likely an absence of choice is to be found.

Assisted living providers have to be extra watchful for unconscionability because residents are often elderly or disabled, need placement right away, do not have much time to meaningfully shop for alternatives, and receive written contracts that are offered on a take it or leave it basis. Facilities may enjoy disproportionate bargaining power, making the contract process one-dimensional. In order to avoid satisfying the first step of unconscionability, facilities should make extra efforts to engage residents in the bargaining process, allowing them to choose services from a menu of options and explaining their rights to seek services at other facilities.

*P**ractice Tip***
A "contract of adhesion" is a contract that is standardized and does not permit the signing party to alter the terms. Adhesion contracts usually include boilerplate language and are offered as take it or leave it agreements. Adhesion contracts are legal but sometimes receive special scrutiny by courts when considering a contract's unconscionability.

The second element of unconscionability is contract terms that are unreasonably favorable to one party. This element is difficult to satisfy as virtually every term of the contract must somehow favor one party. Contracts are not substantively unconscionable unless they are grossly unfair for one party.

A concept somewhat related to unconscionability is when contracts are unenforceable because they violate public policy. For example, a contract where someone agreed to be another person's slave would be void as against public policy. For assisted living facilities, contractual waivers of individual rights could be void for public policy. Such waivers are often found in mandatory arbitration agreements or other forms of limiting a person's right to sue that will be discussed below.

Two other fairness concepts that may void a contract are duress and undue influence. Duress allows a party to void a contract if entering into the agreement was involuntary due to an inordinate amount of pressure. Undue influence happens when a party enters into a contract because a person with extraordinary ability to persuade the party took advantage of their mental incapacity in forcing them to sign the agreement.

Admission Agreements

Admission agreements are the contractual foundation of the assisted living resident relationship. States have different laws about assisted living admissions, but nearly all limit the type of residents a facility may take. State laws also vary on what admission agreements must contain and what is prohibited.

> *P**ractice Tip***
> *Facilities are wise to require residents or their legal representatives to sign an admission agreement prior to admission. If a resident moves in before signing the agreement, they may refuse to sign the agreement or some of its provisions and the facility would likely have to use a burdensome eviction process to remove the resident. Admission agreement issues should be resolved before the resident moves in.*

Who May be Admitted

Nearly all states require that potential residents be formally assessed before they are admitted into an assisted living facility. New York law requires all residents have a health examination performed by a physician within 30 days prior to admission (NY Soc. Serv. Law § 461-c[7][a]). Other states, such as Ohio, Pennsylvania, and South Carolina require that residents be physically assessed at least annually (OH Admin. Code § 3701-17-58[D]; 62 PA Stat. § 1057.3[a][2]; SC Code Regs. R. 61-84-1101[A]). Maryland, New Mexico, and a few other states use standardized forms for assessments. Even if state law does not require an assessment, providers should require them. Aside from assisting in care planning and provision, such physician assessments can give providers a useful tool in identifying a resident's potential problems, as well as a baseline for judging changes in condition.

Prohibited Conditions and Waivers

State laws invariably limit the type of resident to whom assisted living facilities may provide care. Facilities must be especially careful in ensuring that residents with prohibited conditions are not admitted or allowed to remain if they have developed a prohibited condition. Admitting or keeping a resident with a prohibited condition can lead not only to trouble with the state licensing authority, but could impose significant liability exposure to a facility.

Generally, assisted living facilities are considered nonmedical facilities. Residents with significant medical or nursing needs usually cannot reside in assisted living. Prohibited conditions vary from state to state but some common conditions include:

- Intravenous therapy (IVs), including feeding tubes;
- Ventilator assisted breathing;
- Stage III or IV bed sores;
- Bed bound;
- Catheter care;
- Not oriented to person and place;
- Nonambulatory;
- Danger to self or others

Many states that list prohibited health conditions also include waivers allowing facilities to care for residents with the foregoing conditions or needs. Waivers are typically allowed to enable a current resident to remain in the facility despite the development of a serious medical condition. They are not often available for admitting new residents who already have such conditions. In waiver cases, the facility or resident must actively request permission from the state licensing agency. Waivers are more likely to be granted if the facility has made arrangements with suitable medical professionals to provide the necessary care at issue, usually in the form of a staff nurse or home health care providers. Some states allow facilities to obtain hospice waivers in order to care for terminally ill residents using a hospice care agency (e.g., CA Health and Safety Code § 1569.73[a]; FL Stat. Ann. § 429.26[9]).

Admission Agreement Elements

Like most other things, state laws vary on what may and may not be included in assisted living admission agreements. Many of the common requirements are listed below. Even if certain elements discussed below are not required in your state, providers should nonetheless consider including them to protect against possible contractual disputes.

Fees

Some states mandate that certain elements be included in assisted living admission agreements. Nearly all state laws on the subject require that the contracts carefully specify the nature and costs of the services that will be provided to the resident. The base monthly rate should be explicit, along with the costs of any additional services the facility provides. The listing of services and costs must often include details about the charging, usage, and refunding of pre-admission fees or resident deposits. Admission agreements should also detail third party payments if such payments are contemplated at the time of admission. Remember, from the previous discussion of contracts and consideration, the contract should specify the benefits that third parties receive by the provision of care and supervision of the resident. Third party payment agreements may be subject to special state laws, as in Maine, where an admission agreement "may not require or encourage anyone other than the [resident] to obligate himself/herself for the payment of the [resident's] expenses" (Code ME R. 10-144-113, § 3.25.3.7). Maine does allow voluntary third party payment agreements if they are raised by the third party and are written in a separate agreement.

The admission agreement might also need to explain exactly how rate increases will be conducted, stating how the amount of a rate increase will be calculated, and what the resident can expect to receive in terms of advance notice. Some states, like Alabama and Utah, require that all assisted living fee increases be preceded by at least 30 days' notice to the resident (AL Admin. Code § 420-5-4-.05[3][g][19]; UT Admin. Code R. 432-270-10[8][b]). Even if a state does not require advance notice specific to assisted living, general landlord-tenant laws almost always require notice in advance of an eviction, ranging from 3 to 60 days, depending on the circumstances. Providers should not ignore their state landlord-tenant laws as they may be more stringent than those for assisted living facilities. State law may also limit the circumstances under which fees can be increased. New York, for example, limits additional charges in some circumstances to when the facility has experienced "increased cost of maintenance and operation" (N.Y. Soc. Serv. Law § 461-c[2]).

Termination

Many states require that the grounds and procedures for termination of the admission agreement be specified in the contract. The termination provisions should explain the process for facility-initiated terminations as well as resident-initiated terminations. State landlord-tenant laws may be applicable. Facilities should also include a careful discussion of refunds and returns of pro-rated rent and security deposits. Some states, like California, also require the contract to detail what the resident can expect if the facility has to close (CA Health and Safety Code §§ 1569.884, 1569.886).

Negotiated Risk

In an effort to minimize liability to lawsuits and enforcement actions and to retain residents with exceptional care needs, some facilities are using "negotiated risk" agreements. Negotiated risk is a relatively new concept and is not universally understood. From a facility's perspective, negotiated risk allows residents to waive the provision of care to remain in the facility when their care needs would otherwise require they move out. The waiver allows residents to exercise their personal choice for their own level of care and accept the risks of doing so, just as they might acknowledge the inherent dangers of skiing or hang-gliding. Negotiated risk agreements are used for potentially problematic care issues such as resident falls, diabetes management and dietary needs, bed sores, and wandering.

Negotiated risk agreements are quite controversial and their legality is dubious. The agreements purport to allow the assisted living standard of care to be set by contract, foregoing state legal minimums in some cases. Courts may be skeptical of negotiated risk agreements and may void them as contrary to public policy. Voluntarily agreeing to inadequate care is inapposite to the nature of assisted living. People go to assisted living facilities to receive care and supervision. Negotiated risk agreements undercut this arrangement.

At this time, there is no definitive legal treatment of negotiated risk agreements. Some states, such as Illinois, have explicitly outlawed the use of negotiated risk that purports to waive a facility's regulatory requirements (77 IL Admin. Code § 295.2070[e]). Other states, like Kansas and Ohio, require facilities to document any necessary services the resident has refused, including an explanation of the potential risks of the refusal, and express acceptance by the resident (KN Admin. Regs. § 26-41-202[f]; OH Revised Code Ann. § 3721.012). Facilities can certainly consider using negotiated risk agreements, but they should be sure to avoid any agreements that attempt to lower the standard of care below state minimums. The agreements should also not be used to retain residents who have obvious care needs that necessitate greater care than is provided in assisted living. Even when the agreements are used appropriately, providers should be prepared for the possibility that negotiated risk may be found unenforceable by a local court.

Arbitration Clauses

Another controversial contract clause in admission agreements call for mandatory arbitration of legal disputes between the facility and residents. A mandatory arbitration clause holds that any legal dispute between the facility and the resident will be submitted to a private arbitrator instead of a court. Arbitration is a less formal and often, a less costly method of resolving legal disputes. Arbitration clauses are fairly standard in many service contracts but are subject to some important rules in assisted living.

No states currently prohibit the use of mandatory arbitration agreements in assisted living facility admission agreements, but some states do impose limitations on their use. Some states may require a mandatory arbitration agreement be presented as a separate document while others may require the agreement not be required as a condition of admission to the facility. The U.S. Supreme Court recently denied review to an Illinois Appeals Court opinion that the state's ban on mandatory arbitration in nursing homes was legal. Arbitration agreements are thus subject to outright prohibition. In fact, Congress is currently considering a bill that would prohibit the use of mandatory arbitration in any contract for long-term care services. The bill is Senate Bill number 2838 (2009), and entitled "The Fairness in Nursing Home Arbitration Act."

Practice Tip
In order to increase the enforceability of an arbitration agreement, facilities should use clear language explaining that residents are waiving their right to go to court. Facilities may also want to consider including the agreement to arbitrate in a document separate from the admission agreement, and make clear that the agreement is completely voluntary and not a condition of admission.

For facilities that use mandatory arbitration clauses, the signature of the resident or legal representative should be scrutinized. If the resident has any possible capacity problems, the facility should insist on the signature of a legal representative. Legal representatives may not have the ability to waive a person's right to sue by signing a mandatory arbitration agreement. For that reason, facilities should carefully review the document that conveys the representative's legal authority. Spouses and relatives typically do not have the authority to bind residents to arbitration without a document like a power of attorney, specifically authorizing them to do so.

Mobility Devices

A burgeoning problem with assisted living management is the control of resident mobility devices such as wheelchairs and electric scooters. Many facilities are imposing rules that limit the use of mobility devices, but these rules are likely illegal.

Several federal laws, such as the Americans with Disabilities Act, Fair Housing Act, and Section 504 of the Rehabilitation Act of 1973, all prohibit discrimination in housing on the basis of disability. State laws may also prohibit such discrimination. If a resident can demonstrate that he or she suffers from a disability and uses a mobility device to have equal use and enjoyment of the residence, the facility may not unilaterally prohibit the use of a mobility device.

Many facilities have issued rules that are intended to limit the use of mobility devices in their facilities. Some of these limiting rules require residents to:

- Obtain special permission to use a mobility device;
- Obtain a doctor's note or evaluation of safety;
- Obtain liability insurance to operate a mobility device;
- Sign a waiver releasing the provider of any liability for use of the device;
- Pass an operating test;
- Transfer into dining chairs during meals

Generally, rules that limit the use of mobility devices are not legal unless the devices truly pose a threat to others (i.e., violent acts committed towards/against others with a wheelchair). The reason for such a high standard is that the mobility device provides the resident with their only way of maintaining their independence.

The Fair Housing Act does not allow any discriminatory terms to be imposed on residents due to their disability. However, one federal court found that requiring liability insurance for the use of a mobility device could be legitimate if there is a valid business purpose, and the restrictions are narrowly tailored and based on individual inquiries of actual threats posed by specific individuals. A facility may not impose a blanket restriction however, based on a broad stereotype that assumes the general dangerousness of mobility devices. A facility also may not impose restrictions on device use if the resident does not pose a risk to anyone other than themselves.

Signing Authority

The issue of who signs the admission agreement is frequently overlooked to the detriment of assisted living facilities. Residents, regardless of their capacity, should always be asked to sign the admission agreement. If they do not sign the agreement and are later determined to have had capacity, the agreement may not be enforceable. There is no harm in asking a resident with questionable capacity to sign the agreement. The key is to make sure that a legally authorized surrogate also signs the agreement. Surrogates are discussed below. Facilities can rely on the signatures of relatives, but ideally would obtain the signature of a court-appointed guardian or agent under a power of attorney with the ability to contract for services on behalf of the resident.

For residents who have no capacity to sign an admission agreement and no surrogates, facilities should be exceptionally cautious. Such a resident may not be bound to pay rent, comply with facility rules, or other issues that are covered in an admission agreement. The plight of unrepresented residents is discussed at the end of this chapter.

Locked-Door Care

Facilities that use secured perimeters or locked doors to prevent residents from wandering, must be particularly careful about contracts and resident autonomy. In short, locking residents into a facility requires legal authority to do so. Legal authority must come from a court or other legally authorized surrogate. Generally, the law does not provide surrogates with the power to lock up the principal. Court-appointed guardians may have such power, but agents under powers of attorney usually do not. Even if a power of attorney purports to give the agent the ability to lock the principal in a facility, it may not be enforceable. This limitation on the power of surrogates is widely misunderstood and rarely talked about among providers, attorneys, and lawmakers. In California, state law explains that only conservators or residents themselves may sign for an admission to a locked-door facility (CA Health and Safety Code § 1569.698[f]). Despite this explicit policy, providers throughout the state permit agents or family members to sign locked-door admission agreements. Facilities that do so are rarely reprimanded but are risking significant liability for false imprisonment at some point in the future.

New Admission Agreements

Some facilities require residents sign new admission agreements following a temporary hospitalization, an ownership change, or some other change in residency. Providers are legally free to seek new admission agreements at any time provided the elements of a valid contract are satisfied. However, they should be careful about insisting. Many states limit the reasons for evicting a resident, and failing to sign a new admission agreement is not one of them. Providers should check with an attorney about their local laws before undertaking any punitive action against residents who refuse (or whose representatives refuse) to sign a new admission agreement following some change in residency.

EVICTIONS

Evicting residents from assisted living facilities is a common problem and is fraught with legal concerns. Almost all states have laws that limit the reasons for evicting a resident and prescribe a series of procedures that must be followed. In addition, general landlord-tenant laws may apply. Providers must be wary of many laws when pursuing an eviction of a resident.

Grounds for Eviction

Most states limit the grounds for legally evicting a resident. Some common reasons include:

– The resident's medical needs exceed what can be provided by the facility;
– The resident engages in conduct that is harmful to the resident, other residents, staff members, or facility property;
– The resident violates the terms of the admission agreement or other documented rules of the facility;
– The resident violates state or local law;
– The resident can no longer pay for services;
– The state or a physician orders the resident be transferred;
– The facility is closing;

Practice Tip
If a resident is unable to pay for services, the facility should warn the resident, in writing, that eviction proceedings may be commenced. The facility should NEVER withdraw services that jeopardize the health or welfare of the resident.

The mere satisfaction of one of the foregoing eviction reasons may not be sufficient to justify an eviction. Many state laws, regulations, and eviction oversight processes require that the proposed eviction be the absolute last resort for resolving the problem at hand. Therefore, facilities should carefully document every attempt at resolving the problem and efforts to avoid eviction. Physician assessments should be used whenever possible. The facility should give plenty of warning to a resident who is violating the admission agreement or rules. A resident who has failed to pay should be given ample advance notice of the impending consequences. The facility's documentation should not only illustrate that the resident eviction is merited but also that it has exhausted every other method for resolving the issue.

State-Ordered Relocations

Some states have a process by which residents can be ordered to move into a higher level of care by the assisted living oversight agency. In such situations, the state usually has a fairly detailed procedure by which it will ensure the resident is transferred; however, facilities may also be required to undertake action, especially if the resident refuses to leave. The state relocation orders are often directed to the facility not to the resident, so the facility may have the burden of physically sending the resident to another home. Providers should learn their local laws and have policies and procedures in place for dealing with state ordered relocations.

Eviction Procedures

Aside from having satisfied the reasons for eviction, facilities must also comply with any required procedures. The initial procedure for an eviction is usually providing legally sufficient notice to residents that they are being evicted. The notice usually has two components, the format and the timing. Some states prescribe one or the other or both.

The format of the notice is actually specified in a handful of states. New York is one such state (18 NY Compilation of Codes, Rules and Regs. § 487.5[f][3]). Even if the form of notice is not mandated, many states require that certain information be included. Many states require the proposed date and reasons for the eviction be set forth. California requires that details such as facts and witnesses be included so that the resident has a fair ability to oppose the proposed eviction (22 CA Code of Regs. § 87224[d]). Many states also require residents be told of their right to appeal the proposed eviction through a state appellate process.

The required timing of an eviction notice varies from state to state, but is generally 14 to 30 days. Some states, like Texas, allow the timing of the notice to be accelerated if there is an emergency situation requiring immediate action for the safety of the resident or other residents (TX Health and Safety Code § 247.065[b][P3]). While the law may allow for relatively short notice of eviction, providers should be aware that residents may have a difficult time finding alternative housing and should consider working closely with residents to assist them as best they can.

No states explicitly require an assisted living facility to help a resident find a new home. Facilities can proceed with evictions regardless of whether a resident has found new housing or not, but explicit legal requirements and pragmatic liability concerns are often separate notions. Any facility that evicts a resident with no place to go by casting them into the streets or to a homeless shelter with nothing but bus fare is risking significant legal problems if the resident suffers an adverse outcome. Again, facilities should be very careful about post-eviction plans of residents. Providers are certainly not responsible for finding the best alternative housing possible, but the level of resident dependence coupled with the care services universally offered in assisted living, seem to suggest that facilities do have more responsibility to evicted residents than standard landlords.

Appeals

A few states augment their eviction laws with an administrative appeal process to weigh the merits of proposed evictions that are opposed by residents. State processes are all that is available to residents as there is no federal constitutional right to a hearing to contest an eviction from an assisted living facility. Missouri, North Carolina, and Ohio have administrative hearing processes for resident appeals. Rhode Island also offers administrative hearings but prior to the eviction the facility is required to make "a good faith effort to counsel the resident if the resident shows indications of no longer meeting residence criteria, or if service with a termination notice is anticipated" (RI Gen. Laws § 23-17.4-16[a][2][xviii][E]). New Jersey and Utah specify methods for appeal but they are most likely not very meaningful. New Jersey allows individual facilities to establish their own appeal procedures and directs residents to appeal a proposed eviction to the facility administrator (8 NJ Admin. Code § 8:36-4.1[a][40]). Utah limits residents to an informal conference with facility representatives (UT Admin. Code R. 432-270-11[5]). Appeals decided by facility administrators or staff are doubtlessly difficult for residents to win.

Landlord-Tenant Requirements

Beside laws that are specific to assisted living eviction procedures, facility operators may have to be watchful of landlord-tenant laws as well. Landlord-tenant laws do not typically make explicit exemptions for assisted living facilities. Therefore, an argument can be made that landlord-tenant laws apply to facilities. Wisconsin assisted living laws use the term "tenant" to refer to residents while Iowa law explicitly applies the state's landlord-tenant law to assisted living (WI Admin. Code § DHS 89.24; IA Admin. Code R. 321-25.42[231C]).

State landlord-tenant laws and even local ordinances may limit the reasons for discharge to a small number of "just cause" reasons that are more narrow than those found in assisted living laws. The landlord-tenant laws may also mandate additional procedures for evicting residents, prescribing more information that must be in the notice and longer periods of time for providing it.

Even if general landlord-tenant laws do not apply to assisted living facilities in a particular state, evicting residents almost certainly requires a court order if the resident refuses to leave past the period of time provided in the notice. Physically removing a resident is patently illegal in all circumstances, unless a court order has been obtained and is executed by an authorized law enforcement representative. If residents hold over past the times in their eviction notice and administrative appeals have been exhausted, providers should seek the counsel of an attorney to learn about landlord-tenant evictions. The judges involved may be unfamiliar with assisted living facilities and the laws governing their operations.

Housing Discrimination Laws

Resident evictions may also be subject to federal and state housing antidiscrimination laws. Such housing laws may be unfamiliar to the average provider but recent academic focus has been placed on evictions as a form of disability-based discrimination. Many of the legal theories involved are untested, but there is some likelihood that future evictions may be scrutinized for discrimination. If a facility allows a resident with a prohibited health condition to stay by obtaining a waiver, it may have some explaining to do if it chooses not to seek a waiver for the next resident with that condition. Federal and state disability discrimination and housing law may preclude assisted living facilities from refusing a resident's admission based on a disability. In such a case, the resident may elect to file a lawsuit seeking an order to compel admission, or may file a complaint with the federal Department of Housing and Urban Development or a state housing agency.

Readmission Following a Hospital Stay

Facilities frequently contemplate resident evictions after a resident has been hospitalized. Hospitalizations often indicate a significant change of condition in a resident that may necessitate additional care that either the resident cannot afford or the facility cannot provide. Medically clearing a hospitalized resident to leave the hospital does not necessarily mean that the resident's needs may be managed in assisted living. A facility's reaction in such situations may be to refuse to readmit the resident until their condition has improved. State laws however, usually do not permit facilities to lock residents out of their homes, regardless of whether they have been hospitalized or not. A few states permit quick evictions in emergency situations, but even those states may require advance notice be provided to those residents, and they may have legal rights to appeal the move. In addition, a state's landlord-tenant laws likely strongly discourage landlords from locking residents out.

Returning residents pose a legal dilemma for facilities. On one side, the law usually directs facilities to allow residents to return to their home at the time of their choosing. Landlords simply cannot lock tenants out of their homes. On the other side however, facilities have a limited range of services that may not meet the care needs of a resident returning from a hospital. If a facility were to accept the return of such a resident, it risks liability if the resident suffers neglect or other form of harm. One possible compromise is to allow the resident to return to the facility, engage the legal eviction process immediately, and write a letter to the resident or their representative explaining the facility's reservations in detail. That way, the facility has complied with the law while also undertaking everything it can do to warn the resident of the risks of returning.

ESTATE PLANNING

Estate planning means different things to different people, but it always includes advance planning for the disposition of a person's property at the time of their death. Estate planning can be accomplished in a few different ways: through wills, trusts, or by operation of law in the absence of any formal documents.

Wills

Wills are written documents that specify the division of a person's property at the time of their death. The formalities of wills varies from state to state but usually require the maker of the will (the testator) to sign the document in front of witnesses and make a formal declaration that the document is intended to be a last will and testament. Wills may also include the testator's wishes regarding the disposition of their remains and a designation of an executor, the person(s) in charge of ultimately distributing the testator's property according to the division directed in the will.

> **P**ractice Tip
> *In most states, when a person dies without having executed an estate planning document, the distribution of their property is governed by state law. This process is known as "intestate succession." Intestate succession usually distributes property to spouses and close relatives first, and then moves out to more distant relatives. The beneficiary of last resort, in the absence of any family, is usually the state itself.*

As an estate planning device, wills have several advantages, but also a couple of important disadvantages. One, they are well known among all people as perhaps the primary method for distributing property after death. Two, they are relatively easy to draft and execute, often costing modest amounts for preparation by an attorney, and can even be done using a computer program, or simple form found on an internet web site. Another advantage to wills is that they are relatively easy to change or terminate, as long as the testator retains the mental capacity to do so. The only disadvantages of wills is that they do not provide any mechanism for handling an estate prior to the testator's death, even if they become incapacitated, and they do not help an estate avoid probate. Probate is the generic name for the process by which the distribution of an estate via will is supervised by a court. Each state is different, but states often require that estates of a certain size ($100,000 or more in California) require court supervision of the property distribution to ensure no fraud occurs. The probate process is often cumbersome and costly, reducing the value of an estate by up to 10% after paying state fees and court costs.

Trusts

Trusts are another form of written estate planning. Much like wills, trusts allow the person creating the trust (trustor) to direct the distribution of their property at the time of their death. A trust is a legal entity, apart from the trustor, so only property that is actually placed in the trust is distributed at the time of the trustor's death. The trustor's valuable property, such as houses, cars, and large financial accounts must be formally re-titled into the name of the trust. While the trustor is alive, the property in the trust is usually at their disposal just as if it were not in a trust. At the time of the trustor's death however, the trust terminates, and the property is distributed to beneficiaries as it would be in a will.

The primary advantage of a trust is that it usually allows the property in trust to avoid the state's probate process. Since the property in the trust does not technically belong to the trustor at the time of death, the trustor's "countable" property is below the probate threshold. Another significant advantage of trusts is that they almost always include a financial management component, whereby the property in trust can be managed by a substitute "trustee" if the trustor ever becomes incapacitated. The disadvantage of trusts is that they are often fairly complicated - even simple trusts run over 20 pages - and thus require an attorney's assistance, which can be costly. Trusts' complexity also increases the difficulty of amending or terminating the documents.

> **P**ractice Tip
> *Trusts fall into one of two categories: irrevocable or revocable trusts. Irrevocable trusts are permanent and cannot be changed once they are executed. Irrevocable trusts are often created for tax purposes or to exert control over property after the trustor's death. Setting up a college fund for a grandchild is a popular goal of irrevocable trusts, for example. Revocable trusts, as their name suggests, may be altered or terminated by the trustor at any time as long as they retain capacity. Because revocable trusts may be changed as long as the trustor is alive, they are often called "living" trusts.*

Totten Trusts

Totten trusts are an older name for an arrangement where a particular account is paid to a beneficiary at the time of death of the original owner. Such arrangements are also called payable on death ("POD") or transferrable on death ("TOD") accounts, and supersedes a contrary designation in a will or trust. POD or TOD accounts are not included in a person's probate estate and can be a simple method for estate planning.

Rep Payee

For incapacitated beneficiaries of Social Security or SSI benefits, a representative payee or "rep payee" may be appointed to manage the money that is paid out each month. State laws do not prohibit assisted living providers from becoming rep payees but facilities should be cautioned against such an appointment. Providers acting as rep payees create an obvious financial conflict of interest. Many states have local agencies that will act as rep payees for incapacitated beneficiaries for free or for a minimal cost.

Providers as Beneficiaries or Executors

Assisted living facilities should be aware that the law frowns on providers acting as beneficiaries in wills and trusts. Most states do not expressly prohibit providers as beneficiaries or executors, but all states do consider "undue influence" when the validity of a will or trust is contested. Providers usually have a relationship of limited duration but exceptional intensity with residents. If providers are named as beneficiaries in a resident's will or trust the presumption may be that the designation must be the product of undue influence exerted on the testator. Providers should be particularly wary of being named or having staff named in wills or trusts, particularly if the resident's family members do not know that such a designation has been made. Providers may want to consider personnel policies that prohibit staff from being named as beneficiaries, as well as discussing such matters with residents at the time of admission.

ADVANCE PLANNING

Aside from estate planning, people may also engage in other forms of advance planning that allows them to account for the management of their estates or health care while they are alive but incapacitated. There are many methods for creating such advance planning, and they are quite important to residents of assisted living facilities.

Trusts

As previously mentioned, trusts almost always include estate management provisions that allow a substitute trustee to handle all property that is in the trust if the trustor loses the capacity to do so. Property that is not in the trust may only be managed by a substitute decision maker if there are other forms of estate management in place.

Powers of Attorney

Powers of attorney are documents that designate a substitute financial decision maker (agent) to serve if the creator of the power of attorney (principal) loses the capacity to do so. Powers of attorney must be in writing, signed by the principal, and witnessed or notarized. Powers of attorney can be very broad or extremely limited; the breadth of the document can be tailored according to the principal's needs. The power that can be granted ranges from control over financial accounts and insurance policies, to retirement and government benefits, lawsuits, and real property. Usually, the principal may grant or withhold powers from a menu of options.

The agent's ability to manage the various granted powers usually do not begin until the principal loses capacity. In these circumstances, the power of attorney is said to be "springing" because the powers are dormant at the time of execution and then "spring" into effect if capacity is lost. The loss of capacity is typically determined as specified in the power of attorney form, but usually requires a doctor to state the principal has lost capacity to manage their financial affairs. Other power of attorney forms become effective immediately, as soon as the principal signs them. These forms are more risky to the principal because it allows the agent to immediately begin handling their financial affairs, with or without the principal's knowledge.

Practice Tip

Powers of attorney are often called "durable" powers of attorney. Long ago, powers of attorney had very limited usage and would expire at the time a person lost capacity to manage their affairs. Now, powers of attorney are completed specifically to cover periods of incapacity. For that reason, the powers granted continue despite incapacity, making the form durable.

Providers of assisted living facilities should be wary of acting as agents under a power of attorney. Oregon for example, explicitly prohibits any facility staff members from acting as a resident's guardian, trustee, or agent (OR Admin.Code § 411-054-0027[2]). Other states' laws may not prohibit such a relationship, but it could create substantial conflicts of interest that subject the facility to allegations of fraud, undue influence, or elder abuse.

Joint Ownership

Another method of providing for financial management is adding a joint owner to property or a financial account. This method, less formal than a power of attorney, allows the joint owner to undertake property management. However, joint owners have full access to the property and are not bound to exercise fiduciary responsibility, meaning they may sell, withdraw, or spend any funds just as any owner would. For that reason, joint ownership is a risky form of advance planning, and not recommended in most situations.

Health Care Planning and Decision Making

Informed Consent

Any understanding of health care decision making begins with the legal and ethical principle of informed consent. Informed consent doctrine holds that every person has the right to determine what health care treatment they receive or not. Unsurprisingly, there are only two elements of informed consent: 1) information provided to the patients, and 2) consent. The right to give or withhold informed consent is grounded in constitutional principles of privacy and self-determination. If the patient does not have capacity to make health care decisions, state laws allow surrogate decision makers to provide or withhold consent. When a patient lacks capacity and a surrogate decision maker, state laws vary on how informed consent requirements are satisfied.

The information necessary to obtain informed consent varies from state to state, but prominent state law cases have set a functional baseline. Before consent can be considered "informed" the health care provider must tell the patient or surrogate decision maker the:

1) Diagnosis;
2) Nature and purpose of the proposed treatment and the desired outcome;
3) Risks and benefits of the proposed treatment;
4) Alternative treatments and their relative benefits and risks (including the likely results of doing nothing)

Right to Refuse Treatment

A corollary to the right to informed consent is the right to withhold consent, or the right to refuse proposed treatment. The right to refuse proposed treatment is extensive, recognized by the U.S. Supreme Court to include the ability to refuse life-sustaining treatment. If the patient does not have capacity, surrogates may generally refuse treatment, although the refusal of life support sometimes requires procedural safeguards be satisfied. Patients, or their surrogates, may also refuse proposed medications at any time and may refuse placement in long-term care facilities, including assisted living. Treatment and placements may be forcibly applied at times, although the circumstances are rare and court intervention is almost always required.

One legal issue that is often intertwined with a patient's right to refuse treatment is physician-assisted suicide. Active measures undertaken by a patient or physician to end a life (i.e., euthanasia) is treated much differently under the law than the withdrawal of life-sustaining treatment. The U.S. Supreme Court has addressed physician-assisted suicide, and held that a state law ban was constitutional. In doing so, the Court found that the right to assisted suicide is neither fundamental nor traditional. Since that case, only two states, Oregon and Washington, have legally authorized physician-assisted suicide. Both states use a highly detailed process for limiting suicides to people who are terminally ill and have decision making capacity.

Advance Directives

All states provide legal mechanisms by which people can express their wishes regarding health care treatments in advance. These efforts were reinforced by Congress when it passed the Patient Self-Determination Act of 1990. The idea of an advance directive is to allow any adult to declare their preferences regarding certain health care treatments, particularly regarding the provision of artificial life support, to guide health care decisions if the person ever becomes unable to make decisions. Advance directive laws were in direct response to well-publicized medical cases where young people were victims of terrible accidents that left them in persistent vegetative states. In these cases, courts were asked to authorize the withdrawal of artificial life support, often receiving great resistance from religious groups and state officials. In an effort to avoid such controversy, state lawmakers adopted advance directives to clear up confusion about the decision making preferences of the person lacking capacity and to allow them to exercise their constitutional right to refuse treatment in advance.

Every state authorizes advance directives by using a written form. Some states have the forms written into the law, other states simply list some requirements and let lawyers or health care providers draft the forms. The forms almost always include an expression of preferences regarding the provision of artificial life support in situations where the principal is in a persistent vegetative state, or has a terminal condition that is likely to result in their death in a short period of time. Some forms allow the principal to state other preferences, including anatomical gifts, placement in a long-term care facility, and disposition of remains. The forms must be signed by the principal and often have very specific witnessing requirements. Assisted living providers should learn the basic requirements for advance directives in their states and consider stocking some forms for residents to execute while residing in their facilities. Advance directives can make a critical difference in health care provision, particularly for elderly people, yet they remain largely underutilized.

Practice Tip
Advance directives are often called "living wills" which can be confusing to people who have also heard of wills and living trusts. A living will is an advance directive, limited to advance health care decision making. Wills and living trusts, on the other hand, deal exclusively with property, primarily to designate a distribution of property at the time of death. Living wills deal exclusively with health care and have nothing to do with property.

Other Forms of Advance Health Care Planning

Besides advance directives or living wills, many states allow people to designate their health care preferences in advance in other formats, often after a person has been diagnosed with a terminal condition. Physician orders regarding life-sustaining treatment ("POLST") are methods for a doctor and patient to address specific types of life-sustaining care, including the administration of CPR, artificial nutrition and hydration, and ventilators. A similar document, known as a "do not resuscitate order" ("DNR"), also allows advance declarations about life-sustaining treatment, although they tend to be more narrow in scope than POLSTs.

Whenever a person has failed to make advance written expressions of their wishes regarding health care, courts will nonetheless allow evidence of a person's verbal expressions in cases to determine whether treatment should be initiated or terminated. Even seemingly unimportant conversations about artificial life support can serve as evidence to assist a court in deciding what a currently incapacitated person would want in their current situation.

SURROGATE DECISION-MAKING

With medical science continually improving, the ability to preserve life even after a person has lost decision making capacity; the need for surrogate decision makers is increasing. States have devised several methods for allowing surrogates to make health care decisions for incapacitated people.

Powers of Attorney

Much like financial powers of attorney, state laws enable surrogate decision makers (agents) to handle health care whenever a person loses the capacity to do so. The designation of the agent must be performed in writing on a document that must be signed by the principal and comply with witnessing requirements. The principal may designate a surrogate and substitute surrogates in case the first person cannot serve. Health care powers of attorney are often combined with advance directive forms so that an agent is designated and instructed on the principal's wishes regarding specific health care treatments. The extent of the agent's authority over the principal's health care is as broad or limited as the document states.

Guardianships and Conservatorships

For people who have not named an agent in advance, the courts can be asked to name a surrogate decision maker. This process is known as guardianship in most states, conservatorship in California. Petitioning for guardianship is often a complicated and time-consuming process, engaging piles of paperwork, attorneys, and court hearings. Once a guardianship is awarded, many states require constant court reviews. Since the process is so burdensome, many people treat it as a last resort only, to be used only after every other form of surrogate decision making has been exhausted. If a person in need of guardianship does not have a relative or other person willing to act as guardian, states have public guardians whose job is to act as guardian in such cases.

Guardianship law was designed mainly to name surrogates for people who did not nominate a surrogate in advance of losing capacity. Since that time, some states have created new laws that permit family and others to circumvent guardianship. These far less formal devices are legal when state law has expressly permitted them; however, many states have not addressed informal surrogacy. In these states, guardianship is still legally necessary. In reality however, illegal surrogates are often allowed to make health care decisions for a person who has allegedly lost capacity.

Some states have created a formal mechanism for health care decision-making under court supervision that does not require the appointment of a guardian. These methods are used to make a one-time health care decision and thus do not require the same number of procedures that guardianship does. This alternative court process is often used to make critical health care decisions regarding such things as surgery and the withdrawal of artificial life support when the proposed patient has not made an advance directive.

Informal Forms of Surrogacy

A few forward-looking states have passed laws allowing people to designate health care surrogates in advance without having to execute a written document. These oral surrogacy designations must usually be made to a health care provider who is instructed to document the designation. The oral designation may be of limited duration and scope but is a practical alternative in an emergency situation.

Another informal method for assigning health care surrogacy status is based on simply having a close relationship with the person who has lost capacity. Most states allow spouses and domestic partners, by mere existence of their relationship, to act as surrogates when one has not been designated formally. These states also often include family members as informal surrogates if the person who has lost capacity has no spouse or partner.

Unrepresented Residents

One national study estimated that 3 to 4% of nursing home residents have lost capacity, have no formal or informal surrogates, and have not executed any advance directive (Karp & Wood, 2003). These residents are sometimes called "unrepresented residents." Assisted living facilities are also sites where unrepresented residents can be found. The provision of health care to such residents is nearly impossible to figure legally in most states as their laws are silent regarding an applicable informed consent process. Iowa, New York, and Texas have state-authorized decision making committees to provide informed consent for unrepresented people. These states are the exception however, as most states are left with a completely unregulated process by which health care providers are left to their own internal policies and procedures or seeking the assistance of the local public guardian.

> **P**ractice Tip
>
> *Careful assisted living facilities will not have unrepresented residents because they will require someone with legal authority to sign the admission agreement. Providers should not admit any residents who have neither capacity to sign an admission agreement or a legally authorized surrogate. Providers cannot contract with unrepresented residents.*

Assisted living facilities should adamantly avoid acting as health care surrogates for their unrepresented residents. The law is clear that informed consent is required before any health care can be provided. Most states have a hierarchy of potential surrogates to provide consent if a person has lost mental capacity. If a resident does not have capacity or a surrogate, no consent can be legally given and any provider who does so may be guilty of battery, false imprisonment, or other crimes and torts. The local public guardian should be engaged for unrepresented residents.

Practice Tip

A recent study performed in San Francisco revealed that informed consent laws are often violated for unrepresented patients of health care services. (White, 2007). Doctors routinely make health care decisions unilaterally for their unrepresented patients despite state law and professional guidelines requiring much more process. And these decisions have fatal consequences: one-third of the studied physicians have withdrawn life support for at least one unrepresented patient. In the study, 37 unrepresented patients required life support decisions. For 30 of the 37 patients, physicians and other direct care providers made the life support decisions without formal court or even internal hospital review. In some cases, the providers did not even follow their own hospital's internal policies. Hospital policies provide guidelines designed by organizations such as the American Medical Association, and state laws were not followed despite a supposed belief by physicians that they are in legal jeopardy when they make life support decisions for unrepresented patients. Any concern about legal liability was not enough to dissuade physicians from ignoring state law and recommended best practices.

CONCLUSIONS

This chapter has provided the reader with a comprehensive overview of legal concepts and issues pertaining to assisted living facilities. It is evident that elder law and liability are important concerns for assisted-living administrators. This chapter illustrates the need for assisted living administrators to be well informed about tort law; contracts; estate planning, advance planning, and surrogate decision-making. It is important to be mindful that the law can, and should, be an ally of assisted living administrators in their pursuit to address the concerns and needs of both residents and staff.

REFERENCES

Carlson, E. (1999). *Long-term care advocacy*. New York: Mathew Bender & Co.
Carlson, E. (2005). *Critical issues in assisted living: Who's in, who's out and who's providing the care*. Washington, DC: National Senior Citizen's Law Center. Retrieved from http://www.assistedlivingconsumers.org/state-specific-information/State%20Summaries%20-%20NSCLC.pdf
Karp, N., & Wood, E. (2003). *Incapacitated and alone: Healthcare decision making for unbefriended older people*. Washington, DC: ABA Commission on Law and Aging.
Mollica, R. (2006). *Residential care and assisted living: State oversight practices and state information available to consumers* (AHRQ Publication No. 06-M051-EF).
Polzer, K. (2009). *Assisted living state regulatory review 2009*. Washington, DC: National Center for Assisted Living. Retrieved from http://www.ahcancal.org/ncal/resources/Documents/2009_reg_review.pdf
White, D., et al. (2007). Life support for patients without a surrogate decision maker: Who decides? *Annals of Internal Medicine, 147*(1), 34–41.

CHAPTER **11**

Accessibility, Fire Safety, and Disaster Preparedness

Learning Objectives

Upon the completion of Chapter 11, the reader will be able to:

- *Describe selected federal regulations, laws, and statutes related to accessibility, and disaster preparedness.*
- *Describe the National Fire Protection Association (NFPA), the International Code Council, and the NFPA Life Safety Codes.*
- *Identify accessibility issues relevant for assisted living administrators.*
- *Identify fire safety issues relevant for assisted living administrators including current life safety codes.*
- *Identify selected workplace safety issues relevant for assisted living administrators.*
- *Discuss disaster preparedness issues relevant for assisted living administrators.*
- *Discuss strategies for disaster preparedness including disaster preparations, disaster protection, and recovery from disasters.*
- *Describe selected best practices in fire safety and disaster preparedness.*

INTRODUCTION

Assisted living administrators must have a comprehensive understanding of current federal, state, local laws, and regulations that relate to accessibility, fire safety, and disaster preparedness within assisted living facilities. Awareness of landmark federal laws and agencies are an important first step in this process. Federal legislation which includes the Americans with Disabilities Act of 1990 as amended by the Americans

With Disabilities Amendment Act of 2008, the Occupational Safety and Health Act of 1970, and the creation of the Federal Emergency Manpower Agency, is presented and briefly discussed in this chapter. Also identified are important national fire safety codes. Selected issues related to accessibility, fire safety, and disaster preparedness are discussed and presented as important components of the work of administrators. Best practices in selected areas associated with fire safety and disaster preparedness will be presented at the conclusion of this chapter.

REGULATIONS, LAWS, AND STATUTES

While there are numerous laws, regulations, and statutes that administrators must address on a daily basis, administrators should be able to identify landmark federal legislation. Additionally, administrators should have an understanding of national fire and safety codes. Both federal laws, along with national fire and safety codes are briefly reviewed and discussed.

Americans With Disabilities Act of 1990

Signed into legislation by President Bush in 1990, and amended in 2008, is a wide ranging civil rights law designed to protect Americans with disabilities from discrimination in any setting. Disability is defined in this legislation as "physical or mental impairment that substantially limits major life activity" (Americans With Disabilities Act, 2009). Title I of the legislation notes that discrimination should not occur against any qualified individuals with disabilities, and applies to job applications, hiring, advancement, and the discharge of employees. Discrimination is defined here to include limiting or classifying job applicants in adverse ways, denial of employment to qualified applicants, failure to make reasonable accommodations to address physical or mental limitations of disabled employees, failure to provide training accommodations, and failure to advance employees with disabilities. Title II of the legislation covers in part access to all programs offered by specific entities. Physical access to facilities is more fully described in the Uniform Federal Accessibility Standards and the Americans With Disabilities Act Standards for Accessible design and access. Title III of this legislation states that no individual may be discriminated against based on disability, and is entitled to full and equal enjoyment of all services, facilities, and accommodations of any place of public accommodation. Public accommodations are defined to include most places of lodging, transportation, recreation, dining, stores, and care providers. Of special note is the application of Title III to existing facilities. One definition of discrimination in this area is the "failure to remove" architectural barriers in existing facilities.

Awareness of this important legislation is important because assisted living facility administrators will need to provide services to elders residing in assisted living facilities that are nondiscriminatory. Additionally, administrators must also be prepared to create work environments that prevent employee discrimination, and will thus benefit from review of the disability laws.

Occupational Safety and Health Act of 1970

The Occupational Safety and Health Act of 1970 (as amended in 2004) was authorized by the United States legislature to ensure safe and healthful working conditions for working men and women, to assist states in assurance of safe and healthful working conditions, and to provide information, education, training, and research in the field of occupational health. Additionally, this legislation is designed to encourage employers and employees to reduce the number of occupational safety and health hazards, as well as to institute new and improve existing programs for safe and healthful working conditions, and for the development and dissemination of occupational and health safety standards.

Administrators working in assisted living facilities must have an awareness and understanding of current health and safety legislation as it serves to protect both employers and employees from a number of potential problems that may occur in settings designed for elder care.

Federal Emergency Management Agency

The Federal Emergency Management Agency (FEMA) was initially created by Presidential Order in 1979. As an agency of the United States Department of Homeland Security, FEMA has been designed to coordinate disaster responses that are not controlled by local or state agencies. This new federal agency included services from a number of federal departments including the National Fire and Prevention Control Administration, the Federal Disaster Assistance Administration, and the Department of Defense Civil Preparedness Agency. FEMA currently offers a number of emergency response services as well as training programs for emergency personnel in the United States.

Administrators in assisted living facilities should be aware of FEMA and the role that this agency plays in local, state, and federal emergencies and disasters. While most administrators will hopefully not have to utilize these resources, awareness of what is available before emergencies or disasters occur, is an essential component of comprehensive emergency preparedness.

National Fire Safety Code

Assisted living facility administrators must adhere to a number of fire safety codes, many of which are determined by state laws and regulations. Administrators can benefit however, from an understanding of two national associations dedicated to national fire protection.

National Fire Protection Association

The National Fire Protection Association (NFPA) is a United States organization developed in 1896 to standardize the new market of fire sprinkler systems. Originally composed of insurance underwriting firms, the NFPA now consists of fire departments, insurance companies, unions, trade organizations, and manufacturing organizations. The current work of this organization involves the development and maintenance of over 300 fire safety codes and standards. Many state and local governments incorporate these standards and codes into legislation. The association standards and codes are accepted by many courts and exist as the standards currently in use in the United States. Evidentiary use of these codes can be found in the 'life safety regulations' sections of assisted living facilities in a number of states. The Assisted Living Workgroup Report to the U.S. Senate Special Committee on Aging (2003) Topic Group Recommendations on Operations noted that assisted living facilities should comply with the most current versions of the NFPA Life Safety Code. The codes are created by groups of experts in fire safety, and are regularly updated to reflect current standards of fire safety professionals (Wolf, 2002).

International Code Council

The International Code Council (ICC) was established in 1994 in the United States, and focuses on building safety and fire prevention. This association develops codes used for residential and commercial building construction, and are adopted in many U.S. cities, counties, and states. The International Codes or I-Codes are designed to provide minimum safeguards for individuals in homes, schools, and institutions, and include coordinated building safety and fire prevention codes. All 50 states have adopted the use of I-Codes at either the state or local level. The Assisted Living Workgroup Report to the U.S. Senate Special Committee on Aging (2003) Topic Group Recommendations on Operations noted that assisted living facilities should comply with applicable state and local building codes. States, however, should in part adopt the most current national versions of building codes to ensure that the most current perspectives on building safety are incorporated into state requirements.

ISSUES RELATED TO ACCESSIBILITY, FIRE SAFETY, AND DISASTER PREPAREDNESS

There are a number of issues related to accessibility, fire safety, and disaster preparedness that are of relevance for assisted living facility administrators. Selected issues in each of these areas will be presented and further discussed.

Accessibility Issues

Each state has individual regulations and codes that govern many aspects of accessibility within assisted living facilities. Administrators should be familiar with their state specific requirements. Additionally, administrators should note that accessibility is also legally mandated throughout the Americans with Disabilities Act of 1990. The construction and design of new facilities must ensure that buildings are readily accessible for disabled individuals. Regulations and codes are also applicable to older facilities. Existing facilities undergoing alterations must be designed whenever possible to ensure access to altered areas by individuals with disabilities, including wheelchair access. Paths of travel through such altered areas should ensure access to bathrooms, telephones, and drinking fountains whenever possible for individuals with disabilities (Americans with Disabilities Act, 1990).

The Assisted Living Report to the U.S. Senate Special Committee on Aging (2003) recommends that environmental management in assisted living facilities should include the maintenance of safe conditions for all residents, staff, and visitors in compliance with all applicable federal, state, and local laws. Resident needs should be accommodated, and common areas should be accessible to residents using a variety of assistive devices. Administrators need to assess their use of environmental management to ensure that all residents have access to accommodations within the assisted living facility. The Assisted Living State Regulatory Review of 2009 (Pelzer, 2009) describes assisted living regulations in each state as well as the District of Columbia. Information is provided for regulations detailing physical plant requirements, including a summary of the square foot requirements for resident units, the number of residents maximally allowed per resident unit, and bathroom requirements including the number of toilets, lavatories, and facilities required for each resident. As administrators review and adhere to the regulations for their state, accessibility issues should also be addressed. For example, in California, physical plant requirements allow for private or semiprivate resident rooms that must be of sufficient size to allow for easy passage of wheelchairs, walkers, and any required equipment such as oxygen. (Polzer, 2009). In Hawaii, physical plant requirements state that residents must be provided with an apartment unit that includes in part a refrigerator and cooking capacity, along with a separate and complete bathroom, having a sink, shower, and toilet. This would include accommodations for the physically challenged and wheelchair bound persons as needed. (Polzer, 2009).

Administrators working in states where regulations do not specify accessibility requirements will need to review and implement resources required to accommodate residents with disabilities. Assisted living facility administrators should refer to the regulations, codes, and laws that are relevant to their state, as they work to ensure that all residents in their facility are provided with accessible accommodations.

Fire Safety Issues

Administrators in assisted living facilities are responsible for ensuring that their facilities are safe from fire hazards and workplace fire safety issues. As previously noted, the National Fire and Safety Codes, and the National Fire Protection Association provide information and regulations on a national level for fire and safety protection. Administrators are responsible for adhering to state and local fire safety regulations and codes that vary within each state, and the District of Columbia. The Assisted Living State Regulatory Review (Polzer, 2009) described the regulatory category of life safety to summarize fire safety requirements and other standards to ensure residents' physical safety. Variation is noted among each of the state regulations in the area of life safety. For example, life safety regulations for the state of Delaware are comprehensive, noting that assisted living facilities must comply with all applicable state and local fire codes, and must implement fire safety plans through staff training and drills. These plans must be approved by the jurisdictional fire marshal, and must include an evacuation route posted on each floor and unit. At minimum, fire drills must be conducted annually. Additionally, the Delaware regulations require that specified incidents must be reported within an 8 hour period to the Division of Long-Term Care Residents Protection, including in part any fire or resident burns greater than first degree. This regulation exists in contrast to states such as Iowa, where life safety regulations require the use of sprinkler systems and smoke detectors that comply with the National Fire Protection Association (NFPA) 101, 2003 Edition, and NFPA 72, National Fire Alarm Code. Additionally, sprinkler systems must comply with the NFPA 13 or 13R standards (Polzer, 2009). As demonstrated, state regulations differ widely, and administrators should clearly understand and implement their states' regulations to protect assisted living residents from fire and safety problems.

The importance of understanding and implementing life safety regulations is underscored by reports from the National Fire Protection Association (NFPA) regarding board and care facilities, with senior assisted living facilities falling under the designation of board and care facilities according to the Life Safety Code (Wolf, 2002). The NFPA documented 23 multiple death fires (three or more fatalities) for a total of 122 deaths in board and care facilities from 1990 to 2003 (Kaspar, 2008). NFPA analysis of the fires revealed that major contributing factors to fire deaths included a lack of automatic sprinklers, unprotected vertical openings, doors open in the room of fire origin, and an insufficient staff and resident training response to disasters.

Updated Life Safety Codes (2006) address two main concepts: (1) larger buildings are more difficult to evacuate than smaller buildings, and thus require more fire protection; and (2) occupants who are more difficult to move and evacuate will require more built-in fire protection than individuals who require less assistance during evacuations (Kaspar, 2008). The 2006 codes stress a "defend in place" approach through the use of fire and smoke barriers in combination with automatic sprinkler systems. These strategies allow for the evacuation of residents to safe locations within the building's structure. Fire sprinkler systems are required in new assisted living facilities and should be either quick response or residential sprinklers.

Assisted living administrators must maintain a safely engineered environment for all residents. All floor surfaces, hallways, doorways, stairs, and ramps must be accessible for residents with decreased mobility (Kaspar, 2008). Assisted living facilities have specific means of egress requirements as determined by NFPA 101. Hallways must accommodate equipment such as oxygen tanks, and a minimum of 60 inches of clearance must be maintained in all hallways (Kaspar, 2008). Residents must also have an appropriate amount of time to respond to emergencies. Newer assisted living facilities should be designed with travel distances from corridor doors to building exits no more than 100 feet, and overall maximum travel distances should not exceed 200 feet (Kaspar, 2008).

Best Practices in Fire Safety

Assisted living administrators can also benefit from understanding best practices in fire safety. One example of a best practice has been identified in the Harpers Joy assisted living facility in Brunswick, Georgia (Batiwalla, 2009). The use of fire safety measures in this assisted living facility included not only smoke detectors, fire alarms, and sprinkler systems, but also the institution of training drills for residents. The institution of these combined measures saved the lives of residents when a fire started and destroyed two rooms in the assisted living facility. Fire investigators noted the use of these practices constituted not only a success story for the assisted living facility, but also served as an example of fire safety best practices.

Workplace Safety Issues

Issues related to workplace safety in addition to fire safety, must also be addressed by assisted living administrators. Regulations governing life safety for residents of facilities are identified in state regulations. Many states have regulations regarding the number of staff required on a per shift basis in assisted living facilities. In addition to work hours, many states regulate the training and education required for all staff members to ensure workplace safety. For example, Arkansas addresses staffing requirements for their level 1 and level 2 facilities, and also requires staff education and training in the areas of building safety, appropriate responses to emergencies, communicable diseases, along with food and sanitation safety (NCAL, 2007). Administrators should also follow all state and local regulations designed to provide staff members with safe and effective working environments.

Disaster Preparedness Issues

Administrators in assisted living facilities must be prepared for any number of potential disasters and emergencies, natural as well as man-made. Disaster preparedness begins with preparations for disaster and emergency plans, protection during the actual emergency or disaster, assessment and treatment of problems during an emergency or disaster, and efforts toward recovery and re-building. The information discussed will be of benefit to administrators running assisted living facilities.

Preparations for Disaster or Emergency

Administrators in assisted living facilities must be prepared for any number of disasters and emergencies including hurricanes, tornadoes, floods, fires, earthquakes, pandemics, and acts of bioterrorism. The initial step in disaster preparedness involves risk assessment. As noted by Robertson (2004), good plans begin with an understanding of the risks associated with the area in which the facility is located. Natural risks include storms, earthquakes, high winds, heat waves, and severe weather. Technological risks include electrical fires, toxic spills, computer, and power failures. Security risks include theft, fraud, sabotage, and vandalism. Finally, proximity risks need to be considered. These are risks from problems such as fires, toxic spills, explosions, and accidents that occur outside of assisted living facilities in neighborhoods or nearby communities. Such risks have the potential to create an emergency situation for residents and staff of facilities as a result of close geographic proximity to emergencies or problems (Robertson, 2004).

Once administrators have assessed and determined potential risks, the next step is to ensure that both residents and staff in assisted living facilities have the resources to care for themselves in the initial phase following a disaster or emergency, and also to build on existing relationships and reduce or minimize risks (Grachek, 2006). The disaster plan should include the following: (1) plans for sheltering in place and for evacuation; (2) plans for coordination with community, city, county, and state agencies and emergency management services; (3) discussion of emergency plans with staff and residents; and (4) plans and communication strategies for family members and friends of assisted living residents and staff, including out of town phone numbers for emergency family contacts.

The U.S. Department of Health and Human Services Center for Medicare and Medicaid Services has developed an emergency planning checklist for persons in long-term care facilities (2007). This extensive checklist begins with an understanding of the location of emergency exits, and the need for emergency evacuation plans for residents, staff, and family members. Also included are plans for long-term care Ombudsmen working with assisted living administrators, staff, and residents.

Emergency disaster plans must include evacuation plans for residents and staff. Plans should include verification of emergency evacuation shelters, and strategies in place to transport staff and residents to emergency shelters. Written contracts for bus or transportation services should be prepared in advance, along with emergency supplies and kits prepared to accompany staff and residents as they are evacuated to emergency shelters. Backup electronic pharmacy records should be kept in a separate geographic location to ensure access to this important information during a disaster (Cefalu, 2006).

Effective communication of disaster plans is essential to successful plan implementation. Communication will impact the establishment and maintenance of effective plans, and can in fact mean the difference between life, death, injury, or health for both residents and staff. Everyone involved in the disaster plan must understand the plan, and easily access the plan information (U.S. Department of Labor). This includes administrators, staff, and residents of assisted living facilities. It is important to note that all communication strategies must be effective for staff and residents with disabilities as The Rehabilitation Act of 1973 and the Americans with Disabilities Act of 1990 do not specifically require emergency preparedness plans. Equal access for people with disabilities is required however, and emergency plans must include provisions for individuals with disabilities (U.S. Department of Labor). Effective communication systems should include accessible signage, emergency telephone and TTY numbers, lobby posters, occupant emergency plans, and fire alarm evaluations to ensure that alarm sounds are adequate to warn both staff and residents (U.S. Department of Labor).

Protection During Disasters

Once a disaster or emergency occurs, administrators will need to implement established disaster plans. If plans have been made to evacuate staff and residents to alternative emergency shelters, triage of residents is an essential first step. Ambulatory residents should be evacuated first, followed by residents in wheelchairs, and finally those residents requiring additional assistance and support. Having roommates or close friends evacuate together will help to reduce stress and anxiety for residents. Staff should also plan to carefully check the facility (including bathrooms) to ensure that all residents have been evacuated (Cefalu, 2006). Administrators should plan to maintain facility security during a disaster. Security is needed to prevent the theft of drugs, personal possessions, and food from evacuated facilities, and administrators should also consider business interruption insurance to cover costs of facility mortgages, payroll, and other expenses during a facility evacuation (Cefalu, 2006).

Administrators who develop disaster plans which have residents and staff shelter in place, rather than evacuate the facility should have arrangements to ensure the health and safety of both residents and staff members. Frequently, power outages accompany disasters resulting in loss of heating or air conditioning, leaving residents at risk for dehydration, heat stroke, or hypothermia. A lack of electricity also means a loss of electronic alarms, door locks, and equipment for cooking and laundry. Administrators should plan to have generators available to power refrigerators, keep food cool, and provide residents with ice (Cefalu, 2006). Additionally, emergency equipment including chain saws, hand tools, extraction equipment, and tarps should be available at the facility. Emergency transportation should also be available for staff members who need alternative transportation methods (Cefalu, 2006).

Assessment and Treatment During Disasters

Administrators must be prepared to assess and treat residents for problems that may result from disasters or emergencies. Incontinence can be a major problem for residents who must evacuate their facility. Preparations should include appropriate incontinence, and hygiene supplies (Cefalu, 2006). Administrators should also have information available to address hazards that may result from pandemic or man-made disasters, including biological and chemical attacks.

Recovery

Administrators must develop disaster plans that also focus on recovery from the disaster. Adequate emergency preparations that include adequate supply of resident medications and supplies will enhance recovery following the disaster. Technology and the use of back-up computer systems, will also serve to provide essential medical information that will serve to facilitate recovery efforts following a disaster.

Residents in assisted living facilities can improve their recovery from a disaster or emergency by maintaining a healthy state of mind prior to the disaster. Mental and emotional preparation serves as an effective strategy to counteract the stresses associated with disasters and terrorist acts. The American Red Cross and Centers for Disease Control (2006) identify strategies that elders can use to deal with emotions following a disaster. Strategies include the following: (1) talking about the disaster; (2) sharing feelings with others who have been through the same events or are trustworthy; (3) taking care of physical needs including adequate nutrition, adequate sleep, and regular use of medications; and (4) return to normal routines as soon as possible. Additionally, elders can enhance their ability to recover from disasters through connections with family members, friends, significant others, adherence to regular exercise programs, use of stress management programs, and asking for any help and service they need (American Red Cross, 2006).

Resources for Administrators

As administrators develop disaster plans, their work can be facilitated by using a number of available resources. The American Red Cross, the Federal Emergency Management Agency, The Occupational Health and Safety Agency all have websites with information on disaster preparedness. Administrators may also access a number of resources to assist in the planning of emergency and disaster plans. As earlier noted, the U.S. Department of Health and Human Services (2007) serves as an excellent resource to ensure that disaster plans address necessary emergency services. Administrators must also investigate resources made available by state agencies addressing disaster preparedness and emergency service availability.

Administrators can additionally benefit from review of best practices in disaster preparedness. The Florida Department of Elder Affairs serves to promote best practices in disaster preparedness for elders in Florida and throughout the United States. In his testimony to the U.S. Senate Special Committee on Aging, Douglas Beach, Secretary of the Florida Department of Elder Affairs, identified emergency preparedness plans for Florida elders (2009). This disaster plan is comprehensive and encourages the coordination and integration of federal, state, and local emergency response plans specifically designed for elders. Hallmarks of this plan, important for all elders, including those residing in assisted living facilities, include preparations prior to the onset of emergencies, a focus on the nutritional needs of elders in the development of shelf-stable meals that are specific for elders, development of evacuation plans designed to protect elders, and recovery plans that additionally address the care needs of seniors.

CASE STUDY

CK is a new assisted living administrator of a medium size facility in the eastern United States. Disaster preparedness is an important consideration for CK who understands that preparations for disasters begin with an understanding of the risks associated with the area in which the facility is located. Geographically, CK's facility is in a low-lying area about 3 miles from a small river that floods during seasons with heavy rain or snow falls. This puts the facility at risk for flood related disasters. As CK begins the development of a comprehensive disaster plan, he identifies the importance of communication about emergency evacuation plans if river flooding should occur.

The staff plan a number of information sessions with the assisted living facility residents. The information sessions include a discussion of how residents can inform family members and friends if they are evacuated from their assisted living facility. While all of the residents have phone contact numbers for family and friends and some of the residents use text messaging for on-going communication, CK decided to additionally use social networking sites such as Facebook and Twitter for enhanced communication during potential emergencies. His decision was based in part on the reported successful use of these strategies in a number of disasters including the recent Haitian earthquake.

Interested residents were invited to participate in the social networking emergency preparedness communication project. CK purchased a cell phone with text messaging and social networking capabilities for each of the resident participants. The phones were adapted to ensure that residents with hearing and visual problems as well as arthritis or motor problems were able to use the phones. Facility staff members assisted residents in learning how to successfully use the phones as well as in the creation of a social networking site. Residents then contacted family members and friends and developed emergency communication networks.

One outcome of this project was an overall increase in resident communication with family members and friends as residents reported the use of the cell phones and the social networking sites to be both easy and enjoyable. While CK has not experienced a flood-related emergency to date, he is confident that if a disaster occurs, communication among residents, their families, and friends will be both effective and enhanced due to the use of cell phones and social networking sites. CK has also now started to discuss the benefits of social networking communication in disaster preparedness with other assisted living administrators.

CONCLUSIONS

This chapter highlights the importance of protecting disabled elders and other individuals, by adhering to federal legislation designed to promote access to facilities and services. Protecting elders from residential fires through a focus on fire safety and prevention was discussed, and current life safety codes were reviewed. Issues related to the engineering of residential environments to promote fire safety, from the installation of sprinkler systems, to the numbers of staff on duty during evening and night shifts, were introduced, along with the protection of elders through disaster preparedness. Issues associated with disaster preparedness, along with additional resources for facility administrators during disasters and disaster recovery, were also presented. Assisted living administrators can potentially benefit from ideas discussed in the best practices case study regarding the use of social networking sites to enhance communication during potential disasters.

REFERENCES

Americans Disabilities Act. (2008). *Americans with Disabilities Act of 1990 as amended by the ADA Amendments Act of 2008*. (Pub.L. No. 110–325).

American Red Cross and the Centers for Disease Control and Prevention Preparedness Today. (2006). *Maintaining a healthy state of mind for seniors*. Retrieved from http://www.redcross.org/preparedness/cdc_english/mental health-6.asp

Assisted Living Workgroup. (2003). *U.S. Senate Special Committee on Aging. Final Report*. Washington, DC: U.S. Government Printing Office.

Batiwalla, N. (2009). Sprinklers credited for saving GA. Assisted living residents. *The Brunswick News*. Retrieved from http://www.firerescuel.com/print.asp?act=print&vid=533892

Cefalu, C. A. (2006). Disaster preparedness for long-term care facilities. *Annals of Long-Term Care, 14*. Retrieved from http://www.analsoflongtermcare.com/article/6200

Federal Emergency Management Agency. (n.d.). *Department of Homeland Security*. Retrieved from http://www.fema.gov

Grachek, M. K. (2006). *Community-wide emergency planning involving long-term care: The joint commission approach to enhancing community support of long-term care during disasters*. Retrieved from http://findarticles.com/p/articles/mi_m.3830/is_5_55/ai_nl6485900

International Code Council. (n.d.). *About the ICC: Introduction to the ICC*. Retrieved March 25, 2009, from http://www.iccsafef.org/news/about/Occupational Safety and Health Act of 1970, P.L. 91–596, 2 (2004)

Kaspar, J. (2008, February 1). *Protecting a vulnerable population*. Retrieved from http://www.csemag.com/index.asp?layout=articlePrint&articleID=CA6533630

Polzer, K. (2009). *Assisted living state regulatory review*. Washington, DC: National Center for Assisted Living.

Robertson, G. (2004). *Emergency planning for long-term care/seniors nursing home/residential care facilities.* Retrieved from http://www.onwellness.info/0-services-disaster/

U.S. Department of Health and Human Services. (2007). *Emergency planning checklist.* Retrieved from http://www. hhs.gov

U.S. Department of Labor. (n.d.). *Preparing the workplace for everyone: Implementation, communicating about and distributing the plan.* Retrieved from http:// www.dol. gov/odep/pubs/eppreparing/implement.htm

U.S. Senate Special Committee on Aging. (2009). *Department of Elder Affairs state of Florida. Florida Elder Affairs Secretary Testifies to Senate Committee on Emergency Preparedness for Seniors.* Retrieved from http://elderaffairs.state.fl.us/english/News/ PressReleases/2009/

Wolf, A. (2002). NFPA standards guide life safety for many assisted living facilities. *NFPA Journal, 39–42.*

Models of Care

Learning Objectives

Upon the completion of Chapter 12, the reader will be able to:

- *Discuss the philosophy of service delivery in assisted living facilities.*
- *Identify the Medical Model of Care in assisted living facilities and discuss the roles of staff, administrators, residents, families, and communities within this care model.*
- *Describe the concept of culture change in assisted living facilities.*
- *Discuss the Green House Model of Care including the roles of staff, administrators, elders, families, and communities within this care model.*
- *Describe the Eden Alternative as a care delivery model in assisted living facilities and discuss the roles of staff, administrators, elders, families, and communities within this care model.*
- *Identify benefits and challenges associated with the Medical Model of Care.*
- *Identify benefits and challenges associated with the Green House Model of Care.*
- *Identify benefits and challenges associated with the Eden Alternative.*
- *Describe selected best practices associated with the use of the Green House Model of Care and the Eden Alternative.*

INTRODUCTION

Many assisted living facilities follow one of several models of care with administrators using a medical model to govern administration and facility functions. This is considered to be a traditional approach to care. Recently, advocates for changes in the culture of long-term care delivery, including services provided in assisted living facilities, have proposed a culture shift in approaches to service delivery to older adults. The Pioneer Network, Green Houses, and the Eden Alternative are approaches currently in use in the United States. Assisted living administrators can benefit from an understanding of these newer care models. Information about traditional approaches to service delivery, as well as information about proposed culture changes and current alternative care approaches will be discussed. Potential benefits and possible challenges associated with the traditional and newer care models will also be presented as will selected best practices associated with models of care delivery.

MODELS OF CARE IN ASSISTED LIVING FACILITIES

Current definitions and philosophies of assisted living are applicable to both the traditional and newer alternative care models. The Assisted Living Workgroup Report to the U.S. Senate Special Committee on Aging Topic Group Recommendations (2003) defines in part, assisted living, although no state or federal mandated definition exists. This definition notes that assisted living is a state regulated and monitored residential long-term care option. Services that are required by state law or regulation include the following: (1) 24-hour awake staff to provide scheduled and unscheduled elder needs; (2) health related services; (3) social services; (4) assistance with activities of daily living and instrumental activities of daily living; (5) meals; (6) housekeeping; and (7) transportation. Elders in these facilities have the right to receive these services in ways that promote their dignity, autonomy, independence, and quality of life.

The Assisted Living Workgroup Report to the U.S. Senate Special Committee on Aging Topic Group Recommendations (2003) provided additional information on Assisted Living Facilities. A philosophy of service delivery was articulated and designed to maximize individual choices, independence, autonomy, dignity, and quality of life. Additionally, core principles of assisted living are identified and should be reflected in a setting's mission statement, culture, policies and procedures. The core principles include: (1) creation of a residential environment that is supportive of each resident's right to privacy, choice, dignity, independence, quality of life, and privacy rights as defined by each resident; (2) offer of quality supportive services that are collaboratively developed and individualized for each resident; (3) provision of resident-focused services emphasizing individual needs and incorporating creativity, innovation, and variety: (4) support of an individual's decision-making control whenever possible; (5) fostering social climate that allows individuals to develop and maintain social relationships; (6) provide consumers with full disclosure of service provision and cost prior to and during the elder's stay in the facility; (7) minimize the need to move; and (8) creation of a culture that provides quality environment for elders, staff, administrators, families, volunteers, and the larger community.

Medical Model of Care

The medical model of care is a traditional approach to care delivery in many facilities throughout the United States, and familiar to most assisted living administrators. In this model, the medical problems experienced by elders serve as a focus for service care and delivery. Aging is viewed in terms of a series of changes to both physiological and psychological processes, as well as in changes in functional capabilities, and abilities to perform activities of daily living. Diseases are identified as alterations in physiological or psychological functioning with the goal of treatment and management to improve elder functioning. The Assisted Living State Regulatory Review (Polzer, 2009) identifies the services provided in assisted living facilities in each of the 50 states and the District of Columbia. While facility definitions are variable, many are focused on care delivery from a traditional perspective. For example, the assisted living facility definition used in the state of Illinois notes in part that assisted living establishments provide community based residential care for residents who need assistance with activities of daily living, including personal, supportive, and intermittent health related services to meet scheduled and unscheduled resident needs (Polzer, 2009). Other states have similar definitions of assisted living care that remain centered on a traditional medical care model.

Philosophy of the Medical Model of Care

The focus of care in this traditional model is to promote health, maintain functioning, and improve outcome and quality of life for older adults. Because aging is viewed in part as involving physiologic and psychological changes, the goals of care involve management are to improve existing problems and prevent of future problems.

Elements of the Medical Model of Care

As noted, the medical model of care is focused upon a traditional disease and treatment approach to problems associated with aging. As elders enter into assisted living facilities, initial assessments include information obtained from standardized medical and functional histories, as well as physical examinations. Care plans for elders are determined in part from data obtained from medical evaluations. Frequently, indicators of effective care delivery and effective functioning within the assisted living facility are determined from these initial assessments.

Roles of Staff and Administrators in the Medical Model of Care

Staff and administrator roles are traditional in the medical model of care. Staff is selected to provide services to elders and work in roles that support care for any existing physical, psychological, and functional problems, as well as potential problems in each of these areas. Staff and administrative roles are congruent with the state regulations governing assisted living facilities in the United States. The Assisted Living State Regulatory Review (Polzer, 2009) identifies information from applicable state statutes and regulations in a series of categories that delineate the roles of staff and administrators. Facility scope of care summarizes the nursing and personal care services provided in individual facilities. Resident assessment indicates in part the assessments conducted by staff on residents. Medication management indicates whether medication administration is permitted in facilities and the staff who may be eligible to provide this service. Staffing requirements are based on the number of residents, and staff education summarizes qualifications for different staff positions (Polzer, 2009). While care in assisted living facilities should be focused on resident choices and resident dignity, roles within traditional medical models of care are also delineated to adhere closely to state regulations and statutes. This has the potential to present confusion or a conflict of interest when staff and administrator roles that adhere to regulations, conflict with individualized resident care.

Roles of Residents and Families in the Medical Model of Care

Residents in assisted living facilities select their facilities in part to reflect care that is individually centered and designed to promote healthy aging, well-being, and improved quality of life. Family members of assisted living residents expect to be included in the care process. Facilities that focus on traditional care delivery are designed to provide residents with these services within a structure that emphasizes medical care delivery and the prevention of physical and psychosocial problems. Administrators and staff members also work with family members to provide services that include caring for the well-being of the resident within a framework of medical service provision.

Roles of Community in the Medical Model of Care

The role of the community in a traditional or medical model is often formalized. While connections with members of local communities are encouraged, and in fact desired, many of these interactions occur in more formal programs such as volunteer programs, or those which connect school children with elders in facilities.

CULTURE CHANGES IN LONG-TERM CARE DELIVERY AND ASSISTED LIVING FACILITIES

Administrators working in assisted living facilities should have an awareness of changes being proposed within long-term care settings, especially nursing homes. Understanding new ways of conceptualizing care for older adults and the culture changes that accompany proposed changes is beneficial to administrators in assisted living facilities. Most cultural changes are designed to improve quality of life and well-being for elders, and therefore have relevance and applicability in a number of settings including assisted living facilities.

According to the Pioneer Network (2009), culture change is a common name for a national movement designed to transform services for elders. Culture change is focused on person-directed values and practices with a goal of having older adults and caregivers provide input into care that is respected and valued. The core values related to culture change are dignity, respect, choice, self-determination, and a sense of purposeful living (Pioneer Network, 2009). Culture change is also viewed as a regenerative model designed to increase resident's sense of control and autonomy in what can be identified as a resident-centered care model (Brawley, 2007). Additionally, culture change refers to a progressive view of aging and reformulating the essential meaning of growing older in the United States (Brawley, 2007). As noted by Misiorski (2003), culture change transforms an institutional approach to care into a person-centered approach to care. Culture is seen as a community where individual capabilities are affirmed and developed. Additionally, Farrell and Eliot (2008) identify culture change as person-directed care developed as an alternative to traditional institutional frameworks used in many settings. The goals of culture change are centered in increased resident autonomy, control and life choices, improved quality of life for residents, as well as enhanced community with a continuity of individual social life and individual interests (Kane, 2007).

Much of the literature describes the concept of culture change within nursing homes. In these settings, culture change refers to a transformation of nursing homes as models of acute medical care, to models more towards the person or consumer. Quality of care, quality of life, and positive financial benefits for nursing home administrators are goals associated with the implementation of culture change in nursing homes (Baker, 2007). The National Citizen's Coalition for Nursing Home Reform (2006) describes culture change in nursing homes as a re-thinking of practices, and values that involve changes in working relationships among administrators, staff, residents, and families to create a humane environment supporting resident rights, dignity, and freedom. In essence, culture change involves the de-institutionalization of nursing homes, and supports individualized resident care.

Pioneer Network

The Pioneer Network, based in Rochester, New York, was established in 2000 as an umbrella organization for the nursing home culture change movement. Designed as a loose association of providers, regulators, advocates, and elders who advocate for improvement in the quality of life for institutionalized elders, this network advocates for a process of culture change that brings a sense of community into nursing home settings (Sadden, Deaton, & Gonzales, 2004). The Pioneer Network has been designed in part to: (1) create communication and networking opportunities; (2) participate in community building; (3) identify and advocate for transformation in practice and research; (4) serve an advocacy role in public policy; and (5) develop resources and leadership (Pioneer Network, 2009).

The Pioneer Network works with the National Citizen's Coalition for Nursing Home Reform to disseminate a number of culture change principles and practices. There are a number of key principles that have been framed by the Pioneer Network for use in culture change. As noted in a publication on culture change in nursing homes (National Citizen's Coalition for Nursing Home Reform, 2006), the principles used by the network include the following: (1) know individuals in the institutional setting; (2) recognize that each individual makes a difference; (3) recognize that relationships are the fundamental building blocks of cultures that are transformed; (4) note that responses should be to mind, body, and spirit; (5) identify risk taking as a normal part of life; (6) recognize that individuals and their needs should be put ahead of tasks; (7) recognize that all elders are entitled to self-determination; (8) note that communities can be considered as an antidote to institutionalization; (9) encourage growth and development for all individuals; (10) recognize environmental potential to be used in all aspects including physical, organizational, psychosocial, and spiritual aspects; and (11) recognize that culture change and transformation are a journey rather than a destination, and are always a work in progress.

BEST PRACTICES IN CULTURAL CHANGES

Administrators, staff, and residents in a number of assisted living facilities have been recognized for practices that reflect cultural changes in assisted living care. One example of a changing model of care is identified in BPM Senior Living in Portland, Oregon. This organization received a "Best of the Best" award from the Assisted Living Foundation of America for the development of a Personal Preferences Program (Redding, 2009). The program provided a personal preference coordinator for assisted living community members to promote advocacy as well as to identify each resident's preferences and priorities for care, routines, and activities. This approach is congruent with many of the culture changes associated with the Pioneer Movement, serving as a best practice for resident focused, individualized services within an assisted living setting.

Green House Model

The Green House Model is an alternative care model of nursing home care developed by William Thomas, a geriatrician, to deinstitutionalize the traditional nursing home environment. In 1999, Thomas determined that long-term care facility reform could best be achieved by a major redesign of nursing home architecture and organization. Thomas named his concept "Green House" to signify life and continued growth. Rather than one large building, Thomas' Green House was conceptualized as a community of small homes with a total of six to eight elders living in each home (RWJF, 2007). The model creates a small and intentional community of elders and staff with a focus on fostering relationships among the groups. Radically different from the traditional medical model of care, the Green House model was designed to provide older adults with assistance and support in activities of daily living and clinical care without the assistance, and the care of residents serves as the focal point of all activities and daily existence (NCB Capital Impact, 2009).

Philosophy of the Green House Model

The Green House Model operates on the concept that a community of small homes housing a total of six to ten elders and staff will provide an environment of support and growth for both residents and staff. Clinical services are provided in Green Homes but are de-emphasized in favor of a quality of life focus. The underlying philosophy of the Green House Model is focused on habituation and improved quality of life for elders in a normal and home like environment, rather than a medical or clinical environment (Rabig et al., 2006). The model emphasizes quality of life outcomes without ignoring clinical or therapeutic issues. Quality of life outcomes include a sense of security, enjoyment, meaningful activity, physical comfort, relationships, dignity, functional competence, privacy, individuality, spiritual well-being and autonomy (Kane, 2001). The Green House concept is also designed to emphasize competence through participating in daily activities of living in the effort to reduce the loss of control experienced by many institutionalized elders (Rabig et al., 2006).

Elements of the Green House Model

The elements of this alternative model of care are centered upon architectural changes to the traditional long-term care facility. As noted, the Green House Model promotes the use of small houses with a small number of residents and staff. The units are designed so that each resident has a private room and bathroom. Rooms are designed to receive increased levels of sunlight, and all are situated around an open area containing a hearth, an open kitchen, and open dining area (NCB Capital Impact, 2009). Easy access to all areas of the house, outdoor gardens, and patios are provided for elders who can also access laundry and kitchen facilities. Green Houses are designed to blend into existing neighborhoods. Architectural designs eliminate long hallways, institutional furnishings, overhead calling systems, nursing stations, and medication, as well as other carts (Rabig et al., 2006). The Green Houses are designed not to resemble medical or nursing home units commonly found in traditional medical model facilities.

Roles of Staff and Administrators in the Green House Model

Roles of staff in the Green House Model are significantly different from traditional medical models. Certified nursing assistants are considered to be the key staff members in the Green House Model. Provided with 120 hours of additional training, the nursing assistants have additional work responsibilities. They work in self-managed work teams and assume responsibility for cooking, cleaning, and managing the house, as well as working with and nurturing residents (RWJF, 2007).

Reporting structures are different in the Green House Model. Staff is not supervised by nursing service personnel as is customary in traditional models; staff members report to an administrator who is labeled a guide. Clinical support teams provide services to elders that are required by regulations in long-term care settings. Clinical teams consist of physicians, nurses, social workers, dieticians, and therapists. While the services that team members perform are similar to services in traditional medical model settings, they are expected to behave as guests in the elders' homes, and have no direct supervisory authority over other staff members (Rabig et al., 2006).

The language that is used to describe staff is different as well. Certified nursing assistants are called by a different title, shabaz, which is a Persian term meaning royal falcon. Residents are referred to as elders, administrators are called guides, and members of the community who provide assistance to the elders are known as sages. Convivium is a term used to describe food preparation and dining (Rabig et al., 2006). The rationale for these changes in language is to further delineate Green House operations from those found in traditional medical model facilities.

Role of Elders and Families in the Green House Model

The roles of elders and families are redesigned in the Green House Model. Decision-making is given to elders who do not adhere to fixed schedules. Elders make choices about meal times, sleep and rest times, and the types of activities they wish to participate in during the day. Elders and caregivers have close and informal relationships. Elders are encouraged to interact with staff members in daily activities, household activities such as gardening, cleaning, laundry, and pet care (Rabig et al., 2006).

Family members are also considered to be active participants in the Green House model. Because elders have control over their daily schedules and do not adhere to fixed times for meals, activities of daily living or other activities, family members can be encouraged to fully participate in these more flexibly organized living arrangements.

Role of Community in the Green House Model

The role of the community is viewed differently in the Green House Model. As noted earlier, houses are designed to be integrated into the surrounding community so that elders and staff become part of the neighborhood in general. Open relationships with community members are encouraged, and visitors are also welcomed to work with elders and staff informally, rather than in the more formal volunteer programs seen in traditional settings.

Eden Alternative

The Eden Alternative was developed by William Thomas, a geriatrician, in 1991 in the reformation of the long-term care industry. The goal of this approach to long-term care delivery was culture change, including the improvement of quality of life for older adults through the introduction of pets, plants, and children into traditional long-term settings. These changes were designed to improve and create meaningful relationships among long-term care residents through improvements in social and physical environments (Robert Wood Johnson Foundation, 2007). The addition of pets, families with children, plants and gardening were designed to create an environment that was more normal and less institutional in nature.

Philosophy of the Eden Alternative

The Eden Alternative was designed to create significant culture change in long-term care facilities. Thomas noted that long-term care facilities created a number of problems for elders including boredom, helplessness, and loneliness. The Eden Alternative was designed to eliminate these problems through the encouragement of meaningful relationships. The addition of pets, plants, gardens, and families with children was included in the culture change to provide elders with the opportunity to provide care to others, as opposed to only being passive care recipients. The Eden Alternative was also conceptualized to promote a more meaningful life for elders in long-term facilities through re-distribution of both power and energy (Rabig et al., 2006).

Elements of the Eden Alternative

As noted earlier, the Eden Alternative was designed to create culture change in long-term care facilities. While the Green House Model focused on architectural changes to effect culture change for elders, the Eden Alternative focuses on social and environmental changes to effect culture change.

The addition of nontraditional elements such as pets to what are otherwise traditional long-term care settings, was developed to provide elders with more control over their environment, as well as to promote an enhanced sense of well-being and improved quality of life. The introduction of pets was designed to help elders deal with issues of loneliness through companionship with a variety of birds, dogs, and cats. The introduction of staff members' children, as well as family members into the long-term care facility was designed to provide elders with the opportunity to care for others, and thus alleviate loneliness. Pets and children have been noted to help elders deal with feelings of helplessness. As elders provide care for others, they in fact are making empowering decisions. Boredom is less of an issue for elders who live in an environment that is engaging, constantly changing, and filled with a number of unanticipated events (NCPAD, 2008).

Role of Staff and Administration in an Eden Model

While the roles of staff members and administrators are more traditional in an Eden Model, staff members are encouraged to work with elders in nontraditional activities focused around pets, children, plants and gardening. This is designed to empower staff and to enhance opportunities for staff to engage with elders and family members in ways that have meaning for both groups. While administrative roles are also more like roles in traditional medical model settings, there are opportunities for administrators to work in interdisciplinary teams. Eden Alternative settings have staff working in nursing care teams. Each team is responsible for a small number of residents and the operation of work units. Eden teams consist of all workers who provide services to residents including certified nursing assistants, nurses, rehabilitation specialists, housekeepers, laundry workers, and maintenance staff members (NCPAD, 2008).

Role of Elders and Families in an Eden Alternative

As noted earlier, the roles of elders in an Eden Alternative are designed to be more participatory, more engaged, and more empowered than the roles played by elders in more traditional settings. Elders are encouraged to provide care to pets and to children, to participate in the care of plants and gardens, and to enhance their control and decision making opportunities in a number of areas. Planning in an Eden Alternative facility is focused on the person or individual, as opposed to more central organizational planning in traditional care models. Elders are encouraged to flexibly plan meals, choose the times they sleep, wake, and perform daily activities in an effort to promote decision making, and ultimately improve quality of life.

Role of the Community in an Eden Alternative

In an Eden Alternative facility, the community is considered to be a part of the long-term facility. Community volunteers are encouraged to participate in a number of Eden related projects, and to work directly with residents in the care of pets and gardens.

Issues Related to the Medical Model of Care in Assisted Living Facilities

Many assisted living facilities use a traditional medical model of care. The benefits of using this model are underscored by the state statutes and regulations that govern assisted living facility operations. Most state regulations require facilities to comply with standards that are congruent with traditional care models. Definitions in state regulations include definitions of care, facility scope of care, resident assessments, medication management, physical plant requirements, staffing requirements, and staff education and training, and are traditional in scope (National Center for Assisted Living, 2009). Administrators have a responsibility to adhere to standards and regulations. The development and design of facilities in compliance with existing regulations, offer a number of administrative, economic, and staffing benefits that are not present in facilities using alternative care models.

Resident well-being and quality of life are the primary challenges of traditional models. Elders who reside in traditional assisted living facilities have less control over their environment, schedules, and interactions with family and friends. This has the potential to impact quality of life and well-being for these elders.

Issues Related to the Green House Model of Care in Assisted Living Facilities

While the Green House Model of Care has been developed for use in long-term facilities, many of the benefits of this model can be applied to assisted living facilities. Designed to promote culture change, this care model was initially designed to promote improved quality of life, social involvement, and enhanced well-being for residents. Elders are more involved and engaged in activities within their homes. Families are more involved with elders because they have more opportunities to interact with elders, and both groups have more opportunities to interact with members of the community.

Research applying the Green House Model in Tupelo, Mississippi, in 2006 (Rabig et al., 2006) revealed positive outcomes and experiences for residents, staff members, and family members participating in this project. A 2 year, longitudinal quasi-experimental study was conducted comparing residents in Green Housing to residents in two traditional comparison sites. The study findings revealed statistically significant differences in self-reported quality of life with residents in the Green House Model. These residents reported improved quality of life over residents in more traditional settings. Additionally, residents in the Green House Model experienced improved functional status and quality of care as compared to residents living in more traditional facilities (Kane et al., 2007). These studies provide data to indicate that the Green House Model can impact and improve quality of life and well-being for elders. This model has implications for services provided in assisted living facilities.

Challenges associated with the implementation of the Green House Model in assisted living facilities are fiscal and regulatory in nature. Building and staffing the environment that is required for implementation of a Green House Model is expensive, and may be beyond the resources of many administrators. Because assisted living facilities must be in compliance with state statutes and regulations, conversion of traditional facilities into a Green House Model can involve many challenges and problems that must be addressed by administrators.

Best Practices in Implementation of Greenhouse Approach

Best practices in the implementation of the Green House approach to elder services have been identified. One example of a best practice involving residents with community projects can be found in the work done by community connections. Community connections represent one of a number of "good neighbors" projects conducted by residents in the New Haven, Connecticut Tower One/Tower East facilities (Connecticut Assisted Living News Topics, 2005). Residents supported global relief efforts to aid tsunami victims by collecting donations from facility residents and staff. Residents also participated in a number of community service programs including the Connecticut Food Bank, and an art and craft program conducted in conjunction with children in the New Haven Welch Elementary School. Again, these best practices illustrate the resident focused cultural changes away from the traditional medical care models found in many assisted living facilities.

Issues Related to the Eden Alternative in Assisted Living Facilities

The Eden Alternative has been designed to create culture changes in long-term facilities. This model of elder controlled and focused care can be applied to assisted living facilities as well. Benefits from this model include improvements in elder well-being and quality of life. Implementation of the Eden Alternative in the Chase Memorial Nursing Home in the early 1990s revealed the following research findings: (1) reduction in overall number of drug prescriptions; (2) reduction in the number of overall infection rates; (3) reduction in mortality rates; and (4) decreases in staff turnover (NCPAD, 2008). Administrators in assisted living facilities may wish to consider these findings as they consider implementation of the Eden Alternative in their facilities.

Challenges to implementation of the Eden Alternative are focused primarily on the fiscal costs of implementation and maintenance of this model. Changes to the social structure of facilities, the addition of pets, children, plants and gardens are costly, requiring additional staff resources and funding. Administrators who consider implementation of the Eden Alternative must also make sure they remain in compliance with all state regulations and statutes.

Research conducted in 2002 examined the effects of the Eden Alternative on quality of life of nursing home residents (Coleman et al., 2002). Residents in two nursing homes, one traditional and one using the Eden Alternative, were studied 1 year after implementation of the Eden Alternative. Resident cognition, immune functioning, survival, functional status, and care costs were compared in both study groups. Study findings revealed that residents in the Eden Alternative setting had more falls, experienced more nutritional problems, more staff terminations, and new hires. The researchers concluded that there were no benefits from the Eden Alternative site in terms of functional status, cognition, survival, infection rates, or cost of care after 1 year of implementation (Coleman et al., 2006). Researchers did speculate, however, that it may take longer than 1 year for Eden Alternative models to demonstrate positive outcomes for this model.

Best practices have been identified in the integration of assisted living facilities and local communities, an integral component of the Eden Alternative approach to elder care service delivery. The Greens at Cannondale in Wilton, Connecticut developed a program to connect assisted living residents with the local community. The program, entitled "Intergenerational Connections" received a Best of the Best award from the Assisted Living Foundation of America (Redding, 2009) for partnership with the Wilton High School and local teens. Residents of the Greens at Cannondale judged an art contest open to high school students and also participated in intergenerational talent competitions. Both events were positively received by residents, teens, and local community members, and served to enhance community relationships as well as relationships between elders and teens.

CASE STUDY

DL is a 90-year-old female who has recently moved into an assisted living facility from the home she lived in for 50 years. While DL was able to initially transition into the facility without many problems, she has recently become more withdrawn from the other residents, spending most of her time alone in her room. During a recent evaluation for depression, DL notes that she "lost her will to live" with the move to the assisted living facility and stated that she missed sitting in her kitchen where she could watch the neighborhood cat climb the maple trees in her backyard, and also watch different birds eat from the birdfeeders that her husband crafted prior to his death 10 years ago. DL's physician recommended medication to treat her depression, but the facility staff noted that the medication served to make DL sleepy and confused and did not resolve her depression.

The administrator of DL's facility has been interested in the implementation of culture change to improve the quality of life for elders as noted in work done by the Pioneer Network (2009). The administrator has been working to transform the facility from an institution based exclusively on the medical model to one with a focus on individual values and needs. The administrator worked with the facility staff to identify strategies for decreasing DL's depression. Although the staff were unable to move DL to another room or change the view from her windows, the staff were able to obtain several photographs of the maple trees in her former backyard. DL was able to hang the photographs where she could view them on a daily basis. The staff were also able to obtain birdfeeders similar to those crafted by DL's husband and placed the feeders in the facility garden. DL was then able to sit or walk in the garden at different times of the day to observe both the birds and bird feeders. DL was also encouraged to make recommendations to the staff regarding the types and amount of bird seed that would be best used in the bird feeders.

The assisted living facility also participated in a pet therapy program with a local animal shelter. DL was encouraged to attend regularly scheduled sessions, especially during times when cats were brought into the facility. DL enjoyed the opportunities to spend time with the animals in the pet therapy program, stating that she even enjoyed the opportunity to pet the hamster who accompanied the animal therapist at one of the visits. Both the administrator and facility staff noted that DL was less depressed with the implementation of simple environmental changes. DL was able to discontinue the medications for depression and she became less confused and more outgoing, more engaged in facility activities, indicating that she was "happier in her new home."

CONCLUSIONS

As stated in this chapter, administrators in assisted living facilities must adhere to state regulations in the operation of their facilities. Regulations that paralleled with traditional operations seen in the medical model were identified. This approach was discussed as a more cost efficient method, and more aligned with existing regulations. The challenges associated with the use of the medical model were focused in part on the provision of elder centered and individualized care within a traditional structure. The use of culture changing models as identified in the Pioneer Movement include the Green House Model and the Eden Alternative. It was presented that culture changing model proposed to improve quality of life and well-being outcomes for elders, and designed to provide elders with additional control over daily activities and service provision within residential settings. The benefits of these models were noted and included a focus on improvements for elderly individuals. Challenges associated with culture changing models were discussed, and included increased costs of service provision in nontraditional residential settings. Adherence to regulations in settings that are not traditionally structured, and difficulties in care delivery and provider roles within altered new and different care models was also discussed. The best practices and the best practices case study provided assisted living facility administrators with examples of culture change implementation in a variety of settings. Administrators can then reflect on some of the potential advantages associated with individualized, person-focused care delivery.

REFERENCES

Assisted Living Workgroup. (2003). *U.S. Senate Special Committee on Aging. Final report*. Washington, DC: U.S. Government Printing Office.
Baker, B. (2007). *Old age in a New Age: The promise of transformative nursing homes*. Nashville, TN: Vanderbilt University Press.

Brawley, E. C. (2007). What culture change is and why an aging nation cares. *Aging Today, 28*(4), 9–11.

Coleman, M. T., Looney, S., O'Brien, J., Ziegler, C., Pastorino, C. A., & Turner, C. (2002). The Eden alternative: Findings after 1 year of implementation. *The Journals of Gerontology Series A: Biological Sciences and Medical Sciences, 57*, 422–427.

Connecticut Assisted Living News Topics. (2005). *Residents at Tower One/Tower East "good neighbors" to community, world.* Retrieved from http://www.ctassisted living.com/news_topics.cfm

Farrell, D., & Elliot, A. E. (2008). Investing in culture change. *Provider,* 18–30.

Kane, R. A. (2001). Long-term care and a good quality of life: Bringing them closer together. *The Gerontologist, 41,* 293–304.

Kane, R. A., Lum, T. Y., Cutler, L. J., Degenholtz, H. B., & Yu, T. C. (2007). Resident outcomes in small nursing homes: A longitudinal evaluation of the initial Green House Program. *Journal of the American Geriatrics Society, 55,* 832–839.

Misiorski, S. (2003). *Pioneering culture change.* Retrieved from http://www.ltlmagazine. com/ME2/dirmod.asp?sid=&nm=&type=Publishing& Mod=Public

National Center on Physical Activity and Disability. (2008). *An Eden Alternative: A life worth living.* Retrieved from http: www.indiana.edu/~nca/ ncpad/eden.shtml

National Citizens' Coalition for Nursing Home Reform. (2006). *Culture change in nursing homes.* Washington, DC: U.S. Government Printing Office.

NCB Capital Impact. (2009). *The Green House concept.* Retrieved from http://www. Ncbcapitalimpact.org/default.aspx?id=148

Pioneer Network. (2009). Retrieved from http://www. pioneer network.net

Polzer, K. (2009). *Assisted living state regulatory review.* Washington, DC: National Center for Assisted Living.

Rabig, J., Thomas, W., Kane, R. A., Cutler, L. J., & McAlilly, S. (2006). Radical redesign of nursing homes: Applying the Green House concept in Tupelo, Mississippi. *The Gerontologist, 46*(4), 533–539.

Redding, W. (2009). Best of the Best. *Assisted Living Executive,* 11–19.

Robert Wood Johnson Foundation. (2007). *"Green Houses" provide a small group setting alternative to nursing homes and a positive effect on residents' quality of life.* Princeton, NJ: Author.

Sadden, L., Deaton, L., & Gonzales, M. (n.d.). *Concept paper: Bringing culture change to Louisiana nursing homes.* Pioneer Network. Retrieved from http://www.pioneer. network.net

Universal Design and Aging-in-Place

Learning Objectives

Upon the completion of Chapter 13, the reader will be able to:

- *Identify definitions and philosophy of universal design.*
- *Describe key principles of universal design.*
- *Identify strategies for connecting universal design elements to assisted living facilities.*
- *Identify definitions and philosophy of aging-in-place.*
- *Describe selected elements of successful aging-in-place programs.*
- *Identify the roles of administrators, staff, residents, and families within aging-in-place programs.*
- *Describe selected benefits and challenges related to universal design.*
- *Describe selected benefits and challenges related to aging-in-place.*
- *Describe selected best practices related to aging-in-place.*

INTRODUCTION

Assisted living facilities administrators can best serve the residents and staff of their facilities through an understanding and awareness of universal design, in addition to the physical work done to help elders to age-in-place whenever possible. These two concepts are presented in this chapter, along with selected issues, benefits, and challenges associated with the use of universal design and aging-in-place in assisted living facilities. Best practices in selected areas associated with universal design and with aging-in-place will also be briefly discussed throughout this chapter.

UNIVERSAL DESIGN IN ASSISTED LIVING FACILITIES

Before the implementation of universal design, administrators need to have an understanding of the definitions and philosophy of universal design, the history of universal design, and key principles of universal design. Strategies for connecting universal design to assisted living facilities will also be presented and further explained.

Definitions and Philosophy of Universal Design

Universal design is defined as the development of buildings, housing, and products that can be used by all people in the most effective way possible. The goal of universal design is the creation of buildings, building interiors, and products that can be used by most individuals, including those with disabilities. Designers balance artistic integrity with human needs and environment, which include recent technological design innovations and also address the need for accessible and adaptable environments (Mace, Hardie, & Place, 1991). Adaptable environments are designed with a number of universal features that can later be modified for the needs of specific users or user groups. Adaptable designs frequently include all of the elements required for users in wheelchairs, but in a universal design approach, fixed accessible features are combined with adjustable, and optional or removable elements. This results in the creation of an environment that will be used by many individuals, but can also be tailored to the functional limitations of specific individuals (Mace, Hardie, & Place, 1991).

The philosophy of universal design is to simplify life for everyone through the creation of housing that is more accessible at little or no additional cost to users. The universal design concept is focused on environments that are used by all individuals, and is applicable to all spaces and buildings (Steinfeld, 1988). This concept is in contrast to building codes, regulations, codes, and standards that have been developed to address needs (primarily mobility needs) for selected groups of individuals, usually those with disabilities or those in specialized settings such as assisted living facilities. Universal design also requires the use of universal features, or elements within facilities that can be used by everyone regardless of their abilities, representing standard products that are placed differently or carefully selected. Examples of universal design include: door handles that do not require gripping or twisting to operate; alarm systems that are both audible and visible; and storage space that is accessible to individuals with height differences (Steinfeld, 1988).

History of Universal Design

The movement toward universal design was formed in response to many of the changes experienced by older adults and those with disabilities in the United States. Demographic shifts now show more Americans to be living longer lives. The U.S. Census Bureau estimates that by 2020, nearly 7-8 million individuals will be over the age of 85, and 214,000 will be aged 100 and older (Center for Universal Design, 2000). The numbers of individuals with disabilities also continues to increase as those with disabilities live longer and more productive lives. Many of these individuals either live or will plan to move to assisted living or long-term care facilities, prompting the need for improvements in the design of these settings.

A number of federal legislative changes have influenced the universal design movement in the United States. The Civil Rights Act of 1964 provided a starting point for subsequent legislation to improve the lives of older adults and those with disabilities. The Center for Universal Design (2000) identified a number of these legislative efforts. The Architectural Barriers Act of 1968 required that all buildings constructed, leased, designed, or altered with the use of federal funding, be made accessible to those with disabilities. The Rehabilitation Act of 1973 (specifically section 504 of the act) made discrimination illegal on the basis of disabilities, and was applicable to any agency receiving federal funding including federal contractors, federal agencies, and public universities. The Fair Housing Amendments Act of 1988 served to expand the Civil Rights Act of 1968 to include people with disabilities. This act required that all housing built after 1988 include accessible units in buildings with four or more units. The act is applied to both public and private housing, and is applicable to newly constructed assisted living facilities. Finally, the Americans with Disabilities Act (ADA) of 1990 required the removal of physical barriers that had the potential to impede access, and banned discrimination in access to public accommodations, programs, services, public transportation, and telecommunications. The ADA Standards for Accessible Design was further developed as a result of work done by the Architectural and Transportation Barriers Compliance Board in 1991. This work serves as the federal standard for accessible design in the United States (Center for Universal Design, 2000).

Universal design was influenced in part by the barrier-free movement which began in the 1950s as a response to individuals with disabilities demanding services that would increase employment and educational opportunities, rather than institutionalization for their differences. These individuals recognized that physical and environmental barriers created significant problems, especially for individuals with mobility problems, including a number of older adults. As a result of the barrier-free movement, architects noted that changes to building and space design for those with disabilities would also benefit others without disabilities. The recognition that many design features could be provided in ways that were attractive, marketable, and less expensive was considered by many to be the beginning of the universal design movement. Again, the concept behind universal design was the creation of designs that would address the needs of all individuals with and without disabilities (Center for Universal Design, 2000). The applicability of this design approach in assisted living facilities with older adults is readily apparent.

Key Principles of Universal Design

There are seven principles of universal design. They were developed by a group of engineers, architects, environmental design researchers, and product designers to serve as a guide for members of design disciplines. The principles may also serve to evaluate existing designs, guide the implementation of new designs, and also educate consumers and designers about more usable environments and products (Center for Universal Design, 1997). Each of these principles, with applicability to those working and residing in assisted living facilities, will be briefly addressed. Information about each of the seven principles is obtained from the work done through the North Carolina State University Center for Universal Design (1997). The first principle involves equitable use, with designs that are useful and marketable to individuals with diverse abilities. Guidelines for this principle include development of the same or equivalent means of use for all users to eliminate stigma or segregation of users. Additionally, equitable use must include provisions for security, privacy, and safety for all users. One example of equitable use in assisted living facilities is the use of power entrance doors with movement sensors that are convenient for all users.

The second principle of universal design involves flexibility in use. The goal here is to develop designs that accommodate a wide number of individual abilities and preferences. Adaptability to user pace, user accuracy, and precision are important components of this principle. An example of flexibility in use in assisted living facilities includes the use of scissors that can be used by either right or left handed older adults.

The third principle of universal design is focused on use that is both simple and intuitive. Here the goal is to design products and environmental factors that are simple to use and easy to understand despite the users' knowledge level, experience, language skills, or cognitive abilities. The goal of the simple and intuitive use principle is to accommodate individuals with a wide range of language and literacy skills, arrange information that is consistent with the importance of the information, and eliminate unneeded and unnecessary complexity. One example of simple and intuitive design is the development of emergency plans and guidelines in a manual with drawings and no text, for use by a wide range of residents in assisted living facilities.

The fourth principle of universal design is centered upon perceptible information. Here, objects are designed to effectively communicate necessary information to users, regardless of the environment, or the user's sensory capabilities. The goals of perceptible information are to provide information that is redundant using different strategies (verbal, visual, or tactile), to make instructions easy to understand, and to be compatible with other devices that may be in use for sensory problems. For example, residents in assisted living facilities who can access a thermostat using verbal, visual, and tactile instructions are utilizing designs with perceptual information.

The fifth principle of universal design involves a tolerance for error with designs that minimize hazards, and the consequences of either accidents or unanticipated actions. The design goals of this principle are to provide warnings of potential hazards, provide failsafe features for the designs, and minimize hazards or errors. Providing elders in assisted living facilities with double cut room keys that have been designed for insertion into door keyholes in either of two ways mentioned, serve to create a tolerance for error.

The sixth principle of universal design is low physical effort, or the minimization of fatigue, in which products can be used both efficiently and comfortably with a minimum of fatigue. The goals here are for users to maintain neutral body positions, use reasonable operating forces, minimize repetitive actions, and minimize sustained physical efforts. Those residing in assisted living facilities who use loop or lever handles on faucets or door handles, or use lamps that are operated by touch rather than by a switch, are using products with low physical effort.

The seventh and final principle of universal design involves both size and space for approach and use. The appropriate size and space are provided for reach, approach, manipulation, and used independently of each user's size or mobility. The goals here are to make reach comfortable for all users whether standing or sitting in a wheelchair, provide space for those individuals using a number of assistive devices, accommodate variations in handgrip size and strength, and provide clear visibility for individuals who are either standing or sitting. Assisted living facility residents who have clear space around mailboxes, appliances in their homes, and other elements of their environment, will have easy access for approach and use of these items.

Strategies for Connecting Universal Design to Assisted Living Facilities

Universal design strategies can be used to improve both living conditions and quality of life for both residents and staff in assisted living facilities. As administrators consider the use of existing space or the renovation or building of new spaces, universal design can be employed in all settings. The use of lever handles on room doors can improve entry, especially for elders with arthritis or mobility limitations in their hands and arms. The costs of replacing traditional doorknobs with levers are considered to be reasonable, as the materials for this change are found in a number of hardware stores and equipment centers (Steinfeld, 1988).

Universal design solutions to bathrooms can enhance life for residents in assisted living facilities. Changes to the walls above bathtubs that reinforce the walls with blocking, will allow for the placement of grab bars to facilitate balance and improve mobility as needed. Placement of bathtub faucets close to the outer rim of the tub provides for easy access, especially for elders in wheelchairs or those experiencing mobility problems. The design of new bathroom facilities large enough to accommodate wheelchairs and more than one person at a time, can also serve to improve function and provide a universal feature to such an important living space (Steinfeld, 1988).

There are a number of fixed accessible design features that should be elements of assisted living facility's design. These elements include the following: (1) doorways that provide a minimum of 32 inches of clear opening space; (2) clear pathways at least 36 inches wide that are connections between all accessible living spaces, and the avoidance of stairs and steps at all building entrances; (3) living facilities that must all be on the same level unless all levels are connected by ramps, elevators, or lifts; (4) clear floor spaces, especially around appliances, fixtures, toilets, tubs, showers, and sinks; (5) controls that are easy to reach and easy to operate, including light switches, faucets, and thermostats should be mounted between 9 to 54 inches above the floor, and should also be operable with only one hand; (6) operable windows should have controls that are easy to reach and operate; (7) visual alarms with smoke and fire detectors providing both visual and auditory warnings; (8) tub seats that are either built into the tub; (9) showers that are either a 3 foot by 3 foot size, or the provision of a roll in shower space to provide accommodations for individuals in wheelchairs; and (10) reinforced walls or wood blocking for the addition of grab bars around tubs, toilets, and showers as needed (Mace, Hardie, & Place, 1991).

Administrators may also wish to consider the use of adaptable designs in assisted living facilities. Here, a number of basic and universal features in a number of living spaces can be easily changed or adapted to the requirements of specific users. Adaptable design includes features that are required for wheelchair access. These features can be hidden from sight, added as needed, and adjustable to accommodate users of different heights, sizes, and abilities. Countertop segments that can be raised or lowered, adjustable height closet rods, and cabinet shelving, adjustable toilet, tub, and shower grab bars, and attachable tub seats, are all examples of adjustable design elements that can be installed as needed in assisted living facilities (Mace, Hardie, & Place, 1991).

Best Practices in Universal Design

Administrators, staff, and residents in a number of assisted living facilities have been recognized for work that reflects aspects of universal design. Selected best practices will be briefly addressed. The Assisted Living Federation of America awarded the Best of the Best Strategy to Sunrise Energy Council and Sunrise Senior Living in McLean, Virginia for practices designed to reduce energy consumption (Assisted Living Executive, 2008). Many of these practices employed energy efficiencies such as the use of compact fluorescent products that also served to improve quality of living for assisted living residents.

The Department of Housing and Urban Development awarded an assisted living conversion grant to the Christian Care Manor in Phoenix, Arizona (National Center for Assisted Living, 2006). This funding was designated to the development of a best practice in the conversion of senior housing to assisted living units for elders. The renovations conducted as part of this grant funded project included the use of universal design elements such as lever hardware installation, relocation of closet rods, outlets, electrical switches, and the installation of folding grab bars in shower, toilet, and lavatory conversions. These renovations not only augmented universal design elements into senior housing renovations but also served to improve the quality of this senior housing.

AGING-IN-PLACE

Universal Design serves to improve the quality of life and well-being for elders in assisted living facilities through a careful process of environmental change created primarily through space and product redesign. Aging-in-place also serves to improve life quality and well-being for elders in assisted living facilities through the process of policy and regulatory adjustments, care delivery, along with environmental and space changes that allow individuals to live in an assisted living facility for as long as possible. Definitions of aging-in-place, as well as the philosophy and elements of this approach to living arrangements for older adults, will be briefly discussed. In addition, space allocation and the roles of administrators, staff, residents, and families will be reviewed.

Definitions and Philosophy of Aging-in-Place

Aging-in-place has been defined as the ability of older adults to age in their own homes or in assisted living facilities. Modifications of the living environment are made to include changes that allow elders to compensate for disabilities and limitations, and thus prevent or slow down admission into long-term care facilities. There are a number of long-standing assumptions stating that as individuals age and become progressively frail, they will need to move from one type of facility to another as their needs change. Additionally, there has been acceptance over the past 10 years that elders can modify their living environment through the addition of supportive services and changes to their physical space (Lawler, 2001).

Successful aging-in-place strategies have been found to minimize costs through the ability to minimize inappropriate care, along with the delivery of flexible care that fits individual needs (Lawler, 2001). Aging-in-place also creates health care and housing options that are flexible, and designed to allow individuals with the personal desire to live independently, to do so for as long as possible. It is important to note that aging-in-place works best when it is a component of a comprehensive and holistic approach that supports the needs of older adults (Lawler, 2001).

The philosophy of aging-in-place within assisted living facilities involves resident control over service delivery, including the types of services and ways in which those services are delivered. This is a consumer oriented model where the setting and the delivery of services is organized around the resident as opposed to the assisted living facility. In contrast to a medical model of care delivery where residents are patients cared for in institutional settings, residents are active participants and consumers of health care services (Chapin & Dobbs-Kepper, 2001). The key to an 'aging-in-place' philosophy is for facilities to adjust service provisions and level of care criteria to address the needs of residents, as well as avoid premature discharge to higher level care facilities. Provision of nursing care services and medication management are also elements of aging-in-place (Chapin & Dobbs-Kepper, 2001).

Chapin and Dobbs-Kepper (2001) conducted research to examine the aging-in-place philosophy in the Midwestern state of Kansas. The researchers conducted a survey of assisted living and residential care facilities in Kansas, collecting data from 141 facilities on their admission and retention policies, reasons for resident discharge, discharge destinations, and average length of resident stay in their facility. The study findings note that some of the Kansas facilities had admission and retention policies that supported aging-in-place. Study residents who were able to age-in-place for longer time periods were not ambulatory, had self-managed incontinence, mild forms of dementia, or a number of special nursing care needs including medication administration, medication monitoring, oxygen administration, catheterization, or ostomy care (Chapin & Dobbs-Kepper, 2001). Many administrators used facility policies to limit admission and retention. Residents with severe cognitive impairments, an inability to work with staff to manage incontinence, and residents at risk for running away from the facility, found their options for aging-in-place to be very limited. Thus, the researchers found that resident's ability to age-in-place to be determined by facility policies that were more stringent than state assisted living regulations, and noted that full implementation of aging-in-place in Kansas assisted living facilities would require additional funding and concomitant staffing, as well as more inclusive admission and discharge criteria (Chapin & Dobbs-Kepper, 2001).

There are a number of elements associated with successful aging-in-place programs. One element includes choice, or the provision of both housing and health care options designed to meet the diverse needs of aging individuals. These options should be both available and affordable so that elders as well as their caregivers can make appropriate care delivery choices (Lawler, 2001). A second component of successful aging-in-place involves flexibility, or the provision of care services that can be applied in a variety of contexts. The levels of health care services and housing or living options must be adjustable for elders (Lawler, 2001).

A third component of successful aging-in-place involves the maintenance of mixed generation communities. Here, elders' enhance their ability for self-help through contributions to the community. For example, these contributions can take the form of tutoring, and the provision of day care services for young children. Children in turn, can provide opportunities to engage seniors, and keep them active as they age and become increasing frail. The development of mixed generation communities should be guided by the assumption that these communities should not be prevented from occurring in either natural or planned settings (Lawler, 2001).

Calibrated support is the fourth and final component of successful aging-in-place programs. Here, calibrated support involves the development of both health care and housing infrastructures that assess for and deliver appropriate levels of coordinated care delivery. To ensure the avoidance of under-care or over-care delivery, ongoing assessment of health care and housing needs must occur. Additionally, a wide range of services must be provided to address the changing needs of those elders who are aging-in-place (Lawler, 2001).

Best Practices in Aging-in-Place

Best practices in the area of aging-in-place and care delivery have been identified for use by assisted living administrators. One example of a best practice is for residents in the Albuquerque preferred assisted living facility in Albuquerque, New Mexico (2009), who stay in homes located in a number of residential neighborhoods. Aging-in-place is supported in these facilities and residents are able to receive a number of services, including end-of-life care and hospice care without leaving their homes. An additional best practice representing aging-in-place has been demonstrated by the Orchards at Bartley/Bartley Healthcare in Jackson, New Jersey, a continuum of care assisted living community. Their Cedar Spring Memory Support Program was designed to provide residents with support and care services to maintain independence and an assisted living lifestyle (Orchards at Bartley, 2009). The Orchards was a recipient of the American Healthcare Association and National Counsel on Assisted Living Best Practices award for their programs and assisted living services promoting the concept of aging-in-place.

Factors that influence aging-in-place include state regulatory requirements that determine facility admission, retention, and discharge policies, and thus determine the feasibility of aging-in-place opportunities for frail elders. Also influencing the ability of elders to age-in-place is the availability of services. Facilities with limited staffing and limited service capabilities will be unable to ensure that frail elders are able to successfully age-in-place.

Additionally, there are a number of design influences that impact aging-in-place. Accessibility features such as facility entrances that are at the ground level and do not require stairs, single story facility construction, and the presence of ramps and elevators are needed for elders who age-in-place as they become frail and experience as increase in mobility problems. The presence of wider doorways, lever handles on doors, walk-in showers, grab bars around toilets, tubs, and showers, as well as the presence of handrails on walkways and ramps, also serve to reduce excess disability and reduce problems associated with gait and balance changes, along with associated with grasp changes. Changes in facility design serve to increase independent functioning and enhance safety for assisted living facility residents (Ball et al., 2004).

In a qualitative study conducted by Ball and associates (2004), the process of aging-in-place was investigated in five Georgia assisted living facilities during a 1-year time period. Through a process of purposive, maximum variation sampling, the five facilities were selected to reflect diversity in elderly residents including race and socioeconomic status, size of the facilities, geographic location of the facilities, and resources available for the elderly residents. The researchers found that the ability of elders to age-in-place was primarily a function of "fit" between residents and facilities to manage resident decline. The managing of resident decline was a function of capacity to manage decline at the resident, facility, and community levels. Resident decline was approached through the process of decline prevention. This involved health education efforts as well as an adherence to treatment regimens. A second strategy involved responding to decline through a process of balancing resident needs with available resources. Finally, the researchers noted that resident and assisted living facility fit was viewed as both an outcome, as well as an influence on the decline process with resident and facility risk both a consequence and intervening factor in resident decline. Their findings highlighted some of the complexities associated with aging-in-place and highlighted the need for residents to become well informed about assisted living facilities (Ball et al., 2004).

Roles of Administrators, Staff, Residents, and Families in Aging-in-Place

Assisted living facility administrators and staff play key roles in determining the capacity of individual facilities to successfully offer and support the services needed for aging-in-place. A number of factors determine whether aging-in-place can be offered in a facility, including both state and facility regulations, policies, and the physical environment of the facility, including whether or not changes can be made to make rooms and buildings accessible to residents growing frailer as they age-in-place. Staff members who work in facilities with aging-in-place must be able to provide the services that are needed by elders as they experience physical and mental decline. Staff must be qualified to provide additional nursing services including medication administration and medication management, as well as services to deal with a number of physical problems such as incontinence, reduced mobility, and cognitive problems such as dementia.

Residents and family members play important roles in aging-in-place in assisted living facilities. One key element of aging-in-place is the focus on services. Residents are encouraged to be in control of the services that are provided to them. Family members are also encouraged to become active participants in the care that their family members receive as they age-in-place.

Assisted living facility administrators can benefit from best practices that have been established for aging-in-place in a number of settings. For example, in West Seattle, Providence Mount St. Vincent (PMSV) initiated a change to resident directed care in an assisted living program entitled "Hand to Hand" (Providence Health and Services, 2009). Residents were encouraged to determine how much assistance they required and fees were negotiated for resident apartments rather than on a fee for service basis. Residents were not moved into nursing homes if they developed urinary incontinence or signs of dementia, thus viewing their apartments as permanent homes and effectively aging-in-place.

ISSUES RELATED TO UNIVERSAL DESIGN

There are a number of issues associated with the use of universal design in assisted living facilities. The economic benefits and benefits to residents, administrators, and staff will be briefly addressed. A number of the recognized challenges of relevance to administrators working with the concepts of universal design in assisted living facilities will also be reviewed and discussed in the following section of this chapter.

Benefits Related to Universal Design

As earlier noted, the use of universal design provides a number of benefits. The economic benefits associated with universal design are well described for builders and contractors who use more economical manufactured rather than custom built materials, and for designers using standardized features, spending less time in design activities (Steinfeld, 1988). The benefits associated with the use of universal design for assisted living residents include increased accessibility and potential increases in mobility, functional status, and independence. The benefits to administrators include the creation of assisted living facilities that increase the functioning and overall quality of life for residents. Staffing costs may be reduced in assisted living facilities if resident rooms and spaces are made more accessible with the use of universal design principles. Studies in hospitals indicate that changes that promote patient independence, reducing the use of nursing services, significantly reduce overall hospital costs (Mace, Hardie, & Pace, 1991). Staffing costs in assisted living facilities could potentially be reduced if design changes to resident rooms and facility spaces also served to improve accessibility and resident independence.

Challenges associated with the use of universal design are primarily associated with the costs of designing and building new facilities, or with alterations to existing facilities. Many argue however that the actual costs of assisted living facility spaces are offset by the benefits accrued from increasing resident independence in accessible living spaces.

ISSUES RELATED TO AGING-IN-PLACE

There are a number of issues related to aging-in-place in assisted living facilities. Benefits of aging-in-place include resident and family benefits, alongside benefits in cost. Challenges associated with aging-in-place include resident challenges, facility challenges, and economic challenges. Some of the benefits and challenges associated with state regulations related to aging-in-place are of additional significance.

Benefits Related to Aging-in-Place

A number of benefits related to aging-in-place have been identified. As noted earlier, a major benefit associated with aging-in-place in assisted living facilities is the increased quality of life and enhanced well-being that residents experience when they participate in this care model. Life in these settings should ensure that individuals, who are not fully able to care for themselves, can maintain the highest degree of independence, autonomy, human dignity, and personal fulfillment possible throughout their life span (Miller & Moore, 2006). Those individuals who are in assisted living facilities practicing aging-in-place, are placed at the center of care giving activities and have their needs addressed, as opposed to institutional or structural needs. This also serves to improve quality of life for assisted living facility residents.

Aging-in-place programs offer a number of social benefits to residents in assisted living facilities. Aging-in-place increases resident self-sufficiency and offsets social isolation. Additionally, aging-in-place prevents or defers relocation, which has been shown to involve the loss of friendship, social connections, and interactions with familiar staff and service personnel. Relocation can be associated with a decrease in the quality of life, dignity, and personal control (Lawlor, 2001). Additionally, the negative effects of relocation and moving from one facility to another can be traumatic for residents who are experiencing loss of their functional independence. This may result in a number of negative consequences including depression, dementia, and diminished abilities to perform a number of functional activities.

Lawlor (2001) notes that health care delivery services to the elderly are more expensive when delivered in a production rather than in a customized model. Services that are provided in traditional assisted living facilities provide the same set of services and housing options to all residents, and care is provided to the median needs of the majority of residents rather than to the needs of each individual resident. The production model is more likely to deliver care that may be "too much" for some residents, while other individuals do not receive enough services. Over-care results in the delivery of services that are unnecessary, costly, and of lesser benefit to residents. The restrictions and loss of independence resulting from too much care can result in shorter and less productive lives for residents who may also experience an orientation, increases likelihood of depression, and can cause a diminished quality of life (Lawlor, 2001). Under-care refers to services that are inadequate for residents in assisted living facilities. A lack of necessary and appropriate services can put residents at risk for a number of problems, and is as debilitating for elders as is the provision of too much care.

Aging-in-place in assisted living facilities not only provides physical, social, and emotional benefits to residents, but also provides a number of cost benefits. Chapin and Dobbs-Keppler (2001) noted that the care provided in assisted living facilities when targeted to the residents at the appropriate care level, can be more cost effective than the care that is delivered in long-term care facilities. Aging-in-place programs which keep residents in more cost effective systems such as assisted living facilities can create significant cost savings for individual residents as well as for a number of state programs. Residents who are less impaired and "aging-in-place" in assisted living facilities will use fewer expensive institutional services, again creating savings in overall costs.

Challenges Related to Aging-in-Place

A number of challenges have been identified in assisted living aging-in-place programs. These challenges include aging-in-place in rural versus urban contexts. As Lawlor (2001) indicates, many individuals in rural areas note that elders who are unable to remain in their homes are forced to relocate to nursing facilities at a distance away from their home settings. Rural communities indicated that they would be able to support assisted living facilities, but experienced difficulty in finding developers willing to build new facilities. Those individuals in urban settings reported that they also experienced a lack of housing options for aging-in-place, and additionally experienced concerns about a lack of support services for aging-in-place (Lawlor, 2009).

Understanding the market for assisted living facilities, especially those with aging-in-place care plans can be a challenge for individuals interested in these services, as well as the communities interested in sponsoring such facilities. Traditional market studies that assess indicators such as age, income, housing tenure, and other demographic data, will not accurately predict whether communities can support either the expenses associated with the building of new assisted living facilities or the retrofitting of older facilities (Lawlor, 2001).

State Regulations and Practices for Aging-in-Place in Assisted Living Facilities

State agencies have adopted a number of regulations that allow for a broad level of service delivery to meet the needs of assisted living residents as they age-in-place. According to a study conducted of state assisted living policies and practices by the National Academy for State Health Policy, 29 states and the District of Columbia supported regulations that promote the assisted living model of care that is resident focused rather than facility focused (Mollica, 2005). A report from the General Accounting Office in 1999 stated that assisted living facilities frequently support the concept of aging-in-place, or remain in their residence with declining or changing health care needs. The ability of elders to age in place is therefore reflected in each facility admission and discharge criteria, and also in the stated move-in and move-out policies and regulations (Mollica, 2005). A review of state regulations revealed considerable variability in the admission and retention criteria for residents wishing to age-in-place in a number of assisted living facilities. Assisted living facility administrators will need to review the regulations for the state in which they work.

Future Directions for Aging-in-Place

The demand for aging-in-place programs in assisted living facilities continues to grow as does the number of older adults who are either in assisted living facilities or considering entry into these settings. As the baby boomers age, the numbers of individuals who will need a care services increases and will continue to increase. The benefits of aging-in-place with an emphasis on quality of life and well-being continue to be of great importance to those interested in aging-in-place services. The problems associated with long-term care institutions also are factors driving increased demand for aging-in-place programs. While regulations vary widely from state-to-state, most states now have regulations in place that serve to facilitate aging-in-place programs in assisted living facilities.

Administrators can find resources and additional information about aging-in-place programs from a number of sources. Review of state regulations regarding aging-in-place has been determined an important resource for understanding the parameters for many aging-in-place programs. There are a number of online resources that administrators may find beneficial to obtain information in this area. Resources include but are not limited to include the AARP Public Policy Institute and the National Institute on Aging.

CASE STUDY

HG is a 78-year-old male who recently moved in an assisted living facility after living for 50 years in his suburban family home. The decision to move to the assisted living facility was very difficult for HG who did not want to move to many different facilities as he continued aging. While the assisted living facility that HG selected did not have a formal aging-in-place policy, HG was assured that he could anticipate spending many years in his new home.

Six months after moving into the assisted living facility, HG fell and broke his right hip. Following surgery to stabilize his hip fracture, HG was informed that he also suffered from severe osteoporosis and would probably experience many future difficulties in walking independently and could expect to be spending a great deal of time in a wheelchair. HG became very depressed as he thought of having to move from the assisted living facility and began to refuse to get out of bed, refused to eat, or spend time with his friends and family.

The administrator and staff of the assisted living facility met with HG to develop a plan that would allow HG to remain in the facility. The doorway to his room and his bathroom facilitated wheelchair access, and the staff worked to make adjustments to ensure safety such as the removal of scatter rugs, changing the location of HG's bed and several small room tables, and making sure that HG was able to access the shower in his bathroom. The administrator also worked with specialists including a physical therapist, occupational therapist, and registered nurse to address many of HG's physical and emotional needs.

The administrator and the staff of the assisted living facility understood the importance of aging-in-place for elders such as HG. Their willingness to work with HG to make adjustments to his physical space as well as their work to assist HG emotionally were extremely helpful in HG's physical and emotional recovery from his hip fracture. HG's depression improved as he moved back into the assisted living facility and informed his family and friends that he was living in the "best place on earth."

CONCLUSIONS

The areas of universal design and aging-in-place are relevant for changes that have the potential to improve the quality of living and well-being of elders in a number of settings, including assisted living facilities. This chapter served to present a basic understanding of both concepts as well as some of the benefits and challenges associated with universal design and aging-in-place. Services to residents in a number of assisted living facilities can be enhanced through an awareness of the information provided within this chapter.

REFERENCES

A Place for Mom Inc. (2009). *Orchards at Bartley.* Retrieved from: http://nursing-homes. aplaceformom.com/new-jersey/jackson/the-orchard-at -bartley-bartl

Ball, M. M., Perkins, M. M., Whittington, F. J., Connell, B. R., Hollingsworth, C., King, S. V., et al. (2004). Managing decline in assisted living: the key to aging-in-place. *The Journals of Gerontology Series B: Psychological Sciences and Social Sciences,* 59(4), S202–S212. Retrieved from http://psychsoc.Gerontologyjournals.org/cgi/content/ full/59/4/S202

Best of the Best. (2008). *Assisted Living Executive.* Retrieved from http://www.alfa.org/ alfa/Best_of_the_Best_.asp?SnID=2

Chapin, R., & Dobbs-Kepper, D. (2001). Aging-in-place in assisted living. Philosophy versus policy. *The Gerontologist,* 41, 43–50.

Lawlor, K. (2001). *Aging-in-place. Coordinating housing and health care provision for America's growing elderly population.* (Report, Fellowship Program for Emerging Leaders in Community and Economic Development, October, 2001).

Mace, R. L., Hardie, G. J., & Place, J. P. (1991). *Accessible environments: Toward universal design.* Retrieved from http://www.design.ncsu.edu/cud/pubs_p/docs/Acc

Miller, E. A., & Mor, V. (2006). *Out of the shadows. Envisioning a brighter future for long-term care in America.* Providence, RI: Brown University Center for Gerontology and Health Care Research.

Mollica, R. L. (2005). *Aging-in-place in assisted living: State regulations and practice.* Washington, DC: American Seniors Housing Association.

National Center for Assisted Living. (2006). HUD awards Assisted Living Conversion grants to six state projects. *Focus, 11*(12), 1–6.

Providence Health and Services. (2009). *Resident directed care at the Mount*. Retrieved from http://www.providence.org/long_term_care/mount_st_Vincent/e75resident.htm

Steinfeld, E. (1988). *Universal design: Housing for the lifespan of all people*. Washington, DC: U.S. Department of Housing and Urban Development.

The Center for Universal Design. North Carolina State University. (1997). *The principles of universal design*. Retrieved from http:// www.design.ncsu.edu/cud

CHAPTER 14

Diversity Issues

Learning Objectives

Upon the completion of Chapter 14, the reader will be able to:

- *Define the concepts of culture ethnicity, and heritage consistency.*
- *Describe the concept of diversity and cultural groups within the United States.*
- *Identify elements of selected cultural elder groups including:*
  African Americans
  Hispanic Americans
  Asian Americans
  Native Americans
  Gays and Lesbians
- *Discuss diversity issues.*
- *Understand selected diversity issues for selected elder groups including:*
  African Americans
  Hispanic Americans
  Asian Americans
  Native Americans
  Gays and Lesbians

INTRODUCTION

Assisted living facilities administrators both represent but also work with residents and staff from diverse cultural and social groups. Understanding of these differences can be beneficial for both administrators and for seniors. Information about the concepts of culture, ethnicity, and heritage consistency is provided to aid in this process. Additionally, diversity is explored in this chapter through a discussion of selected cultural groups including African Americans, Hispanics, Asian Americans, Native Americans, and gays and lesbians. Issues and challenges related to caring for diverse elders in several cultural groups will be presented as will select best practices in service provision to diverse elders including African Americans, Asian Americans, Native Americans, and members of gay and lesbian communities.

CONCEPTS OF CULTURE, ETHNICITY, AND HERITAGE CONSISTENCY

Ebersole, Hess, and Luggen (2004) report a marked increase in ethnically diverse seniors within the United States and projects that this trend will continue for the next 30 years underscoring the importance of an awareness of the concepts of culture, ethnicity, and heritage consistency serving to facilitate the understanding of diversity for administrators and members of assisted living communities. Culture can be viewed as the total of characteristics that are inherited by humans in varied groups and transmitted from one generation to the next generation. It includes the sum of beliefs, habits, norms, customs, rituals, likes, dislikes, and practices that are handed down through generations (Spector, 1991). The essential components of culture are frequently modified or altered by social, political, and economic forces and by the society in which individuals reside (Spector, 1991).

Ethnicity refers to social groups within social or cultural systems accorded status on the basis of variable and complex traits (Spector, 1991). Ethnicity can also be viewed as characteristics common to and shared by members of a specific group. These characteristics include the following: race; common geographic origin; language and dialect; shared traditions; religious faith; shared traditions and values; common literature, music, and folklore; food preferences; migration status; political special interests; institutions that provide specific group services; the internal sense of distinctiveness; the external perception of distinctiveness; and the presence of ties that transcend family and community boundaries (Spector, 1991). Cultural background is also noted to be an important component of the concept of ethnicity.

Spector (1991) notes that heritage consistency is a concept developed by Estes and Zitzow to describe the connections between an individual's lifestyle and their cultural background. The values associated with heritage consistency exist on a continuum and range from a traditional or consistent heritage to an acculturated or inconsistent heritage. Heritage consistency is also identified by a number of defining factors. These factors include the following: (1) childhood development occurring in either the individual's country of origin or in an immigrant neighborhood in the United States that represents the individual's ethnic group: (2) individuals return frequently to their country of origin or their immigrant neighborhood; (3) family homes are in ethnic communities; (4) individuals participate in ethnic and cultural events; (5) they are raised and visit regularly in extended families: (6) individuals have knowledge of their culture and language of origin; (7) they engage in social activities with others of the same ethnic background; and (8) individuals possess a sense of personal pride in their ethnic and cultural background (Spector, 1991).

The concepts of culture, ethnicity, and heritage consistency are inter-related and interconnected. An awareness of these concepts can provide administrators with information needed to provide services that are both sensitive and relevant for elders residing in assisted living facilities.

Diversity and Cultural Groups

There are multiple cultural groups residing in the United States. Demographic changes in the United States occurring recently reveal that fewer than 75% of Americans are considered to be non-Hispanic Whites, in contrast to the early 1900s when 87% of Americans were considered to be White (Aronson, 2002). Additionally, the numbers of African Americans, Hispanics, Asian Americans, and Middle Eastern Americans are increasing and experts project that by the middle of this century, all cultural and ethnic groups will be considered to be minorities (Aronson, 2002).

Assisted living administrators may have interactions with both elders and staff reflecting one or more of many cultural or social entities. Information about elders residing in selected groups including African Americans, Hispanic Americans, Asian Americans, Native Americans, and members of the gay and lesbian communities can enhance understanding necessary for the provision of adequate or enhanced senior services to these individuals. Data regarding aspects of each of these cultural groups, including ethnicity, family, and health will be discussed further.

African Americans

African Americans constitute about 12.4% of the total United States population according to United States census data (U.S. Census Bureau, 2000). Increases in overall diversity during the late 20th century have resulted in increases in African Americans, and this group remains larger than other non-White groups in selected regional areas including the Northeast, Midwest, and Southern United States (NKI Center of Excellence, African Americans, 2008). Although there has been geographic dispersion of African Americans, many of these individuals remain regionally concentrated, especially in the southern United States. It is important to note that many African Americans identify themselves as Black in combination with one or more races, indicating a significant interracial and diverse population (NKI Center of Excellence, African Americans, 2008)

The age composition of African Americans, while described as being a relatively "younger" population, reflects general trends toward aging with projections of the numbers of elders increasing by 102% through 2020 (NKI Center of Excellence, African Americans, 2008). Increases in aging African Americans are tempered by statistics indicating shorter life expectancies for this cultural group as compared to the general population in the United States. African Americans have a life expectancy of 73.2 years as compared to the general population life expectancy of 77.8 years.

Historical factors contribute to an understanding of African Americans. The Transatlantic Slave Trade resulted in the forced immigration of approximately 500,000 individuals during the 15th through the 18th centuries. Most of these individuals worked on plantations in the southern United States. Many African American slaves also moved west with the Westward Expansion of the United States and continued this western migration following the Civil War. During the 20th century, many African Americans moved from rural to urban areas in both northern and mid-western United States (NKI Center of Excellence, African Americans, 2008).

For many African Americans, slavery formed the basis for their culture within an essentially White, European American society. Effects of slavery evident in this culture include discrimination, poverty, social obstacles, and psychological barriers (Miller, 2009). Continuing elements of racism continue in the United States in the present day, contributing to many of the problems experienced by African Americans.

The values held by African Americans are widely varied and may reflect cultural practices from a number of African societies, from adapted American cultural norms, or from personal experiences (NKI Center of Excellence, African Americans, 2008). A history of slavery served to influence the cultural beliefs for many of these individuals, creating a heterogeneous cultural group. Many older African Americans place great value in connections with their churches. The Black church serves an important function in African American culture and communities, providing social and economic connections for elders as well as other members of this group.

Miller (2009) additionally reported data indicating that older African Americans identify with a specific culture. This culture can be characterized by elements including: (1) economic status that is moving from lower income to middle and upper income levels; (2) increases in the numbers of professionals with children who are also professionals; (3) wide ranging educational achievements from minimal education to doctoral level education; (4) religious affiliations with a range of religious groups; and (5) family connections with some elders receiving care from children and others providing care to both their children and grandchildren.

There are variations in African American family structures representing both married couple families, single parent families, many headed by females, and intergenerational families. As noted, many older African Americans serve as grandparent caregivers for their families or for unrelated children as necessary (NKI Center of Excellence, African Americans, 2008). Education, social structure, cultural identity, and personal experiences are also determinants of African American families and changes in families also reflect changing views on racism and discrimination in the United States (NKI Center of Excellence, African Americans, 2008). It is also important to note that in many of the traditions evolving from African American experiences in the southern United States elevate the status of elders in both families and society. Elders are thought to possess wisdom and knowledge as the result of prior experiences and are given elevated status in their homes, churches, and communities. Family caregiving for African American elders is both encouraged and valued in the African American culture (National Association of State Units on Aging, 2009).

Hispanic Americans

The United States classifies Hispanic Americans as members of a specific ethnic group, and not as a specific race. Hispanic is the term used to refer to individuals with Spanish heritage who originate from Spain or Spanish countries in the Americas, and who speak the Spanish language. This is in contrast to Latino Americans who originate from Mexico, Central America or South America and may also speak the Spanish language. Currently, these terms are used interchangeably to identify those individuals representing groups from all geographic areas.

Hispanics or Hispanic Americans represent the largest minority group in the United States, comprise about 14% of the total population, and are estimated to make up nearly 30% of the total population by the year 2050 (NKI Center of Excellence, Hispanics/Latinos, 2008). Currently, Hispanic Americans number more than 35 million individuals, representing an extremely diverse, dynamic, and rapidly growing ethnic groups in the United States (National Association of State Units on Aging, 2009). The Hispanic American older population is expected to increase by over 500% in the next 30 years compared to a less than 100% increase in White elders (NKI Center of Excellence, Hispanics/Latinos, 2008).

There is significant variability in the origins of this ethnic group in the United States. Individuals from Puerto Rico live in the northeastern United States and are more likely to have been born in the United States than other ethnic groups. Mexicans are more likely to live in the western United States and are more likely to hold lower socioeconomic status. Cubans live primarily in the southern United States and hold higher levels of education and socioeconomic status than other Hispanic Americans (Alegria et al., 2008).

Historically, many Mexicans immigrated to the United States to build railroads in the southwestern areas of the country. During the time period from 1940 to 1960, experienced agricultural laborers immigrated to the United States to work in the agricultural industries. Currently, many farm workers are undocumented, and while representative of younger age groups, these individuals will increase the numbers of aging Mexicans residing in the United States (Miller, 2009).

Many Cubans immigrated to the United States during the 19th century to work in the tobacco industry, and a large number of Cubans came to the United States between 1959 and 1979 for political reasons. These Cubans came primarily from middle and upper middle-class families, and represent a significant population of aging individuals, primarily residing in the southern United States. Puerto Ricans, granted citizenship status in the United States in 1917, moved for primarily economic, social, and family reasons, and have mainly stayed in the northern parts of the United States (Miller, 2009).

Many Hispanic Americans encounter a number of socioeconomic barriers and are considered to be overrepresented in low paying jobs, and underrepresented in professional and higher paying employment (NKI Center of Excellence, Hispanics/Latinos, 2008). Many Hispanic Americans work in lower paying agricultural or service jobs, and are much more likely to live in poverty than non-White Hispanics (NKI Center of Excellence, Hispanics/Latinos, 2008). Socioeconomic disadvantages create a number of problems for Hispanic Americans in many of the different ethnic groups.

Many Hispanic Americans hold strong family ties and family values. The emphasis on family connections and collaborative efforts to protect and provide for all family members are characteristics held by this ethnic group (NKI Center of Excellence, Hispanics/Latinos, 2008). The needs of individual family members are placed above the needs of individuals within these ethnic groups. Many older Hispanic Americans are more likely to live with family members or with family support than to live in institutional settings.

Hispanic American women comprise over 50 % of the total Hispanic population in the United States, and are most likely to work in low-paying occupations including restaurants, factories, or clerical positions (U.S. Bureau of the Census, 2000). Unemployment rates are much higher for Hispanic American women than for White women who also encounter many socioeconomic disadvantages, including higher poverty levels, single parenthood, and lower educational levels (NKI Center of Excellence, Hispanics/Latinos, 2008). Much of the family caregiving responsibility resides with Hispanic American women.

Asian Americans

The term Asian Americans refers to many diverse sub-groups of individuals living in the United States. The term "Asian" refers to those individuals from the Far East, Southeast Asia, as well as the Indian subcontinent that includes China and India (Miller, 2009). Chinese Americans represent the largest number of individuals residing within this cultural group and account for about 30 % of Asian elders. Japanese and Filipino elders each comprise about 24 % of the total Asian elder population with individuals from Korea, Vietnam, Cambodia, and Asian India comprising many remaining elder groups (Miller, 2009).

Many Chinese migrated to the United States during the 19th century in response to population overcrowding in China, inter-village conflicts, and the onset of the Gold Rush in the western United States (NKI Center of Excellence, Chinese Americans, 2008). Many Chinese laborers worked on the transcontinental railroad, in factories, or in agricultural settings, but were declared ineligible for citizenship in 1871 and subjected to other discriminatory practices that halted migration from China to the United States (NKI Center of Excellence, 2009). Immigration from mainland China and Taiwan resumed during the late 1960s and 1970s with many Chinese students, families, and professionals entering the United States (NKI Center of Excellence, Chinese Americans, 2008). Early immigrants lived together in communities called Chinatowns, many of which still exist in a number of urban settings. Currently, many of these well educated professionals live in urban areas in California, Hawaii, New York, Texas, and Illinois.

Japanese immigrants came to the United States in the mid 19th century. In 1942, all Japanese Americans were relocated into internment camps. Immigration increased in the mid-1960s when many immigration restrictions were relaxed (Miller, 2009). Filipinos and Koreans immigrated to the United States initially to assume positions as laborers in agricultural settings. Current immigrants are much more likely to be students, college educated, and professionals. Vietnamese and Cambodian immigrants have entered the United States fairly recently as political refugees, many coming from war zones or refugee camps (Miller, 2009).

The concept of family is of critical importance to Asian Americans. The family is considered to be the backbone of Chinese society and the family functions as a collective unit where family members assume interdependent roles (NKI Center of Excellence, Chinese Americans, 2008). The Confucian concept of filial piety or xiao is central to the Chinese family with children expected to provide their elders with respect, loyalty, provision of material goods, obedience, and physical care (Heying, Guangya, & Xinping, 2006). Chinese family members rely on the family for support and assistance and problems and conflicts are expected to be resolved within the family unit as opposed to outside the family (NKI Center of Excellence, Chinese Americans, 2008). In general, Asian American older adults are less likely to live alone than elders in the general United States population. Language barriers are variable with many Asian Americans born in the United States exhibiting bilingual capabilities and many elders and immigrants able to speak only their native language.

Women in Asian American families have traditionally assumed roles that demonstrate respect for male dominance in both family and cultural settings. These roles are now changing as women assume responsibilities not only for family caregiving, especially for children and elderly family members as well as for careers outside of the home. The current responsibilities of these women frequently add to increased stress levels for both the women in question, but also for others within family settings.

Native Americans

The terms Native American and American Indian are used to refer to individuals who are direct descendents of indigenous peoples residing in North America prior to the arrival of European settlers. A number of these indigenous groups, identified as tribes or nations, hold cultural practices that are influenced by geographic, regional, and socioeconomic factors and vary from group to group (Reynolds et al., 2006; NKI Center of Excellence, Native Americans, 2008). Currently, an estimated 4.5 million Native Americans and Alaska Natives reside in the United States, and about 325,000 of these individuals were aged 65 and older (NKI Center of Excellence, Native Americans, 2008). It is important to note that about 60% of Native Americans currently live in urban settings rather than rural or tribal land settings (Yurkovich & Lattergrass, 2008). Many Native Americans reside in the western United States, but there are Native Americans currently living in Texas, Michigan, New York, Florida, and Alaska (Miller, 2009).

Demographically, many Native Americans are poor, living either with their family members or alone. Younger Native Americans are likely to speak English; older Native Americans speak either English or one of a number of indigenous languages. Many Native Americans have low educational levels with a high school education or less (Miller, 2009).

In general, Native Americans hold cultural beliefs that are holistic in design, and view humans as connected physically, mentally, spiritually, and emotionally. The mind-body splitting that is common in western thought is viewed as adverse to many Native Americans (Yurkovich & Lattergrass, 2008). Group membership, connections to nature, respect for the environment, respect for elders, and honor are all viewed by many Native Americans as essential for sustaining their culture. Spirituality and trustworthiness are important to Native Americans who place importance and value on the community as a whole and group success as opposed to individual successes (NKI Center of Excellence, Native Americans, 2008).

Family structures and roles are varied among Native American tribes. The concept of extended family is very strong within Native American culture, providing a network of relationships beyond individual families and tribal groups. In many Native American communities, extended families support children and this is viewed positively for the development of social relationships and supportive environments (NKI Center of Excellence, Native Americans, 2008). Extended families and communities take precedence over the demands of individuals, and frequently include a connection to ancestors through tribal history. Additionally, families are usually multigenerational, including caregiving for both children and for elders (NKI Center of Excellence, Native Americans, 2008).

The roles of many Native American women are significant in many tribes and societies. Women serve important roles in the preservation and transmission of culture and values. Women are regarded as life givers, teachers, healers, doctors, and seers with many viewing women and women's roles as essential for the health of communities (Walters et al., 2006).

Gays and Lesbians

The numbers of gay and lesbian elders aged 65 and older in the United States are thought to be in the range of 1 to 3 million according to the Policy Institute of the National Gay and Lesbian Task Force (Cahill, South, & Spade, 2000). Estimates are that these numbers will increase the next two decades with approximately 4 million elder sexual minority members in the United States (Cahill, South, & Spade, 2000).

Many older gays and lesbians are well educated, middle-class, employed, and involved in a committed relationship. Recent study of 1,000 gay and lesbian baby boomers revealed that about 78% of study respondents had either a college or graduate degree and about 69% of respondents lived in households with annual incomes ranging from $50,000 to over $150,000 (Lourde, 2009).

While gays and lesbians come from a number of different cultural and ethnic backgrounds, many of these individuals noted prior experiences as caregivers for family members or friends and about 80% of these individuals noted that they planned to provide caregiving services at some point in the future (Lourde, 2009). Many of these individuals are concerned that they will not have family members, friends, or children to care for them as they age.

Geographically dispersed throughout the United States, additional data on the culture of older gays and lesbians is difficult to obtain, mainly because these individuals are invisible in many settings and to many individuals. Older gays and lesbians note that they experience discrimination in a number of areas including housing, employment, legal protection, and benefits for partners (Anetzberger, Ishler, Mostade, & Blair, 2004). Additionally, fear of discrimination has been identified as a major barrier for many of these individuals who are afraid to seek health or social services. Many older gays and lesbians also identify fears for personal safety in institutional settings including assisted living facilities or skilled nursing facilities. These fears also involve concerns about the care or services that will be received if these elders seek care in institutional settings.

DIVERSITY ISSUES

While assisted living facility administrators do not provide direct care services to elders, they can improve elder care services and also enhance staff care delivery through an understanding of diversity and diversity issues. Selected diversity issues faced by older African Americans, Hispanic Americans, Asian Americans, Native Americans, and gays and lesbians will be identified and discussed further.

African Americans

Diversity issues faced by many aging African Americans are focused in the areas of family values, as well racial disparity, poverty, and prior history of discrimination. For many African Americans, family members are expected to provide caregiving services to elders and the use of assisted living facilities or other institutional settings remains limited or not used in many communities. Additionally, many African American elders are the primary caregivers for children or grandchildren making it difficult for them to receive care as needed.

While there are services and assisted living facilities dedicated to service provision specifically for African Americans, issues related to the number and location of these facilities have been identified. As Howard and colleagues (2002) noted, African Americans tend to seek services in facilities utilized by African Americans while Whites resided in facilities primarily for White elders. Facilities for African Americans were located in primarily rural African American communities. These facilities also tended to have lower cleanliness and maintenance ratings (Howard et al., 2002). Despite these limitations, African Americans may actually benefit from care received in assisted living facilities with predominately African American residents and staff. The major reasons for potential benefits include: (1) African Americans require services that address many of their unique physical and social problems; and (2) African American care providers have a better understanding of the cultural and social context of many of the illnesses within this community (Howard et al., 2002).

Issues related to poor health status as a result of poverty, inadequate access to health care services, and underutilization of health care services, have been identified in African American communities. African Americans have higher rates of morbidity, disability, and mortality than do Whites in similar age groups. Poverty for many African Americans does not occur with aging but rather is the result of lifelong patterns of discrimination and many disadvantages and this is unique for African Americans (NKI Center of Excellence, African Americans, 2008).

Issues related to financial barriers experienced by many African Americans also have origins in lifelong poverty and disadvantaged backgrounds. Issues related to location and time barriers contribute to decreased care delivery for many African Americans who do not have easy or appropriate access to necessary care services or assisted living facilities located near to family members (NKI Center of Excellence, African Americans, 2008).

Best practices for care delivery to African American elders will need to be developed and focused on care that focuses on the social, cultural, and fiscal issues faced by this population. As previously noted, facilities have been designed for this population but remain geographically limited. Many facilities do not meet current or minimal care standards, making care for this cultural group a future priority.

Hispanic Americans

There are a number of diversity issues experienced by Hispanic American elders. These issues include; communication problems, family structures, poverty, and the presence of a number of chronic illnesses.

Many of these elders experience significant communication problems related to an inability of elders to speak English, and an inability of care providers to communicate in Spanish. These language barriers create problems in the delivery of safe and effective care, and increase frustration and difficulties for Hispanic American seniors.

For many Hispanic Americans, cultural values are associated with strong family connections. Family members are expected to provide care when needed to their elders. Problems and issues develop when families are unable to help family members and must use other options. There are a limited number of assisted living facilities providing culturally relevant services for Hispanic American seniors, creating problems not only for seniors and their families, but also for staff members and facility administrators.

The poverty experienced by many Hispanic American elders is an issue for many of these individuals experiencing many of the problems and chronic illnesses connected to inadequate health care and poor nutrition. Many of these illnesses result in increased morbidity and mortality for Hispanic American elders. Rates of obesity, diabetes, metabolic syndrome, heart disease, and hypertension are increased in this ethnic group as opposed to members of other ethnic and cultural groups. Additional issues of decreased care access are identified in Hispanic American elders. This is related in part to a lack of health insurance and in part to the costs of health insurance. Hispanic Americans are considered to have the highest rates of medical insurance in the United States (NKI Center of Excellence, Hispanics/Latinos, 2008).

Asian Americans

Diversity issues impacting many aging Asian Americans include language barriers, family values, the role of elders in society, and poverty. Many Asian American elders have communication problems because they do not speak English and frequently must rely on care services from non-Chinese-speaking providers or translators. These language difficulties exacerbate existing problems and create new problems for elders both in the community as well as in assisted living and other long-term care facilities. Assisted living facility administrators must take language barriers into consideration as they plan services for many Asian American residents.

The family values held by many Asian Americans give elderly family members great respect and status within family units. Many elders expect to receive caregiving services from family members and do not plan for aging in institutional settings. This creates potential problems when family members are not available to provide care services or when family members have to work both inside the home as well as hold outside jobs. Because many of these cultural groups stress social responsibilities to the family over individual rights, care for aging family members can create increased family stresses, especially when elders are placed in assisted living facilities or other institutional settings.

Poverty is another issue that contributes to many of the problems experienced by Asian American elders. Poverty creates an environment where elders are at increased risk for health issues related to inadequate nutrition, inadequate health care delivery, and poorer health care outcomes. Elders working in substandard working conditions during their lifetimes are also at increased risk for number chronic illnesses that increase morbidity and mortality.

Administrators and staff in a number of assisted living facilities and organizations can benefit from the identification of best practice for service delivery to Asian American elders. One such best practice can be found in assisted living facilities designed specifically to address the diversity of this population. Aegis Gardens in Fremont, CA offers services for Asian American elders in a for-profit facility. Facility staff speaks Chinese, the facilities have been designed with Chinese decorations and gardens, and Chinese food is served to residents who access services specific to their culture (Gokhale, 2007).

Another example of a best practice in caring for Asian American elders is located in the Self–Help for the Elderly, operates facilities for Chinese elders in San Francisco, Santa Clara, and San Jose, CA. These facilities provide residents with staff who are multi-lingual and able to communicate in several Chinese dialects. Residents are also able to access culturally specific services including games such as Mahjong, arts and crafts, and festivals as well as Chinese food (Self-Help for the Elderly, 2009).

The Paolo Chinese Home in Hawaii has been providing assisted living services to Chinese elders in Hawaii since 1896 and represents another best practice in elder care for Asian Americans. This facility focuses on the delivery of culturally relevant services including meals and social services to a predominantly Chinese population. The focus of these services is also on progressive elder care through culturally relevant services for Asian Americans living in Hawaii (Hawaii Business, 2004).

Services for Southeast Asians provided by the AristaCare Health Services in Perth Amboy, NJ represent another example of a best practice in elder care for Asian Americans. This organization developed the "AristaCare Indian Program" to provide culturally sensitive care to Indian American seniors. Services to Indian American elders include Indian food, access to Indian television stations, and care services delivered by Indian physicians and nurses. Elders participating in this program are also able to participate in a number of Hindu festivals and ceremonies (Gokhale, 2007). Elders in this group are thus able to participate in activities that promote physical, social, and religious well-being.

Native Americans

Diversity issues identified in this population include access to culturally relevant assisted living facilities, challenges associated with cultural differences, prevalence of chronic illnesses, and past history of discrimination.

There are very few assisted living facilities available in the United States providing culturally relevant and appropriate services for Native Americans who represent a heterogeneous group of individuals. The United States Indian Health Service is designated as the primary health care service provider for Native Americans. Most of these services are in the form of clinics providing acute or crisis-focused services, and most clinic facilities are located on reservations (NKI Center of Excellence, Native Americans, 2008). Access to these services is limited for many Native Americans who live in urban areas rather than on reservations.

Beliefs in holism and the connection of physical, emotional, spiritual, and cognitive aspects of humans are central to Native American culture. These beliefs are frequently in conflict with the mind-body approach associated with western health care. Many assisted living facilities use a medical model of care that is in direct conflict with Native American beliefs and values. Also, many Native Americans rely on spiritual and traditional healing methods which are incongruent with traditional medical interventions. These cultural conflicts must be addressed by assisted living administrators and staff as they work to provide care to Native American residents.

Native Americans as a group are at risk for a number of significant chronic illnesses. Rates of diabetes, obesity, heart disease, hypertension, and metabolic syndrome are increased in this population, increasing in severity as Native Americans age (Spector, 1991). Major psychiatric problems for Native Americans include alcoholism, substance abuse, pathological gambling, depression, stress, and anxiety with some researchers noting a 70% lifetime diagnosis for alcoholism (NKI Center of Excellence, Native Americans, 2008). Assisted living administrators and those caring for Native Americans must have an awareness of the risks associated with these problems, and must also be prepared to provide services needed to combat these severe and chronic illnesses.

A final diversity issue facing those caring for Native American elders is the history of past discrimination faced by Native Americans as part of a history that included forced relocation, oppression, and both community and individual trauma (NKI Center of Excellence, Native Americans, 2008). For many Native Americans, prior United States laws and governmental practices have created a climate of mistrust for any services provided by agencies or institutions whether they are private or government sponsored. This mistrust creates barriers for those caring for Native American elders and present challenges for administrators and staff members who must work with these individuals.

While administrators and staff working in assisted living facilities and organizations will need to provide culturally relevant services to be providing services to support Native American elders, few of these facilities currently exist. A best practice for the care of Native American elders can be found in an assisted living facility in Dillingham, Alaska. The identified 10-unit assisted living facility has been named Marralut Eniit or "Grandma's House" in the Yupik language. Based in a fishing community of 3,000 individuals, the facility provides a number of services valued by Eskimo, Aleut, and Yupik elders. These services include a steam bath and the provision of culturally specific foods (Native American Report, 2006).

Gays and Lesbians

Diversity issues of importance when addressing care for gay and lesbian elders are focused around stigma, discrimination, and access to housing that is culturally relevant for these individuals. Each of these issues will be briefly discussed.

Stigma is a very significant issue faced by aging gays and lesbians who describe many years of dealing with homophobia or the fear and hatred associated with homosexuals (Cook-Daniels, 2003). Stigma related to sexual orientation for these individuals has been both wide spread and pervasive and has been encountered by many of these individuals throughout their lives. One serious consequence of this stigma is the invisibility that many older gays and lesbians have adopted in many areas, especially in the health care arena. Sexual identity is concealed in an attempt to prevent abuse or substandard care resulting in impeded care access to vitally important services. Stigma creates a climate of fear and mistrust that causes these individuals to avoid situations and services that are viewed to be potentially damaging or abusive and in effect increases problems, especially health care problems. Assisted living administrators must be aware of the stigma faced by older gays and lesbians who may reside in assisted living facilities but have not disclosed their sexual orientation to either staff or other residents. Culturally sensitive services cannot be provided to these individuals if identities are hidden or not readily disclosed. Administrators must work with staff and residents to create an environment that promotes understanding, and welcomes elders who may be gay and lesbian.

Discrimination is an important issue for aging gay and lesbian elders. Many of these individuals have experienced discrimination in all aspects of their lives, especially in the areas of health care and housing. Recent changes in legislation have improved the status of partnerships, but a lack of formal recognition of personal relationships has created inequities for gay and lesbian elders. These inequities include discriminatory treatment in hospital visitation rights, health decision making, pension and tax regulations, housing rights, Medicare and Social Security coverage, and Medicaid regulations (Funders for Lesbian and Gay Issues, 2004). Additionally, many gays and lesbians, in relationships face discrimination in institutional care settings because their relationships many times are not formally recognized or legally protected. Risks of separation from partners occur for gays and lesbians and there is evidence in the research literature identifying prohibitions on same-sex couples living together in many elder care institutions (Funders for Lesbian and Gay Issues, 2004). It is important to note that in 2003, the Joint Commission on the Accreditation of Healthcare Organizations adopted respect for resident's rights (including rights for lifestyle choices connected to sexual orientation) as important requirements for assisted living facilities (Funders for Lesbian and Gay Issues, 2004).

Despite recent advances at both federal and organizational levels, discrimination continues to seriously impact the health and quality of life for aging gays and lesbians. Assisted living administrators must be prepared to work with older gays and lesbians to ensure that discriminatory practices do not occur within their facilities. Staff and residents should be educated to understand both the history and the consequences of discrimination experienced by gays and lesbians and strategies to avoid discrimination implemented for both residents and staff members within assisted living facilities.

Housing for aging gays and lesbians remains a significant issue across the United States. There are very few facilities designed to address the cultural needs of these elders. Many older gays and lesbians do not have family or social networks to provide needed care services, and they are afraid to access existing services and facilities because of prior discrimination. There are emerging models for housing, including assisted living facilities, that are being developed across the United States, but many of these facilities are expensive. Housing for low-income gays and lesbians remains limited making access to affordable, convenient, and safe housing limited or nonexistent for many gays and lesbians.

An example of a best practice in the delivery of elder care services for gays and lesbians includes Openhouse in San Francisco. Openhouse is a nonprofit community organization designed to develop and promote an inclusive residential community especially welcoming for older gays and lesbians. The community includes supportive services for low-income to upper-income gays and lesbians, and focuses on services that are culturally sensitive and supportive for this group of previously disadvantaged seniors (Funders for Lesbian and Gay Issues, 2004).

CASE STUDY

FC is the administrator of a small assisted living facility located in a small southern community who has been asked to mediate a dispute between the assisted living facility staff and MG, a 74-year-old male and facility resident for the past 10 years. The staff is complaining that MG has his male friend spend the weekends with him on a regular basis. While the facility has a policy encouraging married couples to spend weekends together, there is no policy in place for single couples. Several staff members note that two men who would be "sleeping together" should be removed from the assisted living facility community. MG discloses to the administrator that he is gay and would like to have his partner of 5 years spend weekends with him at the facility. Because married couples are encouraged to spend weekends together, MG feels that it is appropriate for his partner to spend weekends at the facility. MG additionally notes that the assisted living facility is his home, that he is unable to manage the stairs in his partner's home and can't live with his partner, and if he is not allowed to stay at the facility he will become homeless.

FC recognizes that there are many issues related to elder care of diverse groups, and is committed to the provision of culturally competent care involving care that is acceptable and useful to elders' cultural background and cultural expectations. She also notes that culturally competent care involves an awareness of provider personal biases, knowledge of population specific cultural values, and provider skills in working with diverse populations (McBride, 2010). FC arranges for a member of the local gay and lesbian community to speak to the facility staff regarding issues important to their community. Additional sessions are also arranged for the staff to discuss their feelings about care of gay residents. FC additionally reviewed and modified the facility policy to include significant others in weekend visits. Following these changes, FC notes that many of the facility staff has a better understanding of how to care for gay elders and more importantly, MG is now happily spending weekends with his partner.

CONCLUSIONS

Assisted living administrators can improve their work with elders through improved understanding of culture and cultural issues identified in a number of diverse groups. As noted in this chapter, awareness of selected cultural differences noted in aging African Americans, Hispanic Americans, Asian Americans, Native Americans, and aging gays and lesbians can provide assisted living facility administrators and their staff members with valuable information. This knowledge can then be used to enhance important services to elderly residents.

REFERENCES

Alegria, M., et al. (2008). Prevalence of mental illness in immigrant and non-immigrant U.S. Latino groups. *American Journal of Psychiatry, 165*(3), 359–369.

Anetzberger, G. J., Ishler, K. J., & Blair, M. (2004). Gay and gray: A community dialogue on the issues and concerns of older gays and lesbians. *Journal of Gay and Lesbian Social Services, 17*(1), 23–45.

Aronson, D. (2002). *Civil Rights Journal.* Retrieved from http://findarticles.com/p/articles/mimOHSP/is_1_6/ai_106647784/

Cahill, S., South, K., & Spade, J. (2000). Outing age. Public policy issues affecting gay, lesbian, bisexual and transgender elders. *The Policy Institute of the National Gay and Lesbian Task Force Foundation.* Retrieved from http://www.thetaskforc.org/downloads/reports

Ebersole, P., Hess, P., & Luggin, A. S. (2004). *Toward healthy aging: Human needs and nursing response* (6th ed.). St. Louis: Mosby.

Funders for Lesbian and Gay Issues. (2004). *Aging in equity. LGBT elders in America.* New York: The Press Room.

Gokhale, K. (2007, August 3). *Experts say assisted living stigma needs to be overcome. India West.* Retrieved from http://www.indiawest.com/view.php?subaction=showfull&id=1186012652&archieve=&start_from=&ucat=11(1of3)8/3/2007 11:50:20

Heying, J. Z., Guangya, L., & Guan, X. (2006). Willingness and availability: Explaining new attitudes toward institutional elder care among Chinese elderly parents and their adult children. *Journal of Aging Studies, 20*(3), 279–290.

Howard, D. L., Sloane, P. D., Zimmerman, S., Eckert, J. K., Walsh, J. F., Bule, V. C., et al. (2002). Distribution of African Americans in residential care/assisted living and nursing homes: More evidence of racial disparity? *American Journal of Public Health, 92*(8), 1272–1277.

Innovative Assisted Living Project Helps Sell Concept to Alaska Natives. (2006, April 1). *Native American Report.* Retrieved from: http://www.accessmylibrary.com/article-1G1-145283888/innovative-assisted-living-proje. . .

Lourde, K. (2009). Facing discrimination issues. *Provider,* 20–32.

McBride, M. (2010). *Geriatric resources for care of older adults: Ethnogeriatrics and cultural competence for nursing practice.* Retrieved from http://consultgerirn.org/topics/ethnogeriatircs-and-cultural-competence-for-nursing-pract . . .

Miller, C. A. (2009). *Nursing for wellness in older adults* (5th ed.). Philadelphia: Lippincott, Williams, & Wilkins.

National Association of State Units on Aging. (2009, October 15). *America's diversity guide. Chapter 2: Cultural and ethnic diversity.* Retrieved from http://www.nasua.org/issues/tech_assist_resorces/national_aging_ir_support_ctr/diversity

NKI Center of Excellence in Culturally Competent Mental Health. (2008). *African Americans.* Retrieved from http://ssrdqst.rfmh.org/cecc/index.php?q=node/8

NKI Center of Excellence in Culturally Competent Mental Health. (2008). *Chinese Americans.* Retrieved from http://ssrdqst.rfmh.org/cecc/index.php?q=node/24

NKI Center of Excellence in Culturally Competent Mental Health. (2008). *Hispanics/Latinos.* Retrieved from http://ssrdqst.rfmh.org/cecc/index.php?q=node/64

NKI Center of Excellence in Culturally Competent Mental Health. (2008). *Native Americans.* Retrieved from http://ssrdqst.rfmh.org/cecc/index.php?q=node/22

Palolo Chinese Home: Legacy in Action for Elders. (2004, May 1). *Hawaii Business.* Retrieved from http://www.allbusiness.com/north-america/united-states-hawaii/142199-1.html

Reynolds, W. R., Quevillion, R. P., Boyd, B., & Mackey, D. (2006). Initial development of a cultural values and beliefs scale among dakota/nakota/lakota people: A pilot study. *American Indian and Alaska Native Mental Health Research, The Journal of the National Center, 13*(3), 70–97.

Self-Help for the Elderly. (2009). *Kwok Yuen assisted living in San Jose.* Retrieved from http//www.selfhelpelderly.org/services/assisted_living/san_jose/kwok_yuen/index.php

Spector, R. E. (1991). *Cultural diversity in health and illness* (3rd ed.). San Mateo, CA: Appleton & Lange.

U.S. Bureau of the Census. (2000). *The 65 years and older population: 2000* (Census Brief). Retrieved from http://www.census.gov

Walters, K. L., Evans-Campbell, T., Simoni, J., Ronquillo, T., & Bhuyan, R. (2006). "My spirit in my heart": Identity experiences and challenges among American Indian tow-spirit women. *Journal of Lesbian Studies, 10*(1/2), 125–149.

Yurkovich, E. E., & Lattergrass, I. (2008). Defining health an unhealthiness: Perceptions held by native American Indians with persistent mental illness. *Mental Health, Religion and Culture, 11*(5), 437–459.

Physical Aspects of Aging

LEARNING OBJECTIVES

Upon the completion of Chapter 15, the reader will be able to:

- *Describe selected normal physiologic changes associated with aging.*
- *Discuss nutritional assessment in aging individuals.*
- *Describe strategies to maintain healthy nutrition in aging individuals.*
- *Identify elements of mobility assessment.*
- *Discuss strategies to promote mobility in aging individuals.*
- *Identify risk factors and assessment strategies for falls prevention.*
- *Discuss strategies for sleep assessment in aging individuals.*
- *Discuss strategies to improve sleep conditions in aging individuals.*
- *Describe assessment of chronic pain in aging individuals.*
- *Discuss selected treatments for chronic pain in aging individuals.*
- *Discuss selected best practices in mobility, falls prevention, and pain management.*

INTRODUCTION

Although administrators working in assisted living facilities do not usually provide direct clinical services to elders, an understanding of how the normal aging process impacts a number of important body systems can provide useful information used in the decision making needed to effectively provide resident services. Age-related changes to selected systems including the cardiovascular, pulmonary, muscular, orthopedic, gastroenterological, genitourinary, neurologic, skin and lymphatic systems will be identified, as will issues related to physiological aspects of aging. Additionally, nutrition, mobility, falls, sleep, and chronic pain issues will be briefly discussed within this chapter. Strategies and best practices identified in improving and dealing with selected physical aspects of aging will be presented throughout this chapter.

OVERVIEW OF NORMAL PHYSIOLOGIC CHANGES ASSOCIATED WITH AGING

Age-Related Changes to the Cardiovascular System

The cardiovascular system consists of the heart and the vascular system, a series of arteries and veins that carry oxygen and nutrients from the heart to all body systems, and remove carbon dioxide and waste back to the lungs. Structural changes to the heart muscle occur with aging as the heart muscle increases in size, and the heart chambers and heart cells increase in size and thicken. These changes, especially in the left ventricle or major pumping chamber of the heart, cause reductions in muscle flexibility and make the heart a less effective pump. The ability of the heart to contract or exert force to pump blood throughout the body does not appear however to change with normal aging (Mauk, 2006).

As arteries age, the walls of these blood vessels become stiff and twisted. This creates an increased resistance to blood flow requiring increased pressure to pump blood from the heart to arteries throughout the body. Increases in pressure then lead to additional changes and damage to these important blood vessels. Veins, the blood vessels designed to return deoxygenated blood from the periphery of the body, also undergo aging changes. With aging, veins become thicker, more dilated, and less elastic. The valves in veins also become less efficient in returning blood back to the heart (Miller, 2009). These changes make blood return to the heart less efficient, and also cause blood to remain in the extremities. This can result in dependent edema in the lower extremities, especially after sitting for long periods of time.

Age-related changes to cardiovascular physiology are thought to be minimal, and healthy elders have heart muscles that are able to adapt to a number of physiologic changes and stressors. Functional changes associated with aging include decreased adaptive responses to exercise, decreased blood flow to the brain, and increased susceptibility to problems such as hypertension and hypotension (Miller, 2009). Normal cardiovascular changes seen with aging include a moderate increase in blood pressure or hypertension, and an overall increased stiffness of both the heart muscle, and arteries and veins.

Age-Related Changes to the Respiratory System

The respiratory system is composed of organs that assist with breathing including the airways (mouth, nose, and trachea), the diaphragm and chest muscles, and lungs. Aging changes to the airways can cause decreases in the ability to clear mucus and other secretions, especially from the trachea. Age changes to the chest wall include an increase in stiffness, due to a loss of elasticity, and increases in calcium in the cartilage connecting the ribs to the chest wall. This stiffness causes a decline in muscle strength. Decreases in the ability of the chest to expand and contract during breathing means that elders use the diaphragm or the major respiratory muscle located at the bottom of the chest for chest expansion and contraction. The diaphragm may also weaken with age, making breathing more difficult (Mauk, 2006).

Age-related changes in the lung tissue also occur. The alveoli are spongy air sacks located in the lung tissue. The alveoli serve as the site for gas exchange with oxygen exchanged for carbon dioxide within these structures. With aging, the alveoli become more flat and shallow, decreasing the surface area available for oxygen exchange and reducing the amount of oxygen available for consumption. The lung tissue itself is designed to be elastic, expanding, and contracting during inhalation and exhalation. Aging causes decreased lung elasticity. This in turn causes the lungs to close prematurely, trapping air and decreasing the efficiency of oxygen delivery (Mauk, 2006).

Some negative functional consequences of aging include decreased cough and gag reflexes, making choking a greater possibility in elders. Additionally, there is an increase in the energy required for breathing, an increased use of accessory muscles including the diaphragm and other major respiratory muscles, and decreased efficiency of oxygen exchange in the lungs. These aging changes increase elder's susceptibility for a number of respiratory infections (Miller, 2009). In effect, the mechanics of breathing usually change with aging.

Age-Related Changes to the Muscular System

The body is comprised of three types of muscles including skeletal muscles, smooth muscles, and cardiac muscles. Skeletal muscles make up the majority of the body's muscle mass and are also most impacted by age-related changes. Reduction in muscle mass known as sarcopenia occurs with normal aging. This loss of muscle mass is thought to be individualized, due in part to genetics and lifestyle (Mauk, 2006). Loss of skeletal muscle mass involves a decline in the number and size of muscle fibers, a loss of motor units or skeletal muscle fibers, and the motor nerves that innervate the muscle fibers. This condition is influenced by hormonal changes, altered protein synthesis, nutritional factors, and a lack of physical exercise (Mauk, 2006). Additionally, lower extremity muscles will tend to atrophy or shrink earlier than the upper extremity muscles (Tabloski, 2006). These age-related changes may make walking and other functional activities of daily living more difficult for elders.

Loss of overall muscle strength or a muscle's ability to generate force is thought to be influenced by age-related changes in muscle mass. These changes related to age are thought to occur in both men and women, and increase as part of the aging process (Mauk, 2006). Age is also connected with changes in muscle quality or the strength generated per unit of muscle mass. This is variable among men and women (Maul, 2006). Many research studies have demonstrated increases in skeletal muscle mass and muscle strength in aging muscles through the use of resistance exercises and training (Maul, 2006). The benefits of resistance exercises in the improvement and maintenance of skeletal muscle function should be viewed positively, and administrators should consider the addition of resistance training programs for residents in assisted living facilities.

Age-Related Changes to the Orthopedic System

The skeleton consists of a system of 206 bones and joints connecting the bones together, and serves to shape, support, and protect the body. Movement occurs because tendons attach muscles to the skeleton. Bones that comprise the skeletal system serve the function of mineral storage and the maintenance of a balance of mineral homeostasis, where bone is constantly reabsorbed and reformed. Aging alters the balance between the formation and re-absorption of bones throughout the body, resulting in bone mineral density loss. Changes in mineral density of bone are thought to occur starting at around age 30, and increases with age in both men and women. Research has demonstrated that reduction in estrogen levels play a key role in bone demineralization with increases in bone porosity occurring in post menopausal women. Men also undergo age-related changes in bone density. Current research indicates that this loss is due to declining estrogen rather than testosterone levels (Mauk, 2006).

Bone strength is thought to decline as a result of normal aging processes. With aging, bones become more porous and thus more brittle. These changes result in an overall loss of bone strength. Younger bones are more flexible, able to withstand force with resilience. Aging bones are more brittle, less flexible, and therefore less able to withstand force (Mauk, 2006). These changes put elders at increased risk for bone fractures.

Joints are the connections or junctions between two or more bones and there are three types of joints in the body. Immovable joints use collagen fibers to bind bones tightly together and prevent bone movement.

Skull bones are examples of immovable joints. With aging, the collagen fibers that bind bones together actually become coated with bone matrix and the bones fuse or join together. This results in a strengthening of the joints, an example of joint changes that are actually improved with the aging process. Cartilaginous joints allow for slight movement through the use of cartilage which separates two connected bones. Ligaments may also serve to connect the bones together (Mauk, 2006). With aging, both the cartilage and the ligaments become stiff and lose elasticity. This results in a reduction of movement and an increase in overall stiffness.

Synovial joints are the third type of body joints. Bones are connected together by a layer of connective tissue at the bone ends, and the joint capsule is lined with a membrane that secretes a thick and slippery fluid that serves in part to absorb the shock of bone movement. These joints serve to provide a great degree of movement and are located in the arms, legs, shoulders, and hips. Functional decline in synovial joints occurs with normal aging. The cartilage lining these joints become stiffer, thinner, and less resilient. This results in reductions in range of motion and joint function, putting elders at risk for joint injuries, balance changes, and falls. Additionally, aging causes changes in the synovial fluid surrounding the joints. This fluid becomes less viscous and thinner, which in turn causes disease and discomfort with joint movement (Mauk, 2006). The number of joint injuries and decreases in overall activity are also seen as components of the joint aging process.

Age-Related Changes to the Gastroenterological System

The gastroenterological system includes body structures from the mouth to the anus. Age-related changes to a number of these structures will be briefly discussed. The mouth serves to moisten food with saliva in order to enhance the passage of food to the pharynx and esophagus. Age-related changes to the teeth and related atrophy of jaw and mouth muscles can make chewing more difficult. Age-related changes to the esophagus include stiffening of the walls of the esophagus, as well as decreased sensations of discomfort and pain. These changes can make swallowing more difficult, which can potentially lead to serious consequences for elders. While researchers do not find significant age-related changes in either stomach or small intestinal functioning, age-related changes in the large intestine or colon include decreases in colonic motility. These changes result in a lengthening of total colonic transit time, or the amount of time required for both fluid and excrement to travel the length of the colon. This increase in transit time puts elders at increased risk for constipation.

This may be worsened by poor nutrition, lack of exercise, and the use of many different medications. The rectum is located at the end of the colon before the anus. Age-related changes to this structure include an increase in fibrous tissue and a decreased ability to stretch as feces are excreted from the body (Mauk, 2006). Age-related changes to the rectum make excretion of feces more difficult, and in the setting of poor nutrition, lack of exercise, poor hydration, and decreases in colonic transit time may predispose elders to fecal impactions.

The liver serves to secrete bile into the small intestine as well as to filter blood from both the stomach and small intestine for toxins and excessive nutrients. Researchers note that as the body ages, overall liver size and the amount of blood flowing through the liver decreases by at least 30% to 40% (Mauk, 2006). One consequence of these changes is a decrease in the body's ability to remove drugs from the system, creating potential problems for elders taking both prescription and over-the-counter medications. The liver's ability to filter and remove alcohol from the blood stream is also decreased as a result of age-related liver function changes. As noted earlier, this can have a significant impact on elders who consume large quantities of alcohol.

Age-Related Changes to the Genitourinary System

The genitourinary system includes the kidneys, bladder, ureters, and urethra. This system is designed to: (1) remove a number of wastes and toxins from the blood; (2) regulate osmotic pressure in the blood; (3) regulate levels of calcium, potassium, sodium, magnesium, and phosphorus in the blood; (4) regulate blood pressure; (5) controls acid base balance; (6) regulate vitamin D; and (7) stimulate the production of erythropoietin, a hormone responsible for red blood cell production in the bone marrow (Mauk, 2006). Age-related changes in the kidneys include both a decline in organ length and weight, decreased blood flow to the kidneys, as well as diminished glomerular filtration rates (Mauk, 2006). These changes result in age-related decline in kidney functioning, especially in the ability to remove toxins, other wastes, and medications from the blood. This potentially puts elders at risk for problems associated with an accumulation of harmful substances.

Age-related changes to the bladder include an overall decrease in size as well as the development of fibrous changes in the bladder musculature, as well as decreased stretching capabilities. The filling capacity of the bladder declines with age, as it does not have the ability to hold urine and withstand voiding. These age-related changes increase the potential for urinary incontinence, a significant problem for elders in assisted living facilities. Changes in the genitourinary system that occur with aging cause additional alterations in genital structures, changes in hormone levels, changes in voiding behaviors, and decreases in the removal of toxins and medications from the body (Mauk, 2006). These changes can impact the physical, social, emotional, and psychological functioning of elders, especially when changes result in urinary incontinence. Understanding of changes associated with aging is important when considering the receipt of services delivered to elders in assisted living facilities.

Age-Related Changes to the Neurologic System

The nervous system consists in part of the brain and peripheral nerves. Age-related alterations within the brain include the following: (1) a decreased number of neurons and an increased accumulation of changes in brain tissue including plaques; (2) an overall decrease in brain size and weight; (3) decreased blood flow to the brain; (4) increases in sleep disorders and insomnia; and (5) decreases in short-term memory (Tabloski, 2006). Changes in brain function impact a number of cognitive functions including memory and any of these alterations can be of significance in the elderly. Changes in brain function can lead to changes in senses, including vision, hearing, taste, and touch, and profoundly impact the functional status of elders.

    The peripheral nervous system consists of billions of nerve cells and nerve fibers that connect the central nervous system to the rest of the body (Mauk, 2006). The speed of nerve conduction slows with aging, causing changes in overall motor speed, reaction times to a variety of stimuli, and changes in sensory ability such as vision and taste. Changes in these nerve pathways cause movements to become slower, less coordinated, and less accurate. Additionally, elders become slower in their recognition of a number of stimuli making their actions and reactions to these stimuli slower and more difficult (Mauk, 2006). Impaired reaction times, impaired coordination, and decreased sensation to light touch, pain, and joint positioning are also seen in the aging peripheral nervous system (Tabloski, 2006). Again, understanding age-related changes to the peripheral nervous system provides understanding and insight into problems that many elders may experience, or may be at risk for experiencing.

Age-Related Changes to the Skin and Lymphatic System

The skin is the largest body system, as it covers the entire body, and provides protection from trauma, microorganisms, and sun exposure. Additionally, the skin performs the following functions: (1) regulation of body temperature; (2) aids in touch and proprioception; (3) works in the synthesis of vitamin D; and (4) prevents loss of body fluids (Tabloski, 2006). There are a number of age-related changes to the skin representing changes in both function and appearance. Aging is associated with thinning and graying of the hair. Baldness may occur in both men and women. Skin color changes are common in the aging skin with areas of hyperpigmentation and increased pigmentation occurring on the face as well as throughout the body. Decreased elasticity, loss of subcutaneous tissue, and thinning of the dermis or the second layer of the skin, are associated with aging. Decrease in elastin results in an increase in wrinkling, while an increase in skin dryness is seen as the result of decreased secretions from sebaceous glands. Aging also produces an increase in the number of vascular lesions such as petechia and telangiectasia, which are benign and seen throughout the body. Additionally, the aging process decreases the skin's ability to provide photo protection from harmful ultraviolet radiation (Tabloski, 2006).

Elders are at risk for pressure ulcers and skin breakdown in result of decreases in blood flow to the skin and overall skin thinning which occurs as part of the aging process. Additionally, decreased blood supply to the skin with aging can result in decreased responses to injury and reduced thermoregulation capabilities. Age-related decreases to the touch receptors in the skin result frequently in the slowing of reflexes and diminished pain sensation throughout the body. Finally, decreases in skin regeneration may create potential delays in both wound healing and vitamin D production (Tabloski, 2006).

Understanding of the many skin changes that are associated with normal aging is essential for providing comprehensive services to elders in assisted living facilities. Of special importance is awareness that thinning and drying create skin that is fragile and a less effective barrier. This can put elders at risk for potentially lethal skin breakdowns and ulcerations.

A number of factors that are associated with aging can impact functioning of the immune system, a highly complex biological defense mechanism designed to protect the body from foreign bodies, chemicals, microorganisms, and parasites. Stress, co-existing diseases, changes in nutrition, and exercise all have the potential to alter immune functioning. Aging has also been shown to alter immune functioning through: (1) overall decreases in immune responses; (2) decreases in immunity through decreases in B cells, and increases in autoimmune responses to self; and (3) decreases in cellular immunity with impairment of immune system regulation. The aforementioned alterations in immune system functions place elders at risk for a number of acute and chronic illnesses in which the immune system plays a significant role (Tabloski, 2006).

Administrators can benefit from an understanding that changes in immune system functioning can increase risks for infection and illness in an elderly population, especially within institutional settings like assisted living facilities.

Best Practices in Improving Physical Problems Associated With Aging

Administrators, staff, and residents in a number of assisted living facilities have been recognized for practices that are designed to address and improve many of the physical problems associated with aging. Best practices in the area of wellness or disease prevention have been identified in a number of assisted living settings. For example, the Horizon Bay Retirement Communities in Tampa, FL, developed a wellness program for seniors used in 70 campuses in 15 states, and received an Assisted Living Federation of America Best of the Best Strategy award (Assisted Living Executive, 2008). The best practice "Live Well! Program was designed to promote holistic wellness through the concept of whole-person wellness. Programs focus on healthy aging, mind aerobics, fitness and exercise, and religious and spiritual topics. Positive outcomes associated with participation in this program include a reduction in blood pressure medication doses, increased participation in social activities, and greater overall satisfaction with this resident program. The Ridgemont at Edgewood Summit in Charleston, WV, has also been recognized for the development and implementation of a number of wellness services through the Successful Aging Program at Edgewood Summit (West Virginia Health Care Association, 2008). This program, identified as a best practice, was designed to work with residents in goal setting to promote health, increase physical activity, and enhance quality of life.

CASE STUDY

The administrator of a large urban assisted living facility has an understanding of many of the normal physiologic changes that occur with aging but is concerned that facility staff are not adequately assessing residents' abilities to routinely perform many daily activities. This concern was highlighted by an interaction with Ms. S, an 85-year-old female who has been a facility resident for 3 years. As the administrator talked with Ms. S, she noted the very strong smell of urine and also noted that Ms. S's clothes were food stained and that her laces on her shoes were untied. Ms. S seemed unaware of these problems.

A best practice that can be used in this situation is the use of the Katz Index of Independence in Activities of Daily Living (ADL) (Katz et al., 1963). The index includes a list of 6 activities including bathing, dressing, continence, feeding, toileting, and transferring. An elder's ability to perform these tasks are scored either as 1 (independence) or 0 (dependence) with a total score of 6 indicting independence in all ADLs and a total score of 0 indicating significant dependence in all ADLs. Use of the Katz Index of Independence in ADLs can provide staff with valuable information about determining the functional status of elders and can be also used to monitor the functional status of elders over time (Wallace & Shelley, 2008).

When the administrator had staff use the Katz Index of Independence in ADL, Ms. S received a score of 3, scoring in the dependent range in the areas of bathing, toileting, and feeding. Further evaluation revealed that Ms. S had experienced a recent and unidentified stroke. The administrator and staff were then able to work with Ms. S to provide her with assistance in bathing, toileting, and feeding herself thus improving her appearance.

ISSUES RELATED TO SELECTED PHYSICAL ASPECTS OF AGING

Assisted living facility administrators will need to have an awareness and comprehension of issues related to selected physiologic changes associated with aging that are relevant for many elders residing within assisted living facilities. The development of programs and services within these facilities can be enhanced through an understanding of physiologic issues. Five such issues, including nutrition, mobility, falls prevention, sleep, and pain management, will be briefly explored and discussed.

Nutrition Issues

The importance of nutrition in elders residing in assisted living facilities cannot be understated. Good nutrition is essential for well-being and for the prevention and treatment of a number of diseases. Healthy People 2010 (U.S. Department of Health and Human Services Office of Disease Prevention and Health Promotion, 2004) clearly connect nutritional status with health status for all citizens in the United States, especially older adults. While there is agreement that adequate nutrition is essential for elders, many factors exist which influence the presence or absence of good nutrition, and therefore the nutritional status of elders. These include lifestyle, medication use, the presence of chronic illnesses, changes in body function and composition, lifetime eating habits, heredity, socioeconomic status, and social interactions (Linton & Lach, 2007). For many elders, malnutrition or undernutrition is a serious concern as a lack of appropriate nutrients serves to compromise health, and contributes to a number of acute and chronic illnesses. This is sometimes referred to as the anorexia of aging. For other elders, obesity or over-nutrition has become problematic, again creating a number of health risks and increasing complications for many chronic diseases including diabetes, hypertension, and cardiovascular disease.

A number of nutritional-related changes have been associated with aging. Some of these changes include decreases in lean body mass, decreased metabolic rate, decreased bone mineral density, decreased saliva production, decreased taste and smell, and decreased thirst production (Tabloski, 2006). Social factors are also associated with nutritional changes in aging. Some commonly occurring social factors include social isolation, loss, grief, reactions to life changes such as retirement, and changes in financial status can result in altered nutrition. Awareness of age-related nutritional alterations helps administrators in assisted living facilities as they work to ensure that residents maintain adequate diets.

Nutritional Assessment

Administrators can utilize the services of dieticians, nurses, or nutritionists in the creation of nutritional assessments for elders in assisted living facilities. Assessments should include a diet or nutritional history. Dietary recall involves asking elders to recall their total food and beverage intake for a 24-hour time period. Elders are asked a series of open-ended questions to determine the specific foods eaten with the types of food, the amount of the food ingested, and the times that food was eaten during the given time period. Additional questions regarding the use of beverages, including alcohol, are also included in this dietary recall. Additional questions about food preparation, food preferences, and food shopping can provide additional information about nutritional status. Limitations of this assessment strategy include difficulties in recalling total food intake for a complete 24-hour time period. This may influence the accuracy of the data collected. Strengths of this assessment strategy include ease of administration for both elders and clinicians.

Nutritional assessments can also be obtained by asking elders to keep food records. This assessment strategy requires elders to list all food and beverage intake for a specific time period, usually a 3-to 5-day time period. Once the food record is completed, clinicians can review the records to determine the nutritional adequacy of total food intake.

The data from these assessments then serves as the basis for recommendations to improve nutritional status for individuals. Elders must be able to recall food intake for an extended time period. Gaps and difficulties in remembering food intake are limitations of this assessment approach. Strengths of this assessment include the ability of elders to provide information about diet and nutrition that reflect cultural and social preferences.

There are a number of screening tools available for nutritional assessment. Administrators should be aware of one assessment, the Minimum Data Set or MDS. This screening tool is a government-mandated component of the Resident Assessment Instrument used in all Medicare or Medicaid certified health care facilities. Nutritional assessments are completed for elders on admission to facilities, and then updated quarterly and annually, or when there are significant changes in an elder's status. The MDS nutrition-related criteria include the following: (1) an inability to feed oneself; (2) chewing problems; (3) swallowing problems; (4) mouth pain; (5) weight loss; (6) altered taste; (7) hunger complaints; and (8) nutritional approaches such as therapeutic diets, supplement use, and the use of weight gain programs (Centers for Medicare and Medicaid Services, 2002; Tabloski, 2006). This nutritional assessment may be of value in the assessment and on-going screening of elders in assisted living facilities.

Nutritional assessments should also take into consideration a number of factors that impact eating. Physical changes related to dentition, with tooth loss, dentures that may fit poorly, or changes in the ability to adequately chew and swallow food. Sensory alterations should also be assessed. Elders who experience decreased taste and smell will frequently experience eating problems and are at risk for malnutrition.

Strategies to maintain healthy nutrition of elders living in assisted living facilities include the use of diets to promote health. Administrators are required by state regulations to provide food that meets minimal nutrition standards. Understanding a number of diets designed to promote health in aging populations can be used in conjunction with standard diets. A number of diets that can be of benefit to elders will be briefly discussed. Low-caloric diets are of use with elders who are overweight or obese. The goal of these diets is to reduce the total number of calories consumed by elders on a daily basis and thus reduce weight. Reductions in calories of 500 to 1000 calories per day can result in weight loss of 1 to 2 pounds per week. More extensive weight loss is generally not recommended in elders. Low-fat diets are designed to reduce the amount of saturated fat in daily food intake. For elders who have cardiovascular disease, hypertension, or diabetes, diets that reduce fat intake can be of benefit in promotion of improved health.

There are a number of dietary recommendations for elders with diabetes. Nutritional guidelines for patients with diabetes include diets that are low in fat with saturated fat limited to 10% of total daily calories, low in sugar with limits on simple carbohydrates and limits on alcohol. The lowering of sodium consumption is also recommended, limiting sodium to 2 grams or less per day. Diets that are high in fiber are recommended for many elders. These diets are thought to be of benefit to elders with diabetes and cardiovascular disease. Because aging causes decreases in colonic transit time with resulting constipation, diets that increase fiber can improve or prevent the painful complications of constipation.

Malnutrition or under nutrition remains a significant problem for many elders. Poor appetite, muscle wasting, weight loss, and insufficient diet define inadequate nutrition, and malnutrition results in poor health. This decreased quality of life encompasses multiple social and physical factors (Chen, Shilling, & Lyder, 2001). Assessment of malnutrition is needed to determine optimal treatment options for elders with this problem; specific treatment options will depend on the problems causing the malnutrition. Diets that provide adequate amounts of protein and calories should be offered to elders with malnutrition. Underlying social and physical problems should be assessed, and strategies to resolve the problems proposed.

Nutritional supplements are recommended for elders who have specific problems and dietary deficiencies. Vitamin D supplementation is recommended for elders because they have less exposure to sunlight, have skin changes that decrease vitamin D absorption, and frequently have diets deficient in this vitamin. Calcium supplementation is recommended for elders again because many diets are deficient in calcium, and also because elders are at risk for age-related bone loss resulting in brittle bones. Older adults should have a minimum of 1500 mg of calcium supplementation per day in the form of a variety of calcium supplements (Linton & Lash, 2007).

Administrators can obtain information regarding healthy nutrition from a number of resources. Experts in the field of nutrition including dieticians and nutritionists are available for consultation. Physicians and nurses can also play a role in nutritional assessment and recommendations for healthy diets in elderly individuals. Online resources include the websites associated with a number of organizations including the American Heart Association, the American Diabetes Association, the American Association of Retired People, and the National

Institutes of Health. Information from online resources may be current, relevant, and research-based and is also easy for busy administrators to access and review.

Mobility Issues

Mobility is the second issue related to physical aspects of aging. Mobility, or the ability to move and function, is influenced in older adults by age-related changes in muscles, bones, joints, and nervous system functioning. Factors that influence mobility include age-related decreases in muscle mass, degenerative joint changes, thinning or demineralization of bones, and changes in the overall functioning of the nervous system (Miller, 2009). Age-related changes create functional problems including an inability to conduct activities of daily living including walking and balancing, and increasing the risk for serious falls. The presence of decreased mobility with associated loss of independence creates a number of social and psychological problems for elders. Loss of independence results frequently in a lessening in the quality of life for elders with even minimal mobility loss. Depression is a problem associated with decreased mobility.

Mobility assessments will provide information related to both physicality and functioning, and should include a health history that can be obtained by physicians, nurses, geriatric specialists, physical therapists, or other clinicians working in assisted living facilities. The health history should include questions about the muscles, especially if muscle pain, weakness or cramping is present. Questions about bones should be focused upon on the presence or absence of pain, deformities, and a history of prior fractures or bone problems. Information about joints should focus on the presence or absence of pain, decreased mobility, stiffness, and swelling. Questions should also be focused on an elder's ability to perform activities of daily living including bathing, dressing, feeding, moving, shopping, preparing meals, performing housework, and independently physical activities (Linton & Lach, 2007). Data obtained from a mobility assessment can be used to address both current and potential mobility problems in elders.

Exercise is considered to be an essential component of mobility, and the goal of exercise is to maintain or improve musculoskeletal functioning. Linton and Lash (2007) identify a number of exercises that can be easily and effectively implemented in assisted living facilities. Aerobic exercises should be encouraged for at least 20 to 30 minutes per day. Aerobic activities can include walking, swimming, biking, or dancing, and must be individualized for each individual participant. Passive exercises to maintain joint mobility are recommended for elders who are unable to exercise independently or unassisted. Resistive exercises or strength training exercises are now recommended to improve both musculoskeletal and cardiovascular functioning. Research indicates that regular participation in strength training programs increases both muscle strength and muscle mass. Isometric exercises involve muscle contractions without the use of joints, and can be effective in muscle strength training. Balance exercises are used to provide an additional form of strength training for elders. Tai chi is one example of a balance exercise that is successfully used by many elders in both independent and group settings.

There are a number of assistive devices available for elders with changes or impairments in mobility. Understanding how devices including canes, walkers, and wheelchairs can assist walking, and thus improve mobility, is important for administrators working in assisted living facilities.

Canes are mechanical assistive devices that increase balance by broadening the base of support and absorbing body weight when partial weight bearing is required (Elkin, Perry, & Potter, 2007). There are a number of canes available for use including a standard or straight leg cane, a tripod cane with 3 feet and the quad cane with 4 feet (Berman, Snyder, & Jackson, 2009). The canes with 3 or 4 feet provide additional stability for elders with balance problems and also serve to improve security with use of these assistive devices. Walkers are assistive devices that improve mobility by providing additional support, especially for elders who need help with partial weight bearing. Standard walkers are lightweight, made of polished aluminum, and have four legs. Walkers with rollers or wheels do not need to be picked up to be moved forward, but are less stabile than standard walkers. Elders who use walkers must have at least partial strength in hands, wrists, and elbows, as well as strong shoulder muscle depressors (Berman, Snyder, & Jackson, 2009).

There are two types of wheelchairs in use to improve mobility. Manual and electric wheelchairs are commonly in use, and come with adjustable foot and leg rests. The wheels and tires on the front of the wheelchair should be selected according to use. Larger wheels move easily over bumps or obstructions but are harder to turn and also take more room to turn (Berman, Snyder, & Jackson, 2009). Ease of turning wheelchairs and the ability to turn wheelchairs in assisted living environments with space limitations, should be considered when selecting wheelchairs. Additionally, the seat used in a wheelchair should also be considered. Rigid wheelchair backing and solid seating with foam or air cushioning should be considered for those elders using wheelchairs on a long-term basis (Berman, Snyder, & Jackson, 2009).

Administrators working with elders using assistive devices to enhance mobility must make sure that facility physical spaces are designed for the safe use of devices. Flooring must be designed to prevent skids or slips when elders use canes or walkers. Corridors and rooms must be free of furniture and equipment that would create problems or impede the use of walkers and wheelchairs. As noted, elders in wheelchairs must be able to freely move and turn the chairs in rooms and hallways. Administrators can refer to state regulations regarding the development of physical space in assisted living facilities for assistance in developing environments that ease elder mobility, with or without the use of assistive devices.

Best Practices to Improve Mobility

In addition to strategies to improve mobility through exercise and the use of assistive devices as needed, best practices in the area of fitness and mobility will be briefly discussed. The Country Meadows Retirement Communities in Hershey, PA, received a Best of the Best award from the Assisted Living Federation of America for their development and implementation of a fitness walking trail (Redding, 2009). The fitness trail, a flexible and portable indoor fitness course, was created to connect exercises with functional activities. The overall goal of this fitness strategy was the provision of practical and individualized exercises designed to promote fitness, mobility, and physical independence. The fitness trail was also identified as a screening tool for identifying physical challenges and deficiencies.

Administrators have access to a number of clinicians who can provide information regarding mobility for elders. These clinicians include nurses, physical therapists, occupational and recreational therapists, all of whom can assess elders for mobility issues and recommend exercise programs to improve mobility within this population.

Falls Prevention Issues

Falls prevention is a third issue related to the physical aspects of aging. Administrators in assisted living facilities should have an understanding of this important issue to prevent potential problems for residents in assisted living facilities. The importance of falls prevention is underscored by statistics indicating that falls are a major cause of morbidity and mortality in elders. More than 1.6 million older adults were treated for fall-related injuries in 2001 (CDC, 2003). About 13,000 older adults aged 65 and older died from fall-related injuries in 2002 (CDC, 2006; Elkin, Perry, & Potter, 2007). Approximately one half of elders living in institutions will experience falls every year (Mauk, 2006). The economic costs of treating elders who fall and require either hospitalization or treatment, are significant for all segments of the population. The social costs of treating elders who fall are also significant with changes in mobility creating both physical and functional impairments that can impact the quality of life for elders. Fall prevention programs can effectively reduce the economic, physical, and social burdens associated with falls. Currently, the Joint Commission on Accreditation of Healthcare Organizations (2005) recommends the development of fall prevention programs for elders, and refers to data in stating that such programs can reduce fall rates and the significant costs associated with falls.

There are a number of risk factors associated with falls experienced by elders. Commonly occurring risks include the following: (1) poor vision; (2) cognitive impairments including memory changes, poor judgment, confusion and dementia; (3) impaired mobility including changes in gait, balance, and problems with lower extremities); (4) difficulties in movement, especially in getting out of a chair or bed; (5) weakness from illnesses or therapies; and (6) the use of a number of medications that can cause changes in orientation or mobility (Berman, Synder, & Jackson, 2009). Understanding the risks related to falls is important in fall assessment and the implementation of fall prevention programs.

While administrators in assisted living facilities will not conduct assessment for falls, understanding of falls assessment risk is an initial step in the creation of strategies to prevent falls, and the physical, social, and economic problems associated with falls. There are a number of fall assessment instruments that are available for use by clinicians; assessment instruments that focus on physical factors, history of prior falls, medication utilization, and environmental factors. Each area will be briefly presented and discussed.

Assessment of physical factors associated with increased risk of falls includes evaluation of motor and sensory problems, balance problems, along with memory and cognitive problems. Elders with existing medical problems that create fatigue, musculoskeletal weakness, incontinence, changes in cognition or mental functioning, or changes in vision or hearing are at increased risk for falls, and should have these problems assessed. Assessment of prior falls should include questions to assess the presence of any symptoms at the time of the fall, location of prior falls, time at which prior falls occurred, activities that were taking place at the time of the prior falls, and the presence or absence of trauma at the time of the falls (Elkin, Perry & Potter, 2007). Special attention should be paid to the medications used by elders. There are a number of medications which increase fall risks in older adults. Antidepressants, sedatives, sleeping medications, antihistamines, steroids, antihypertensives, diuretics, muscle relaxants, cardiac medications, and hypoglycemics are some of the medications that may be problematic for elders (Elkin, Perry, & Potter, 2007). Elders should also be assessed for use of over the counter medication, as well as the use of vitamins and herbal supplements that may contribute to the risk of falling.

Environmental factors should be evaluated in fall risk assessment. Factors that contribute to falls include the physical environment, and are affected by lighting, flooring surfaces, physical plant design, presence of clutter in rooms and hallways, and safe use of mobility assistive devices. Stairs with uneven step height, absence of railings, furniture with unsteady bases, and bathrooms without grab bars, slippery floors, and inappropriate toilet heights should also be assessed as potential risks for falls. Additionally, the clothing and footwear worn by residents in assisted living facilities is of high importance, and the use of nonskid footwear should be considered.

Fall prevention programs should be implemented following careful fall risk assessment. Effective falls prevention programs include the following elements: (1) medication reviews and medication modification as needed; (2) modification of environmental factors that increase fall risks; (3) use of assistive devices as needed; (4) exercise and strength training to enhance mobility; and (5) education of older adults to reduce fall risks (CDC, 2006).

Best Practices in Falls Prevention

Administrators, staff, and residents in a number of assisted living facilities have been recognized for practices that are designed to address elements of aging through the development of best practices. The Fall Prevention Program developed by Carlton Senior Living received a Best of the Best Strategy award from the Assisted Living Federation of America (Assisted Living Executive, 2008). Located in Martinez, CA, the Carlton project started with a review of best practices. Residents participated in exercise programs that included standing balance classes as opposed to more traditional sitting exercise programs. Fall risks were assessed for residents, and a fall injury action plan developed for all residents at risk for falling. These individualized risk assessment and treatment plans also included assessment and elimination of environmental risks and fall hazards. Administrators can work with nurses and physical therapists in fall assessments and the implementation of fall prevention programs. Use of these experts can assist administrators in the management and prevention of economically and socially costly problems associated with falls and fall risks.

Sleep Issues

Sleep issues occur frequently and exist as a fourth area related to the physical aspects of aging. Sleep is essential for healthy physical functioning. During sleep, a number of physiologic processes occur including increased production of growth hormone, acceleration of protein synthesis and tissue repair, deceleration of metabolic processes, as well as the filtering and organization of cognitive and emotional information. Researchers have noted a number of age-related changes to sleep patterns. Older adults have changes in sleep and rest quantity although overall sleep quantity appears to be unchanged from earlier adulthood (Miller, 2009). A number of sleep disturbances are also seen in older adults. These problems include insomnia, with difficulties in falling asleep or staying asleep, snoring, which may be an indicator of sleep apnea, breathing pauses which may also indicate sleep apnea, and tingling or discomfort in the legs which may indicate restless leg syndrome (Mauk, 2006). Frequent nighttime awakenings, early morning awakenings, and difficulties falling asleep may also be seen in aging adults as age-related sleep changes, or as the result of co-existing medical problems. Additional age-related changes to sleep patterns involve decreased time in deep sleep stages, decreased time spent dreaming, and increased time spent in light sleep stages. Elders may experience a number of functional changes resulting from age-related sleep alterations. An overall increase in the time needed to fall asleep, frequent arousals during the night, increased difficulty in returning to sleep once aroused or awakened, an increase in the amount of time spent in bed with a decreased amount of overall sleep time, and poorer sleep quality also occur in older adults (Miller, 2009).

It is important to note that while assisted living facility administrators will not be conducting sleep assessments, the information obtained from such assessments can be valuable in understanding problems that elders may experience in regards to the design of interventions to assist in the promotion of healthy sleep patterns.

Sleep assessment should involve the assessment of commonly occurring risk factors affecting sleep and sleep patterns, including physiologic factors, psychosocial factors, medications, environmental factors, and pathologic problems such as sleep apnea. There are a number of physiologic factors that can alter sleep patterns such as chronic illnesses like cardiovascular disease and respiratory problems, physical discomfort or pain from chronic illnesses such as arthritis, neuromuscular disorders such as foot or leg cramping, and urinary problems that cause increased nighttime urination such as prostatic enlargement (Miller, 2009).

Psychosocial factors serve as risk factors for sleep disturbances. Problems such as stress, anxiety, depression and dementia are frequently associated with a number of sleep problems. Elders with depression take longer to fall asleep, experience more light sleep, awake more during the night as well as the early morning, and feel much less rested upon awakening. Elders who feel alone or who have few work responsibilities, social demands or environmental stimuli, or who experience increased stress may also be at risk for a number of sleep problems (Miller, 2009). Questions to determine the presence or absence of these psychological risks should be included as part of the psychological sleep assessment.

Medication assessment is an important part of sleep assessment. There are a very large number of medications which that have the potential to alter sleep patterns, including over the counter medications and herbal supplements. Caffeine is a central nervous system stimulant that can lengthen sleep latency as well as increase awakening during the night. Nicotine interferes with sleep because of stimulant and respiratory effects. Alcohol increases the number of nighttime awakenings as well as suppressing REM sleep (Miller, 2009). In older adults, small quantities of caffeine, nicotine, and alcohol can create significant sleep problems.

Sleep assessments should include questions about environmental factors that may create sleep problems. Increased noise, changes in sleep routines, alterations in temperature (rooms that are too warm or cold) may increase the risk for sleep problems. Increased lighting can create sleep problems as well. A lack of bright light during daylight hours can create problems by interfering with circadian rhythms and the production of melatonin, a hormone that regulates sleep, body temperature, and circadian rhythms (Miller, 2009).

Sleep apnea is another problem that should be assessed in elders at risk for sleep disturbances. Obstructive sleep apnea is defined as an involuntary cessation of airflow for a minimum of 10 seconds or longer, and the presence of 5 to 8 of these episodes per hour is an indication of serious problems (Miller, 2009). Assessment data indicating the presence of sleep apnea requires that the elder with this problem be referred to a physician or sleep specialist. Administrators should also note that there are a number of sleep assessment tools available to obtain additional sleep assessment data. Consultation with sleep experts can assist in the use of specific sleep assessment tools.

Once sleep assessment data is obtained, administrators can work with clinicians to develop strategies to improve sleep conditions for elders. Educational programs can provide older adults with information about sleep changes associated with aging. There are a number of strategies that can enhance good sleep hygiene. Older adults should work to structure conditions that are conducive to good sleep. Use of the same bedtime every evening, use of relaxation strategies such as warm milk, warm baths, relaxing music, or relaxing reading, can improve sleep conditions. Environmental changes including soft lighting, cool temperatures, and quiet noise free conditions, are also recommended as is aromatherapy and massage. Use of daytime exercise, relaxation exercises, and stress management strategies can also improve sleep problems for older adults.

There are a number of medications available to treat sleep problems in elders. Hypnotics, antidepressants, and non benzodiazepine sleeping medications may assist elders with sleep problems. While many of these medications are effective in treating sleep problems, there are a number of side effects that accompany the use of these drugs. Elders who use these drugs may be at risk for medication dependence or side effects from interactions with other drugs that may also be used for existing diseases or problems. Use of these medications with alcohol can create problems that are potentially life threatening. Additionally, use of these medications may also put older adults at increased risk for falls and accident-related problems. Elders who require these medications require evaluation and consultation from physicians or sleep specialists.

Elders may also consider the use of herbal remedies for sleep problems. Ginseng and valerian are two remedies used by a number of older adults to promote sleep. Melatonin, a hormone synthesized by the pineal gland, may be used to promote sleep. Research indicates that the use of exogenous melatonin may improve sleep in older adults (Miller, 2009). Nutritional supplements such as L-tryptophan may also assist in improving sleep. L-tryptophan is an amino acid that aids in serotonin production in the brain. Naturally occurring in proteins and dairy products, use of L-tryptophan shortens sleep latency periods in elders who have difficulty falling asleep (Miller, 2009). L-tryptophan can also be taken in supplement form to enhance sleep.

Assisted living administrators can obtain information about sleep problems and the treatment of sleep problems from clinicians who specialize in sleep disorders, and from other health professionals including physicians and nurses. Additional information regarding sleep problems can be obtained from a number of online resources including the National Institute on Aging, the National Institute of Mental Health, and the American Association of Retired People.

Chronic Pain Issues

A fifth and final issue related to physical aging is chronic pain. Administrators must have an understanding of the importance of chronic pain as they work with elders in assisted living facilities. Additionally, administrators must have an understanding of the state regulations that govern administration of medications within assisted living facilities if residents with chronic pain receive these medications as part of a pain management program. Finally, administrators can benefit from information about common causes of chronic, as well as some of the age-related changes that affect pain in older adults.

Chronic pain is defined as pain that persists beyond the usual course of a disease or injury, or lasting longer than a minimum 3- to 6-month time period (Miller, 2009). Some experts now recommend the use of persistent pain rather than chronic pain as a label that evokes a more positive description of this condition (Miller, 2009).

Chronic pain is described as a wide-spread and significant problem for older adults who are at risk for this problem resulting from the presence of many chronic illnesses. Many commonly occurring diseases are accompanied by chronic pain, including arthritis and diabetes. Arthritis is considered to be the most common cause of persistent pain in elders, with 49% to 59% of this population experiencing some form of arthritis-related pain (Miller, 2009). Diabetes is another problem experienced by many older adults that frequently causes chronic pain in the extremities.

There are a number of functional consequences associated with chronic pain including: (1) problems with walking and mobility; (2) decline in overall functional abilities; (3) psychosocial problems including sleep disturbances, depression, anxiety, and fatigue; and (4) increased risk for disability and loss of independence (Miller, 2009). Additionally, age-related changes that may be experienced by older adults are not well understood, and elders may not complain of pain but rather confusion, fatigue, aggression, or restlessness (Miller, 2009).

Assessment for chronic pain should be conducted by clinicians including physicians, nurses, or pain specialists. Assisted living facility administrators can benefit from understanding the assessment process as it relates to residents with chronic pain. While there are a number of pain assessment instruments and scales available for use in evaluation of pain in older adults, basic assessments should focus on a series of questions. Clinicians should focus on questions that provide information about the nature or intensity of the pain, the location of the pain, the duration of the pain, pain frequency, pain movement or radiation, factors that make the pain better or worse, current treatments for the pain, and other poblems that may be associated with the pain. Additional assessment questions should be focused on functional changes that are associated with chronic pain. Elders should be questioned about changes in activities of daily living that result from chronic pain such as an inability to clean, bathe, sleep, perform housework, or shop. Changes in exercise patterns, or inability to exercise, along with a decrease in mobility related to chronic pain should also be noted. Changes in eating patterns including decreased appetite or weight loss resulting from chronic pain should be noted. Changes in emotional feelings including depression, anxiety, or other mood changes should be assessed, as well as changes in socialization with family members and friends that result from chronic pain. Changes in mental functioning also resulting from chronic pain or the medications and treatments used to treat it should be assessed Finally, changes in any other aspects of the elder's life that have been altered as a result of chronic pain should be evaluated as part of a comprehensive pain assessment. Factors such as economic changes, social isolation, or decreased feelings of well-being and life satisfaction as a result of chronic pain, should be explored and discussed.

Administrators can benefit from an understanding of treatments available for chronic pain experienced by elders in assisted living facilities. The benefits of non pharmacologic strategies and some of the challenges associated with pharmacologic pain management strategies will be briefly discussed. Non pharmacologic strategies designed to address chronic pain include exercise. For elders with chronic pain due to arthritis or other musculoskeletal problems, exercise programs such as swimming or yoga have been shown to be of benefit, and may serve to reduce pain. Stress management activities such as relaxation exercises, meditation, aromatherapy, art therapy, music therapy, or guided imagery, can provide benefits in pain modification or reduction. Physical therapy, acupuncture, or acupressure has also been identified as strategies that may be beneficial to elders experiencing chronic pain. Additional benefits may be obtained from the use of herbal or non prescription treatments. Vitamins and herbal supplements may be used by elders to reduce pain. Additionally, the topical use of agents such as capsazacin or anagelsic ointments or creams can provide relief for musculoskeletal pain and joint pains from arthritis.

The pharmacologic management of chronic pain should be managed by physicians, advanced practice nurses, or pain management specialists. There are a number of medications available for chronic pain management including over-the-counter analgesics and a variety of prescription analgesics including opioids. Specialists in pain management are able to identify medication management programs that are tailored to individual elder needs and are also then qualified to monitor and re-assess elders on an on-going basis. Challenges associated with the administration and utilization of opioid medications in assisted living facilities focus on how these drugs are administered and stored. Administrators need to review individual state and local regulations governing medication storage and administration for controlled and regulated medications. Administrators should also review state and local regulations for appropriate disposal strategies when opioids and other controlled pain medications need to be removed from assisted living facilities.

Best Practices in Pain Management

In addition to the strategies for pain management that have been previously described, a best practice in the areas of pain management has been identified. The pain associated with joint problems was addressed by members of the Benchmark Assisted Living Communities in Wellesley, MA, through the development of a partnership with the Massachusetts Arthritis Foundation. This collaboration earned Benchmark Assisted Living with an Assisted Living Federation of America Best of the Best award (Redding, 2009). The partnership allowed 100 Benchmark associates to teach seniors in 42 communities. Associates were then able to teach an arthritis foundation exercise class to over 700 Benchmark residents and community members. Residents with dementia were also included in exercise activities designed to reduce joint pain.

Administrators can access a number of resources to obtain information regarding chronic pain management for elders living in assisted living facilities. Clinical experts in chronic pain management include physicians, nurses, pharmacists, pharmacologists, pain specialists, and psychologists. Additionally, administrators can access current and accurate information regarding chronic pain management from a number of online resources including the National Institute on Aging and the National Institute on Mental Health.

CONCLUSIONS

Assisted living administrators can benefit from an awareness of some of the many physiologic changes that normally occur in the body systems of elders. Changes to the cardiovascular, respiratory, muscular, orthopedic, gastrointestinal, genitourinary, skin, lymphatic, and neurological systems that occur as part of the aging process presented in this chapter can also place older individuals at risk for a number of problems that are both acute and chronic. Staff in assisted living facilities will need to identify and address functional alterations and problems resulting from normal age-related physical changes. Administrators can facilitate these processes with a basic understanding of some of the physiologic changes that are aging related. Commonly occurring issues related to nutrition, mobility, fall prevention, sleep, and chronic pain management were identified and briefly discussed. Administrators can work to improve services to elders through an understanding of these important issues.

Administrators can also benefit from a review of the best practices that are in use in different settings. Examples of programs that facilitate exercise and promote improved balance for elders through standing rather than sitting exercises, or through the use of a portable fitness trail rather than the use of exercise equipment are of potential benefit to administrators in many settings. Additionally, the best practice case study highlights the value of measuring activities of daily living as a measurement of functional status and abilities.

REFERENCES

Best of the Best. (2008). *Assisted Living Executive*. Retrieved from http://www.alfa.org/alfa/Best_of_the_Best_.asp?SnID=2

Berman, A., Snyder, S., & Jackson, C. (2009). *Skills in clinical nursing* (6th ed.). Upper Saddle River, NJ: Pearson Education, Inc.

Centers for Disease Control and Prevention. National Center for Injury Prevention and Control. (2003). *Web-based injury statistics query and reporting system*. Retrieved from http://www.cdc.gov/ncipc/wisqars

Centers for Disease Control and Prevention. National Center for Injury Prevention and Control. (2006). *A toolkit to prevent senior falls*. Retrieved from http://www.cdc.gov/ncipc/pub-res/toolkit/toolkit.htm

Centers for Medicare and Medicaid Services. (2002). *Minimum data set manual, version 2.0*. Retrieved from http://www.cms.hhs.gov/medicaid/mds20/mds0900b.pdf

Chen, C. C., Schilling, L.S., & Lyder, C.H. (2001). A concept analysis of malnutrition in the elderly. *Journal of Advanced Nursing, 36*(1), 131–142.

Elkin, M. K., Perry, A. G., & Potter, P. A. (2007). *Nursing interventions and clinical skills*. (4th ed.). St. Louis, MO: Mosby Elsevier.

Joint Commission on Accreditation of Health Care Organizations. (2005). *Comprehensive accreditation manual for hospitals*. Chicago: JACHO.

Katz, S., et al. (1963). Studies of illness in the aged. The index of ADL: A standardized measure of biological and psychosocial function. *Journal of the American Medical Association, 185*, 914–919.

Linton, A. D., & Lach, H. W. (2007). *Concepts and practice. Gerontological nursing* (3rd ed.). St. Louis, MO: Saunders Elsevier.

Mauk, K. L. (2006). *Competencies for care. Gerontological nursing*. Sudbury, MA: Jones and Bartlett Publishers.

Miller, C. A. (2009). *Wellness in older adults* (5th ed.). PA: Wolters Kluwer Lippincott Williams & Wilkins.

Redding, W. (2009). Best of the best. *Assisted Living Executive,* 11–19.

Tabloski, P. A. (2006). *Gerontological nursing.* Upper Saddle River, NJ: Pearson Education, Inc.

U.S. Department of Health and Human Services. (2004). *Office of Disease Prevention and Health Promotion. Healthy People 2010.* Retrieved from http//: www.healthy people.gov/About/

Wallace, M., & Shelkey, M. (2008). Monitoring functional status in hospitalized older adults. *American Journal of Nursing, 108*(4), 64–71.

West Virginia Health Care Association. (2008). *Meeting the needs of assisted living residents.* Retrieved from http://www.whca.org/pdf/Issue_2_2008.pdf

Psychological Aspects of Aging

Learning Objectives

Upon the completion of Chapter 16, the reader will be able to:

- *Describe selected normal psychological changes associated with aging.*
- *Discuss issues related to memory and cognition in aging individuals.*
- *Describe strategies to maintain memory and cognition.*
- *Define and describe types of dementia.*
- *Describe strategies to maintain optimal functioning for aging individuals with dementia.*
- *Define depression and describe strategies for assessment of depression in aging individuals.*
- *Identify strategies to maintain optimal functioning in aging individuals with depression.*
- *Define alcohol and substance abuse and strategies for assessment of alcohol abuse.*
- *Describe strategies for dealing with alcohol and substance abuse.*
- *Identify best practices in addressing dementia and depression.*

INTRODUCTION

While assisted living facility administrators are not serving as clinicians to elders within their facility, an understanding of selected normal psychological changes related to the aging process will enable administrators to perform their work more effectively. Understanding many of the normal aging-related changes in neurological functioning, mental health functioning, memory, and cognition can be important in understanding how elders in assisted living facilities function. Furthermore, issues related to memory changes, dementia, depression, alcohol, and substance abuse can be commonly experienced by the elderly. An awareness and understanding of these issues can be beneficial to assisted living administrators and will be discussed further in this chapter. Best practices in selected areas associated with psychological aspects of aging have been identified and will also be presented throughout this chapter.

OVERVIEW OF NORMAL PSYCHOLOGICAL CHANGES ASSOCIATED WITH AGING

Neurologic Changes

Arking (as cited in Mauk, 2006) notes that researchers have identified changes in brain weight and size associated with aging (Arking, 1998; Mauk, 2006). Brain volume remains stable in adults until about age 60 with volume losses of 5% to 10% occurring after age 60. Men have a greater volume of brain loss than women, especially in the temporal and frontal lobes of the brain. Numbers of neurons within the brain decrease with age, and this loss may also be accompanied by the presence of senile plaques within brain tissue (Tablowski, 2006). Lipofuscin, a pigment associated with aging, becomes deposited in nerve cells and amalyoid is also deposited in brain cells and blood vessels (Ebersole & Hess, 1998). Additionally, decreased blood flow to the brain may also occur as adults age. Each of these chemical and physiologic changes results in changes to the brain and cognitive functioning.

Slower reaction times are seen in aging adults as a result of changes in the central nervous system. These processing changes are associated with changes in cognitive functioning (Miller, 2009). Changes in vision, hearing, touch, taste, and sensation are also associated with changes in the functioning of the central nervous system. Structural changes in the nervous system result in a decreased ability to respond to stimuli, and changes to the autonomic nervous system make quick recovery from stressors such as heat, cold, and environmental stresses more difficult with aging (Linton & Lach, 2007).

While physiologic changes within the brain have been documented, Cohen (as cited in Miller, 2009) reported that research conducted during the past 20 years indicates that aging brains can perform as well as younger brains in a number of areas. There is evidence that new brain cells form throughout the lifespan as a part of prior learning and experiences, and are used by the brain in reorganizing efforts. Left and right hemisphere functions become more integrated in aging brains, and emotional functions become more mature and balanced in the aging brain (Cohen, 2005).

Mental Health Changes Associated With Aging

Some authors note that the prevalence of mental illness is lower in the elderly than in the general population (Mauk, 2006). Depression is one problem that occurs frequently in aging populations due to multiple factors including medical problems, life transitions, loss of family members and friends, and support systems (Mauk, 2006). Depression in the elderly may also be related to biologic aging factors, sleep changes, and alterations in neuroendocrine substances (Ebersole & Hess, 1998). Anxiety, a feeling of distress, fear, or worry may be seen in elders in a number of settings including assisted living facilities. Presence of generalized anxiety may impact health and quality of life for these elders (Miller, 2009).

Memory and Cognitive Changes Associated With Aging

Mental health and cognition are normally thought to remain stable throughout life with changes in cognition associated with physical or mental illnesses. Tablonksi (2006) identifies some of the age-related changes to cognition. Changes in cognition include: (1) the speed for information processing; resulting in slower learning rates, and an increased need for information repetition; (2) the ability to divide attention between two or more tasks; (3) the ability to switch attention from sources of auditory input; (4) the ability to sustain and maintain attention; (5) abilities to filter out irrelevant information; (6) visual spatial task abilities; (7) mental flexibility and abstraction abilities; (8) short-term or primary memory remains unchanged throughout life; long-term or secondary memory does decline; and (9) accumulation of practical experience or wisdom continues throughout life.

Gerontologists have developed new theories to understand memory and cognition. Contextual theories indentify a number of factors that affect memory. Some of these factors include motivation, expectations, personality, education, learning skills, learning habits, sociocultural background, physical health, emotional health, and style of processing information (Miller, 2009). Psychological developmental theories reveal that the thinking of elders increases in complexity with aging, especially in the area of problem solving. Mariske and Margrette (2006) have noted: (1) motivation is a strong predictor in decision making in elders; (2) elders are more selective in the information they use to make decisions; (3) elders need more time for decision making; (4) task expertise and experience improve decision making especially for elders; and (5) increased task complexity results in more errors and inconsistencies for both elders and younger individuals.

ISSUES RELATED TO PSYCHOLOGICAL ASPECTS OF AGING

Assisted living facility administrators will benefit from an understanding of some of the issues related to psychological aspects of aging as they work with elders in their facilities. While there are a number of psychological problems that administrators must face as they deal with elders residing in assisted living facilities, many problems are commonly seen in a variety of settings. A basic understanding of memory and cognition, dementia and strategies to assist elders with dementia, depression and strategies to assist elders with depression, and alcohol and substance abuse can provide assisted living administrators with information to enhance services for elderly residents. Each of the issues noted above will be briefly described.

Memory and Cognition Issues

Many individuals associate memory changes and problems as an inherent part of the aging process. As noted earlier, research supports some physiologic changes in memory, but overall learning and remembering abilities are not changed in healthy elders (Miller, 2009). A number of factors may alter overall memory and cognition. These factors include: (1) worry and anxiety; (2) stress; (3) physical illnesses; (4) visual, hearing, and functional impairments that preclude information processing; (5) sadness or depression; and (6) the use of medications or alcohol (Miller, 2009). These factors may cause changes in the way individuals' process information.

Assessment of memory and cognition is an important evaluation activity for elders entering and residing in assisted living facilities. While assisted living facility administrators will not administer assessment tests, understanding basic testing and how the tests provide information can be of benefit in understanding issues related to changes in memory and cognition. Two tests of memory assessment, the Mini-Mental Status Examination, and the clock test will be briefly explained.

Mini-Mental Status Examination

The Mini-Mental Status Examination (MMSE) was developed in 1975 by Folstein and others (McGee, 2007). The test consists of 11 items that can be administered within a short time period of 5 to 10 minutes in an elder's room or hospital room. The MMSE contains questions that are both highly specific and highly sensitive. Questions in the MMSE include questions in five categories. Orientation questions elicit information regarding the ability to understand the day, date, month, year, and season as well as location (room, city, state, and country). *Registration* questions ask elders to name three objects and continue to repeat the object names. *Attention and Calculation* questions elicit information about an elders' ability to count backwards from 100 by 7 or to spell words backwards. *Recall* questions elicit the ability to remember information. Finally, *language* questions ask elders to follow three-stage commands, write a sentence, or copy a picture of two intersecting pentagons. The MMSE is scored by giving a point for each question answered correctly for a total of 30 points. Normal scores are considered from 24 to 30. Scores of 23 or less are indicators of memory and cognitive decline. Very low scores on the MMSE suggest dementia. The MMSE can also be used to monitor changes in cognition. Re-administration of the test with a decline of four or more points serves as an indicator of cognitive change and decline.

The Clock Test

The clock test is another simple test that can be administered within assisted living facilities. The test requires that the elder draw a clock face on a pre-printed circle that is 4 inches in diameter. The ability to draw a correct clock face requires that the elder can follow directions, comprehend language, visualize the proper orientation of objects, and execute normal movements. Clock drawings are normal if the elder has included most of the 12 numbers in the correct clockwise orientation. Changes in the ability to accurately draw a clock face strongly indicate the presence of dementia (McGee, 2007).

Strategies to Maintain and Improve Memory in Elders in Assisted Living Facilities

Assisted living administrators can work with staff and elders to maintain and improve memory for elders residing in assisted living facilities. A number of these strategies will be briefly discussed.

Maintaining Memory Through Educational Programs

Miller (2009) noted that the educational process itself serves to maintain memory and cognitive functioning. Cognitive wellness then can be maintained through elder participation in adult education programs. Use of group education programs as well as computer-based educational programs, can work to enhance memory. Additionally, elders can be encouraged to participate in local community college and university continuing education programs. The Institute for Learning in Retirement is a community-based organization designed to develop and implement educational programs for retirement-aged workers (Miller, 2009).

Strategies to Improve Memory Skills

There are a number of simple memory enhancement skills that can be used for elders in assisted living facilities. Writing down information in journals, calendars, and lists, assigning specific places for specific items, and placing reminders in specific places can be used to improve memory. Use of auditory cues and visual reminders, as well as rhyming and first letter associations, also help improve memory. Additionally, there is current evidence which suggests that memory can improve with the regular use of mind-enhancing games and puzzles including crossword puzzles and computer games.

Maintaining Memory Through Aerobic Exercise

A number of researchers have noted the relationship between physical or aerobic exercise and memory enhancement (Mauk, 2006). Elders who regularly engage in exercise through formal programs or informal activities such as walking have been found to have increased cognitive functioning.

Music Therapy

Ebersole and Hess (1998) note the value of music therapy for elders to improve connections through touch as well as cognitive enhancement. While music therapy has been used in the treatment of Alzheimer's disease, benefits of improved cognition through exposure to music may also help elders in assisted living facilities.

Nutritional Supplements

There is literary information suggesting that memory and cognition can be improved through the use of nutritional supplements and herbal remedies. There are a number of vitamins associated with improved memory including vitamin B12, along with a number of herbal remedies associated with memory and cognition, one of which is gingko biloba (Tabloski, 2006). Assisted living administrators should work with health care professionals, and with individual elders to determine whether supplements can be of benefit in memory enhancement.

Best Practices

In addition to the memory enhancement strategies identified in this chapter, a best practice in enhancing memory has been identified. Aegis Living Facilities located in Washington and California (2009) has developed a number of communities designed to assist residents with memory loss. Best practices in use within these facilities include a memory box which is placed outside of the resident's apartment. Each box contains photos, mementos, and stories that can be used by providers and friends as they interact with each resident. An additional best practice to enhance memory in these facilities includes the use of a specific room or portable cart containing lights, aromas, music, colors, and specific shapes and textures. Use of these items increases sensory stimulation for relaxation and sensory redirection.

Resources Available to Assisted Living Administrators

As administrators deal with issues related to the maintenance and improvement of memory and cognition in elders, health care professionals can provide additional consultation and information. Psychologists, neurologists, gerontologists, social workers, geriatric case managers, and geriatric nurses are some of the specialists whom administrators can consult regarding issues related to memory and cognitive improvement. Consultants serve to initially assess elders in assisted living facilities and can also work to provide on-going evaluation of mental status. Assisted living administrators can also use online resources for memory and cognition information. Up-to-date research based resources are available to administrators from a number of organizations including the American Association of Retired Persons, the National Institute on Aging, and the National Institute on Mental Health.

Dementia Issues

Assisted living administrators must have a basic understanding of dementia, how dementia is identified and assessed, and how elders with dementia can be assisted to function optimally in assisted living facilities. While each state has specific regulations and requirements for elders with dementia and Alzheimer's disease that assisted living administrators must adhere to, additional information on this problem can be beneficial.

Dementia in Assisted Living Facility Populations

Dementia is a progressive illness that causes impairments in social and occupational functioning. According to the American Psychiatric Association (1994), dementia is characterized by the following: (1) cognitive deficits and memory problems; (2) impaired motor activities; (3) language disturbances; (4) failure to recognize or identify common objects such as keys; (5) disturbed executive functioning including planning, organizing, sequencing, and abstracting problems; and (6) changes in personality and behavior. Dementia refers to a syndrome rather than a specific disease process, and impaired cognition is the resulting brain dysfunction (Miller, 2009). A common problem experienced by older adults is the increasing likelihood of dementia as one ages. Thirty percent of adults over age 85 are at risk for dementia (Linton & Lach, 2007). Dementia is characterized by a slow progressive onset, and a continuation of cognitive decline that is not connected to other problems (Tabloski, 2006). A diagnosis of dementia requires the loss of intellectual abilities which impact social and occupational functioning, as well as awareness that delirium is not present (Tabloski, 2006).

Delirium is an acute state of confusion, characterized by diminished attention, clouded state of consciousness, physiologic disturbances, and possible hallucinations (Miller, 2009). Delirium is usually reversible, as opposed to dementias which are progressive and nonreversible. Delirium is also viewed as a syndrome of multiple factors including: (1) altered mental status with a reduced ability to focus, shift, or sustain attention; (2) confusion, disorientation, and memory loss; (3) disorganized thinking and speech; (4) fatigue and sleep problems; (5) personality changes; (6) behavior changes; and (7) hallucinations and delusions (Peterson et al., 2006). The risk factors for delirium include advanced age, pain, medications, dementia, surgical procedures, and physiologic problems (Miller, 2009). Because delirium is an acute problem that can be reversed, it is important for administrators and those assessing elders in assisted living facilities, to be able to identify and differentiate delirium from dementia.

Dementia Assessment

While assisted living facility administrators are not in roles designed to assess for dementia, understanding the components of this assessment process are valuable in facilities with elders who have or are at risk for this syndrome. Regulatory requirements for dementia and Alzheimer's assessment vary by state, but again, an understanding of assessment components can facilitate this important process. Elders being assessed for dementia should complete a comprehensive health history. This information includes a history of prior neurological problems, prior cognitive or memory problems, and prior acute and chronic medical problems such as diabetes, heart disease, stroke, cancer, liver, or kidney disease. Past educational background, past employment history, past hospitalizations or surgeries should also be obtained. It is also necessary to include information about family and social functioning. Many times, family members serve as important informants and can provide information about changes in memory or cognitive functioning that an elder may miss or be unwilling to disclose. Additional information should be obtained about all medication use, including the use of nutritional supplements, vitamins, and herbal supplements. Use of alcohol or other illegal substances should also be discussed and included as part of the assessment. Mental status tests such as the Mini-Mental Status Examination or the Clock Test can also be used in dementia assessment.

Because dementia causes changes in life functioning, a functional assessment that includes an ability to adequately perform activities of daily living should also be part of the dementia assessment process. Elders who are unable to provide for daily needs such as care for face and teeth, or grooming needs, may have early signs of dementia.

Types of Dementia

Assisted living facility administrators may benefit from an understanding of the most common types of dementia that may be present in elders residing in assisted living facilities. While dementia is a syndrome or cluster of problems, identifying characteristics of specific dementias including Alzheimer's disease, Lewy body disease, vascular dementia, and dementia associated with alcohol or drug use is helpful. Each of these dementias will be briefly discussed.

Alzheimer's Disease

Data from the 2000 US Census indicated that 4.5 million Americans have Alzheimer's disease (Miller, 2009). Age is considered to be a risk factor for this type of dementia, with the likelihood of developing the disease increasing from 53% in those aged 75 to 84, and 40% in those aged 65 and older (Morris, 2005). The hallmark signs of Alzheimer's disease are seen on autopsy, and include neuritic plaques and neurofibrillary tangles in the neocortex of the brain (Miller, 2009). Mild cognitive impairments associated with Alzheimer's disease include short-term memory loss, difficulties with complex cognitive skills such as arithmetic, and also impairments in the ability to perform daily activities (Miller, 2009).

Theories about the causes of Alzheimer's disease are varied at this time, and include familial or genetic risks for the disease inflammatory processes, vascular risk factors including smoking, prior head trauma, exposure to environmental toxins, and psychological factors such as depression (Morris, 2005). Currently, there are no cures available for Alzheimer's disease.

Lewy Body Dementia

Lewy body dementia is now recognized as the second most common form of dementia in the United States. Forming proteins in the brain, Lewy body dementia may be a variant of Alzheimer's disease, Parkinson's disease, or a disease that combines elements of both diseases (Morris, 2005). Characteristics of this dementia include the following: (1) impaired cognition, especially executive functioning; (2) widely fluctuating cognition; (3) recurring visual hallucinations; (4) parkinsonism with motor symptoms; and (5) falls, apathy, sleep problems, and depression (Morris, 2005). Individuals with this dementia are considered to be very medically frail, and may have significant problems with the addition of minor illnesses or environmental changes (Miller, 2009).

Vascular Dementia

Caused by the death of nerve cells that do not receive adequate blood flow, vascular dementia also occurs with other types of dementia such as Alzheimer's disease (Miller, 2009). Causes of vascular dementia include changes to arteries caused by diseases such as diabetes, hypertension, or arteriosclerotic disease, and overall decreases in perfusion from problems such as congestive heart failure, hypotension, or cardiac arrhythmias (Miller, 2009). Elders with vascular dementia often have cognitive impairments such as aphasia and memory loss, behavioral changes including depression, and changes in sensory motor functions including changes in gait, sensation, and urinary incontinence (Miller, 2009).

Dementia Related to Alcohol and Drug Use

Chronic abuse of alcohol or drugs may produce symptoms of dementia similar to those seen in early Alzheimer's disease. A comprehensive history of prior alcohol or drug use should serve as an indicator of the cause of this dementia.

Strategies to Provide Optimal Functioning in Elders With Dementia

Assisted living facility administrators can work with staff to provide a number of services that may be of benefit to elders with dementia. Programs that support exercise include formal classes or informal exercise programs such as walking. Music therapy, the use of music to improve cognition or behavioral functioning, has been used in a number of settings. Researchers have noted an improvement in cognition following 30 minutes of music therapy twice weekly (Linton & Lach, 2007). The use of art therapy, dancing, and social activities can also be of assistance in dealing with elders with dementia. The use of therapeutic touch can also be of benefit to those with dementia. Family involvement within the assisted living environment can benefit elders with dementia as can the use of a number of social services. Environmental strategies to provide orientation for those with dementia are also of potential benefit in an assisted living setting. Calendars, and clocks with large, easy to read numbers, are visual aids to help orient elders. Environments that incorporate nature, reduce stimulation though the use of quiet sounds, no television, and moderated lighting, can be used to assist elders with dementia. Additionally, the implementation of strategies to enhance the sensory environment such as massage, therapeutic touch, and aromatherapy can be used in assisted living facilities.

Resources Available to Assisted Living Administrators

As administrators deal with issues related to elders experiencing dementia, a number of health care professionals can provide additional consultation and support to address problems related to dementia. Psychologists, neurologists, gerontologists, social workers, geriatric case managers, and geriatric nurses are some of the specialists whom administrators can consult regarding issues related to dementia. Administrators should plan to work with selected consultants to provide assessment and on-going services for elders with dementia. Assisted living administrators can also use online resources for current information on dementia. Updated and research-based resources are available to administrators from a number of organizations including the Alzheimer's Association, the American Association of Retired Persons, the National Institute on Aging, the National Institutes of Health, and the National Institute on Mental Health.

Best Practices

Strategies to address dementia have been identified in this chapter. Additionally, administrators, staff, and residents in a number of assisted living facilities have been recognized for best practices in the area of dementia treatment. Five-Star Quality Care in Newton, MA, has received a Best of the Best Strategy award from the Assisted Living Federation of America for the creation of an Alzheimer's memory care program entitled Revelations (Assisted Living Executive, 2008). The Revelations Program applies a Montessori-based program that is based on the understanding that adults with dementia are normal individuals with cognitive deficits. The staff caring for these individuals present all activities at a level that each resident can understand and enjoy, thus returning to activities that they previously found pleasurable. This approach allows residents to engage and become more involved in activities, enhancing experiences for both residents and staff members.

Brookdale Senior Living in Milwaukee, WI, was the winner of an Assisted Living Federation of America Best of the Best award for the development of the Clare Bridge Dining Program (Redding, 2009). This program was developed by experts in the areas of dining services, clinical issues, and memory care with the goal to create a culinary program centered on dementia. Efforts to prolong the use of utensils for eating, to create dining environments that promote dignity, and to enable residents with dementia to stay focused and engaged while dining, are hallmarks of this program that is a best practice in the care of residents with dementia.

Depression Issues

Administrators working in assisted living facilities need to understand issues related to depression, a commonly occurring problem in elder populations. Clinical depression is the most commonly occurring mental health problem in older adults, with an increased prevalence in those adults who reside in long-term care or assisted living facilities (Mauk, 2006). According to the American Psychiatric Association (2000), older adults must experience five or more symptoms during a two week period including: lack of enjoyment in previously enjoyed activities, sadness, sleep disturbances, restlessness, fatigue, feelings of worthlessness, an inability to think clearly, and suicidal thoughts. Depression can be thought of as a group of disorders with variable severity. It is important for administrators to note that elders who are in the very early stages of dementia may feel that there is something wrong, and begin to experience mild depression along with their dementia (Tabloski, 2006). Depressed elders report more cognitive and physical symptoms including apathy, as compared to younger adults. Elders with depression also frequently experience anorexia, weight loss, early morning awakening, and withdrawal from social activities (Miller, 2009).

Because clinical depression may co-exist with dementia, it is important for those working with elders who have either depression or dementia to differentiate between the two problems. A number of distinguishing features exist between depression and dementia. According to Miller (2009), the onset of symptoms differs between depression with rapid, abrupt onset and dementia, with a more gradual onset. Memory and attention problems associated with depression are mostly related to a lack of motivation and an inability to concentrate. Memory and attention problems associated with dementia are usually impaired, especially for recent events. Emotions in those with depression are usually of sadness while those with dementia may exhibit apathy. Elders with depression have little concern about personal appearance because of a lack of motivation, in contrast to those with dementia who exhibit inappropriate dress and actions. Physical symptoms of anorexia, weight loss, fatigue, insomnia, and constipation accompany depression. Physical symptoms are vague, easily forgotten, and inconsistent in elders with dementia. Those with depression have an exaggerated sense of 'doom or gloom,' while elders with dementia frequently deny reality and may use delusions to explain deficits (Miller, 2009).

Assessment of Depression in the Assisted Living Facility

As noted earlier, while administrators may not administer assessment tests or screenings for depression, an understanding of strategies to assess for this problem can be of benefit in the assisted living facility environment. As discussed earlier, routine and comprehensive health history and screening should be conducted on elders who are suspected of depression. Special attention should be paid to the questions about the symptoms associated with depression as identified by the American Psychiatric Association (1994).

There are number of screening instruments designed to measure depression that can be used in assisted living facilities. One of the more widely used screenings includes the Beck Depression Inventory, a 13-item questionnaire that inventories mood, self-image, and somatic complaints (Beck & Beck, 1972). A score of 16 or higher on this instrument indicates severe depression. The instrument has been shown to be reliable and valid, measuring changes in depression intensity over time (Beck & Beck, 1972).

The Geriatric Depression Scale is a widely used self-rated scale designed for use with older adults (Miller, 2009). Elders complete the 30 question form in about 5 minutes with a normal score of 0 to 10. This depression scale has been shown to be accurate, feasible, and acceptable for use in a number of clinical settings. The questions are designed to focus on the psychological aspects of depression as compared to other instruments that include questions about somatic or physical problems (Miller, 2009).

Types of Depression

Administrators can benefit from understanding the types of depression that may impact elders, especially those residing in assisted living facilities. Minor, subthreshold, or subclinical depression occurs with few or minor symptoms. Major depression occurs with a number of serious symptoms, sometimes requiring hospitalization or medication. Current thinking about depression maintains that minor and major depressions are distinguished by symptom severity (Miller, 2009). Suicide is a very serious consequence of late life depression. As noted in Miller (2009), 18% of seniors aged 65 and older constituted 13% of the total population, and 18% of all suicides in the United States. These rates do not reflect unrecognized suicidal acts such as failure to eat, failure to take medications appropriately, and other acts of self-neglect (Miller, 2009).

Strategies to Promote Optional Functioning in Those With Depression

Assisted living facility administrators can work with staff and elders to address depression through a number of strategies. The benefits of exercise to reduce depression are well documented. Educating elders to recognize the benefits of exercise can also serve to prevent depression. In assisted living facilities, group exercise programs may be of benefit to those with depression as well for other elders.

Nutrition is another beneficial intervention to elders with depression. Good nutrition has overall positive effects on general health, mental health, and overall functioning. For those with depression, poor eating habits, anorexia, and negative nutritional status, depression may increase, as well as create a number of other physical and psychological problems (Miller, 2009). Malnutrition can be a consequence of serious depression in elders, leading to a number of serious or life threatening problems. Use of nutritional supplements as well as dietary interventions can be used as nutritional interventions to treat depression. Diets should include foods high in tryptophan, and phenylalanine including meat, poultry, fish, and soybeans (Miller, 2009).

Patient education and counseling services are interventions that can be of benefit to elders with depression. There are a number of therapies that may be used in the treatment of depression. Some of these therapies include behavioral therapy with an emphasis on problem solving, cognitive therapy with an emphasis on restructuring negative thoughts, interpersonal therapy with an emphasis on exploring relationships, supportive therapy designed to facilitate choices to improve coping, and bibliotherapy, with a focus on reading and exercises to reduce dysfunctional thought processes (Miller, 2009). Additionally, elders with depression may also benefit from group therapy sessions. Group therapy sessions can provide elders with information on depression, improve social interactions, improve self-esteem, and facilitate personal development (Miller, 2009).

Health promotion interventions can be used to alleviate depression. These interventions include the use of regular exercise, avoidance of smoking, caffeine, and artificial sweeteners. The consumption of alcohol should also be evaluated and moderate or large quantities should be avoided.

Complementary and alternative therapies may also be of benefit to elders with depression. Bright light therapy used on a daily basis may reduce depression. Aromatherapy including the use of rose, lavender, sage, bergamot, chamomile, basil, and jasmine may also serve to reduce depression. Art, yoga, dance, imagery, meditation, relaxation, stress management, and spiritual healing, are additional strategies designed to reduce depression (Miller, 2009). Some elders may wish to discuss the use of these therapies with their physicians or providers of herbal treatments, such as St John's Wort for the treatment of mild to moderate depression.

Best Practices

In addition to strategies designed to improve depression, administrators, staff, and residents in a number of assisted living facilities have been recognized for practices to support aging individuals with depression. Best practices in the area of depression and suicide prevention will be identified and briefly discussed. Depression and suicide are significant problems for many elders. One best practice developed to address the prevention of these problems is the University of California, San Francisco Institute on Aging's Center for Elderly Suicide Prevention (2009). These services are focused specifically on the needs of older adults at risk for these problems.

The services provided include counseling, assessment, connections with others, and crisis intervention referrals. The center also provides elders with a number of support groups and telephone hot lines for older individuals experiencing grief, traumatic loss, and for survivors of suicide.

Resources Available to Assisted Living Facility Administrators

Administrators have a number of resources available to assist in the provision of services for depressed elders. Psychologists, gerontologists, registered nurses, social workers, and nutritionists can provide assistance in the assessment and treatment of depression ranging from mild to severe. Online resources can also provide current information on best practices in dealing with depression. Some of these resources include the American Association of Retired Persons, the National Institute of Mental Health, the National Institute of Health, and the National Institute on Aging.

Alcohol and Substance Abuse Issues

Assisted living facility administrators need to clearly understand issues related to alcohol and substance abuse in elders residing in assisted living facilities. These are problems that are widespread, poorly understood, and difficult to treat in all age groups, especially in the elderly. A number of authors note that problems with alcohol frequently go undetected in the elderly population. Because many elders are not working or spending time in social settings, they are able to drink without observation. There are current estimates that 20% of nursing home residents are alcoholics (Ebersole & Hess, 1998). Elders are at significant risk for alcohol-related problems because of age-related physiologic changes, where increases in lean body mass, higher body water mass, and changes in liver function influence the body's ability to metabolize even small quantities of alcohol. Elders frequently have a number of chronic illnesses, and use a number of medications that also impact alcohol metabolism. Additionally, dietary changes and smaller body size also influence alcohol metabolism.

Physiologic problems related to alcohol use are frequently seen in elders. Specific problems with nutrition include malnutrition due in part to failure to eat nutritious foods on a regular basis. Weight loss and anorexia may be seen in individuals with heavy alcohol use. Decreases in gastric absorption of nutrients and osteomalacia, or thinning of the bones, also occurs with increased alcohol use. Changes in liver function and cirrhosis of the liver are frequently seen as consequences of increased alcohol consumption. Alcoholic liver disease is one of eight leading causes of death in elderly populations (Tabloski, 2006). A number of neurological changes are associated with increased alcohol use. Changes in gait and motor function increase the risk for accidents, falls and possible fractures, especially hip fractures. Changes in cognitive functioning may cause significant problems with memory, along with the ability to process information. Elders who abuse alcohol may experience problems with depression and may also exhibit symptoms associated with dementia. Because alcohol has a generalized effect on the central nervous system, learning, judgment and reasoning are altered, as are social and emotional functioning. When elders consume large quantities of alcohol, they may experience drowsiness and stupor, leading to serious motor coordination problems and risks for serious falls.

Assessment for Alcohol Abuse in Assisted Living Facilities

Assessment for alcohol abuse in elders residing in assisted living facilities should be performed whenever alcohol abuse is suspected. Descriptions of the criteria for alcohol dependence and alcohol abuse, as well as commonly used assessment strategies, can provide useful information to administrators.

The American Psychiatric Association (2000) criteria for alcohol dependence include three or more of the following problems: (1) tolerance or drinking more alcohol to get the same effects; (2) withdrawal or drinking to prevent withdrawal symptoms; (3) drinking in larger quantities or for longer time periods than expected; (4) unsuccessful efforts to quit drinking: (5) spending a lot of time obtaining or using alcohol, or recovering from the effects of alcohol; (6) giving up social or recreational activities to drink alcohol; and (7) drinking despite the presence of physical or psychological problems. The American Psychological Association (2000) criteria for alcohol abuse include one or more of the following problems: (1) drinking resulting in the failure to complete major obligations; (2) drinking in situations that are physically hazardous for the individual; (3) drinking that results in alcohol-related legal problems; and (4) continued drinking despite social problems that are alcohol-related.

One screening test for alcohol dependency and abuse in wide spread use, is the CAGE questionnaire. This questionnaire is a self-report screening instrument that asks respondents to answer four questions. CAGE is a mnemonic for the questions that include the following: (1) cut down, a question that elicits attempts to cut down on drinking; (2) annoyance, a question related to suggestions by friends and family to cut back on drinking; (3) guilt, a question related to feelings of shame or guilt about drinking; and (4) eye opener, a question related to the use of alcohol in the morning to remain functional (Ewing, 1984). One or more positive responses to the CAGE questions are strongly indicative of alcohol-related problems. The CAGE questionnaire has been found to be both sensitive and specific in recognizing problems with alcohol (Mauk, 2006).

Additional screening questions can be used in conjunction with the CAGE questionnaire, and provide information to identify alcohol dependence or abuse in elders. These questions include the following: (1) indicate the number of days you drink per week; (2) identify the number of drinks you drink per day; (3) indicate the maximum number of drinks you drink per day; (4) note the types of alcohol you drink (wine, beer, or hard liquor); and (5) define your idea of a drink (Tabloski, 2006).

Assessment for alcohol and substance abuse should also include information from screening health histories. Many assisted living facilities require that elders be assessed as they enter the facility, and be evaluated at regular intervals. Questions about drug use should be focused on the number and types of prescription drugs used on a regular basis, as well as the use of over-the-counter drugs, vitamins, and herbal remedies. Elders should also be questioned about their use of illicit or street drugs, the types of drugs used, and the frequency of drug use. It is also important for elders to indicate their reasons for using drugs, especially if these drugs are used in the treatment of pain, depression, sleep disturbances, or other problems.

Factors Influencing Alcohol and Substance Abuse in Elders

There are a number of factors that influence alcohol and substance abuse in elders. Administrators can assist elders in their facilities by understanding some of the factors that cause or contribute to alcohol and substance abuse. Many researchers note that elders use alcohol and prescription medications to deal with chronic pain. Elders with problems such as arthritis, myalgias, and prior hip fractures are at risk for chronic pain. Many of these individuals will use alcohol and other substances in an attempt to reduce and relieve pain. As noted earlier, many elders suffer from depression. The use of alcohol and other medications to self-treat depression are well described in the literature and in fact, depression is considered to be a major risk factor for alcohol abuse (American Psychological Association, 2003). Social changes experienced by elders are a well know contributing factor to alcohol and substance abuse. The changes associated with moving into assisted living facilities may contribute to, or increase the risk for potential abuse. Social isolation can occur among elders living alone or living in institutional settings such as assisted living facilities, and is a problem that is well described in the literature. Also well described is the use of alcohol and other substances by elders as they attempt to deal with significant and serious problems associated with social isolation. Also well described in the literature are problems associated with grieving and loss. Many elders use alcohol and drugs to cope with losses and the depression that frequently accompanies grief and loss.

Strategies to Deal With Alcohol and Substance Abuse in Assisted Living Facilities

Administrators in assisted living facilities can benefit from an understanding of strategies that can be used to address alcohol and substance abuse problems. There are a number of steps in the treatment of alcoholism that may be used in assisted living facilities. Initially, screening tests should be conducted to identify elders with alcohol problems requiring treatment. Secondly, the individual's willingness and readiness to discuss treatment needs to be identified. Thirdly, individuals who need hospitalization for detoxification from alcohol and/or drugs need to be identified. Finally, care plans should be made for elders following post detoxification (Mauk, 2006).

Elders with alcohol and substance abuse should be referred to experts for evaluation and treatment. Referrals to physicians and alcohol treatment specialists are a recommended first step in addressing abuse problems. Psychologists, nurses, social workers, and gerontologists can provide expertise in addressing these problems. Additionally, a number of professional counseling, group counseling, and social support groups have been found to be beneficial. There are a number of local and national alcohol treatment programs that elders can utilize. Of special note is Alcoholics Anonymous, a world-wide self-help group with a well established record of services for alcoholics. Elders in assisted living facilities can benefit from referrals to this organization.

Most experts agree that hospitalization should be required for elders who are dependent on alcohol. Because elders are frail, have diminished physical and psychological reserves, and frequently have a number of co-existing medical conditions, they are at increased risk for problems during alcohol withdrawal and detoxification. Delirium and seizures are more commonly seen in elders withdrawing from alcohol use (Mauk, 2006). Acute agitation and hallucinations may also accompany alcohol withdrawal. These problems are best managed in a hospital setting. A number of medications can be used to assist elders as they withdraw from alcohol. Drugs such as benzodiazepines can be used in the detoxification process. Following the acute detoxification process, elders will need to have supportive counseling services to assist in the recovery process.

Resources Available to Assisted Living Facilities Administrators

Assisted living facility administrators can assess a number of resources in dealing with alcohol and substance abuse issues. As noted earlier, there are a number of professionals who can assist in the assessment of alcohol and substance abuse including physicians, nurses, social workers, and alcohol abuse experts. Evaluation and treatment of elders with alcohol dependence and abuse problems should be conducted by professionals with expertise in this area. Physicians and alcohol abuse experts need to be consulted when elders require detoxification from alcohol. Online resources can provide current and relevant information for administrators. Alcoholics Anonymous and the Council on Alcoholism have websites that provide important information and resources for understanding alcoholism. The National Institute on Aging, the National Institute on Mental Health, and the American Association of Retired Persons also serve as important sites for administrators.

CASE STUDY

SG is a long-term assisted living facility resident with many friends among other residents and facility staff. A retired school teacher, SG has participated in many of the facility events and has contributed to several facility educational programs. Several of her friends have noted that SG has become more forgetful in the past 6 months, forgetting the location of her keys, credit cards, and check book on a regular basis. When her friends commented on her increased forgetfulness, SG became very angry indicating that she was not forgetful but distracted because of the weather and the poor economy. Concerned about SG, her friends asked the staff and the administrator to help resolve her forgetfulness. The administrator worked with staff members to use a best practice to assess SG's mental status. The staff administered the Mini-Cog, a brief screening instrument designed to differentiate individuals with dementia from those without dementia. The Mini-Cog consists of two mental status tests: 3-item recall and the Clock Drawing Test (Doerflinger, 2007).

SG agreed to take the Mini-Cog screening exam and the staff determined that her scores on both the 3-item recall and the Clock Drawing Test strongly indicated that SG had dementia. SG was then referred to her physician who diagnosed SG with early-onset Alzheimer's disease. The administrator and staff were then able to work with SG and to also provide counseling and support for SG's friends. While SG continued with progressively worsening forgetfulness, her friends found the counseling and support from both the administrator and the staff to be extremely helpful.

CONCLUSIONS

Assisted living administrators can improve their work with elders through a comprehensive understanding of normal psychological changes associated with the aging process. As noted in this chapter, an understanding of selected psychological issues including memory changes and the assessment of memory, dementia, depression, and alcohol abuse can also provide administrators with valuable information which can be used to enhance services to elderly residents. Best practices can provide administrators with information and examples of strategies for approaching some of the psychological issues present in aging individuals.

REFERENCES

American Psychiatric Association. (1994). *Diagnostic and statistical manual* (4th ed.). Washington, DC: American Psychiatric Association.

American Psychiatric Association. Committee on Nomenclature and Statistics. (2000). *Diagnostic and statistical manual of mental disorders* (4th ed., text revision). Washington, DC: American Psychiatric Association.

American Psychological Association. (2003). What practitioners should know about working with older adults. *Professional Psychology: Research and Practice, 29*(5), 413–427.

Arking, R. (1998). *Biology of aging: observations and principles* (2nd ed.). Sunderland, MA: Sinauer Associates.

Beck, A. T., & Beck, R. W. (1972). Screening depressed patients in family practice: A rapid technique. *Postgraduate Medicine, 52,* 81–85.

Best of the Best. (2008). *Assisted Living Executive.* Retrieved from http://www.alfa.org/alfa/Best_of_the_Best_.asp?SnID=2

Cohen, G. D. (2005). *The mature mind: The positive power of the aging brain.* New York: Basic Books.

Doerflinger, D. M. C. (2007). The Mini-Cog. *American Journal of Nursing, 107*(12), 62–71.

Ebersole, P. A., & Hess, P. (1998). *Toward healthy aging. Human needs and nursing response.* St. Louis, MO: Mosby.

Ewing, J. A. (1984). Detecting alcoholism: The CAGE questionnaire. *Journal of the American Medical Association, 252,* 1905–1907.

Institute on Aging. (2009). *CESP: Center for Elderly Suicide Prevention and Grief Counseling.* Retrieved from http://www/ioaging.org.wvproxy.com/services/cesp_suicide_prevention_help.html?wvse

Linton, A. D., & Lach, H. W. (2007). *Gerontological nursing. Concepts and practice* (3rd ed.). St. Louis, MO: Saunders Elsevier.

Mariske, M., & Margrett, J. A. (2006). Everyday problem solving and decision making. In J. E. Birrin & K. W. Schaie (Eds.), *Handbook of the psychology of aging* (6th ed., pp. 57–83). San Diego: Academic Press.

Mauk, K. L. (2006). *Gerontological nursing. Competencies for care.* Sudbury, MA: Jones and Bartlett Publishers.

McGee, S. (2007). *Evidence based physical assessment* (2nd ed.). St. Louis, MO: Saunders Elsevier.

Memory Care. (2009). Retrieved from http://www.aegisliving.com/aegis_memory_care

Miller, C. A. (2009). *Wellness in older adults* (5th ed.). Philadelphia: Wolters Kluwer Lippincott Williams & Wilkins.

Morris, J. C. (2005). Dementia update 2005. *Alzheimer Disease and Associated Disorders, 19,* 100–116.

Redding, W. (2009). Best of the best. *Assisted Living Executive,* 11–19.

Tabloski, P. A. (2006). *Gerontological nursing.* Upper Saddle River, NJ: Pearson Education, Inc.

CHAPTER 17

Resident's Rights

Learning Objectives

Upon the completion of Chapter 17, the reader will be able to:

- *Identify federal legislation designed to protect the civil rights of residents in assisted living facilities.*
- *Describe selected state statutes enacted to protect the rights of residents in assisted living facilities.*
- *Understand the importance of protecting the social and ethical rights of residents.*
- *Identify rights of elderly residents including:*
  Religious liberties
  Communication
  Medical care
  Facility transfer
  Complain
  Receive visits from spouses, family members, and friends
  Respectful treatment
  Privacy
  Dignity, respect, and freedom
- *Identify professional resources available to address resident rights in assisted living facilities.*
- *Explain the role of the ombudsman in assisted living facilities.*
- *Identify issues related to the role of the ombudsman in assisted living facilities.*

INTRODUCTION

Administrators working in assisted living facilities must have a comprehensive understanding of the civil, legal, social, and ethical rights of all assisted living facility residents. Elders in assisted living facilities are vulnerable because of multiple physical and psychosocial problems, and thus must be ensured that protections needed are not only for basic safety, but also to enable residents to enjoy quality of life and well-being as they age. A brief description of major federal legislation and state regulations for assisted living facilities designed to protect legal rights of older adults will be presented. A discussion of the social and ethical rights of older adults, including those residing in assisted living facilities, will be addressed alongside a brief discussion of the issues related to resident rights. Finally, a discussion of professional resources, including the role of the Ombudsman in protecting resident rights, will conclude this chapter. Selected best practices in areas associated with resident rights will be presented throughout this chapter.

PROTECTION OF CIVIL RIGHTS

Federal legislation enacted during the latter part of the twentieth century has been designed to protect the civil rights of all Americans. In 1964, Congress passed the Civil Rights Act, legislation banning discrimination on the basis of sex and race in the hiring, promoting, and firing of individuals, and making it unlawful for any employers to refuse to fail, hire, or discharge any individuals, or to discriminate against any individuals on the basis of race, color, sex, religion, national origin, or sex (U.S. National Archives & Records Administration, 2009). The Civil Rights Act sets the precedence for banning discrimination in the admissions process of residents into assisted living facilities.

The Omnibus Budget Reconciliation Act (OBRA) of 1987 included the Nursing Home Reform Act. This legislation was designed to establish regulations for nursing home residents with an emphasis in part on the rights of residents and resident quality of life (Miller, 2009). The OBRA stated that residents in long-term care facilities should be at her or his highest level possible of physical, psychosocial, and mental functioning and most importantly, this should take place within an environment emphasizing the rights of residents (Miller, 2009).

The Nursing Home Residents Bill of Rights was also included in OBRA. The legislation stated in part, that long-term care facility residents have the right to self-determination, a dignified existence, and the right to access and communicate with others, and with services both inside and outside of their facility (Code of Federal Regulations, Title 42, Section 483.10). Resident rights that are included in this legislation require the following: (1) full information including the right to daily communication in the residents' own language, the rights for assistance as needed, and the rights to be informed of all available services and the costs associated with each service; (2) participation in the resident's care, including the rights to receive and participate in appropriate care and participate in care planning; (3) ability to make independent choices including the right to make personal choices and participate in activities; (4) dignity, respect, and freedom including the right of self-determination; (5) security of possessions including the right to manage all financial affairs; (6) transfers and discharges including the right to receive a 30 day notice of transfer or discharge; (7) privacy and confidentiality including the right to confidentiality regarding medical, personal, and financial affairs; (8) complaints including the right to bring grievances forward for review; and (9) visits including the right to immediate familial access, as well as organizations promoting a number of services including health, social, and legal services.

Additionally, this legislation ensures the rights of elders in nursing homes to vote, file lawsuits, practice religion, marry, enter into contracts, make a will, and dispose of property (Tabloski, 2006). While the Nursing Home Bill of Rights was designed to promote the rights of residents in long-term care facilities, these rights are also relevant and applicable to residents in assisted living facilities. A resident's bill of rights is required in all assisted living facilities and must be posted in locations where residents, visitors, and other individuals working or entering the facility are able to easily read the information.

The Patient Self-Determination Act of 1990 (PSDA) details the responsibilities of Health Care Providers. It was developed to ensure that health care providers in a variety of settings, including assisted living facilities, would protect the rights of all individuals. This was accomplished by providing residents at the time of admission the following services: (1) maintain written policies and procedures for all adults receiving medical services; (2) provide written information to residents regarding the individual's rights under state law to make decisions regarding medical care, including the right to accept or refuse medical or surgical treatments; (3) ensure compliance with state laws regarding advanced directives; and (4) provide staff and community education on issues concerning advanced directives (Burke & Walsh, 1997).

State regulations for assisted living facilities serve in part to protect the rights of all residents. While there are federal laws that impact assisted living facilities, state regulations provide oversight for the approximately 1 million Americans who reside in assisted living facilities (Polzer, 2009). Each of the 50 states and the District of Columbia has enacted regulations governing assisted living facility functions. There is variability in each set of state regulations. The Assisted Living State Regulatory

Review for 2009 summarizes information from each state's regulations in a number of categories. A number of these categories describe regulations that serve to protect the civil rights of assisted living residents. Disclosure items include specific information that must be provided to residents before they sign any residence or service contracts. This area of state regulation protects the rights of residents to obtain full information, and to have appropriate communication regarding available services and the costs of such services. Many states do not specify disclosure items, while some states including Idaho, have disclosure statements indicating that each facility must have written admission policies made available to residents and the public (Polzer, 2009).

State regulations specify the facility scope of care, which is a summary of the personal care and nursing services provided by the facility, be readily available. Third-party scope of care describes whether third-parties such as hospice care providers, are able to provide services in the assisted living facility (Polzer, 2009). Information provided in these regulations serves to protect the rights of residents and ensure they receive appropriate communication regarding their care, and the ability to participate in their care. Again, variations in how these regulations are interpreted are noted across states. For example, in Colorado, facility scope of care is defined as the provision of services to meet the needs of residents including room and board, a physically safe and sanitary environment, protective oversight, social care, and third-party scope of care allows facilities or residents to contract with home health agencies for additional services (Polzer, 2009).

Resident rights to information regarding facility transfers and discharges are addressed in assisted living facility state regulations for move-in and move-out requirements. These regulations specify the types of conditions mandating that residents move out of facilities, as well as conditions that would prevent individuals from moving into facilities (Polzer, 2009). Variation among state regulations is again noted, with some states providing minimal information regarding move-in and move-out requirements. The regulations in Delaware, on the other hand are comprehensive, listing a number of conditions that would prevent individuals from moving into facilities including. These regulations include: a need for extensive nursing services, the presence of stage 3 or 4 pressure ulcers, the use of medical equipment such as mechanical ventilators, and the presence of behaviors that pose a threat to the individual or to others (Polzer, 2009).

State regulations regarding resident assessment include provisions for assessment data collection to identify if an individual's needs can be met by providers, as well as to identify the services required by each individual (Polzer, 2009). This regulation serves to protect the rights of residents to participate in their own care, to receive appropriate care, and to participate in care planning activities. Once again, states broadly interpret this regulation with some providing minimal information while other states provide specific data. In New York for example, regulations require that each assisted living facility resident have an individualized service plan that is developed jointly by the resident, the resident's representative if indicated, the assisted living facility operator, and the resident's physician. The state of New York also requires that each plan assess the medical, functional, cognitive, nutritional, rehabilitative, and other needs for each resident, and that each plan must be reviewed every 6 months or when resident care needs change (Polzer, 2009). Again, the state regulations noted here serve in part to protect the civil rights of all assisted living residents.

PROTECTION OF SOCIAL AND ETHICAL RIGHTS

Administrators in assisted living facilities must have an awareness of the social and ethical rights of residents. While many resident rights are guaranteed through federal legislation and state regulations, social and ethical rights must be protected as well. An understanding of autonomy and individual rights, competency, and decision-making capacities, can provide administrators with information regarding residents' social and ethical rights.

Autonomy refers to the personal freedom to take control of one's life without interfering or infringing on the rights of other individuals (Miller, 2009). The autonomous person is able to solve problems through a thought process that is both rational and organized, and thus control many important life decisions. Residents in assisted living facilities have the right of self-determination and to make independent choices, in essence, to take control of their care as autonomous individuals. When residents experience confusion or dementia, they lose not only their autonomy, but also their ability to make reasoned choices regarding their care; many losing independence as well. For many older adults, the loss of independence that accompanies autonomy creates great difficulties, and may create problems in ensuring that their rights remain protected.

Competency is defined as the ability to fulfill one's roles, and handle all of one's affairs in ways that are both adequate and appropriate (Miller, 2009). Legally, all competent adults are ensured rights guaranteed by the U.S. Constitution, as well as by state laws and regulations, and have the legal right to make all decisions regarding health care and medical treatments.

Residents in assisted living facilities who are competent have the right to make independent choices, to manage all of their financial affairs, and to participate in and make decisions regarding their medical care, including the right to refuse medications or treatments. For those residents who have cognitive problems or dementia, competency becomes an important issue. Protection of competency is important for individuals with cognitive problems. If residents are evaluated and declared incompetent or unable to participate in their own decision making, then a legally appointed decision maker can be obtained for the individual. Legally appointed guardians or conservators make either some decision for residents who have limited abilities in appropriate decision making, or all decisions for those residents with significant cognitive problems (Miller, 2009). Court monitoring accompanies the appointment of legal guardians or conservators, and reflects the compounding of legal, social, and ethical considerations associated with the removal of an individual resident's rights.

Decision-making capacity refers to an individual's ability to consent or to refuse specific medical procedures or treatments, and is usually determined by health care professionals or by members of a health care professional team (Miller, 2009). Decision-making capacity is viewed as the ability to both understand and communicate issues related to a specific decision-making situation, and is not related to a resident's age or specific medical diagnoses (Miller, 2009). The concept of capacity is based on a resident's ability to: (1) appreciate the right to make choices; (2) understand the benefits and the risks of proposed medical interventions, as well as the results of no medical interventions; (3) communicate with others about decisions; (4) be stable over time; and (5) be consistent in their values and beliefs (Miller, 2009). Residents with cognitive impairments or mild dementia may be able to participate in decision-making regarding medical procedures if they are able to understand the issues related to proposed treatments. Resident's rights to participate in their own care, as well as participate in care planning, are linked to decision-making capacity. These rights remain important for residents in assisted living facilities.

ISSUES RELATED TO RESIDENT'S RIGHTS

There are a number of issues related to the rights of all residents in assisted living facilities. The Nursing Home Bill of Rights included in the OBRA of 1987 (Code of Federal Regulations, Title 42, Section 483.10) identifies rights guaranteed to all residents in long-term care facilities.

Individual states have also passed regulations to ensure the rights of residents in assisted living and long-term care facilities. While state regulations differ among all 50 states and the District of Columbia, basic concepts regarding individual rights remain similar throughout the country. Issues related to these and other rights include rights associated with religious liberties, communication, medical care, transfers, financial affairs, complaints, spousal and family visits, and respectful treatment. The right to privacy includes a discussion of legislation to protect privacy and communication of medical information. Avoiding the use of restraints on residents within assisted living facilities is of additional importance.

The rights of assisted living facility residents to have religious liberties are guaranteed by the United States Constitution. Next, residents are ensured under the Nursing Home Bill of Rights (Code of Federal Regulations, Title 42, Section 483.10) to make independent choices, and to participate in activities both in and outside of the facility. While residents are entitled to the right of religious liberties, assisted living facility regulations do not require the provision of religious services. While many administrators and facilities work to provide residents with access to religious services, there are no regulatory requirements other than the right for residents to participate in unspecified activities.

The right of communication is well identified in the Nursing Home Bill of Rights (Code of Federal Regulations, Title 42, Section 483.10) Residents in assisted living facilities are entitled to daily communication, as well as the right to privacy and unrestricted communication with any individual. Issues related to communication may include problems associated with language barriers. The federal legislation has been written to ensure that residents have the right to communicate daily in their own language. For administrators in assisted living facilities, this means staffing the facilities to provide all residents with information in their language. Ensuring the rights of residents for clear communication may in fact create challenges and possible cost problems for administrators. Residents are also ensured the right to be fully informed if they have any sensory problems. Administrators must ensure that those communicating with residents who have visual or auditory problems are able to use appropriate strategies such as the use of materials with pictures rather than text, or to ensure that residents have functional glasses and hearing aids to facilitate the communication process. While residents have the right to private and unrestricted communication, certain issues may create challenges in ensuring that resident rights are met. For example, for those residents with roommates, obtaining privacy for communication may be an issue. Some states and facilities impose restrictions on the times that phone calls may be placed, creating potential barriers to the right for unrestricted communication. Administrators must work with residents as needed to make sure that these important rights are maintained.

Best Practices in the Area of Resident Rights

Administrators, staff, and residents in a number of assisted living facilities have been recognized for practices that are designed to support resident rights. Selected best practices have been identified and will be briefly discussed. One example of a best practice includes work done by the Maristone Senior Living community in Nashville, TN. This organization provided a forum for educating seniors about their rights through a monthly senior newspaper column and weekly TV spot, entitled "On Modern Age." This communication provided information about power-of-attorney documents, medical information communication, and legislative updates. Winner of an Assisted Living Federation of America Best of the Best award (Redding, 2009), this project also served to inform and enlighten residents about many of their important rights as seniors.

The rights to medical care are also guaranteed in the Nursing Home Bill of Rights (Code of Federal Regulations, Title 42, Section 483.10). Residents in assisted living facilities are entitled to receive medical care that is both adequate and appropriate, and to participate in the planning and evaluation of care. While there is agreement on the concept of resident rights to medical care, state assisted living facility regulations differ among each of the 50 states and the District of Columbia. Variance exists, for example, in the regulations regarding resident assessment designed to identify services required by residents and medication management, identifying the extent to which medication assistance is possible. Administrators will need to identify regulations specific to their state, in order to ensure that all resident rights are upheld.

Residents in assisted living facilities are entitled to rights related to transfer from their facility. Residents are entitled to at least a 30 day notice if they will be required to relocate or to transfer to another facility. It is important to note that there are differences among state regulations for assisted living facilities. While the regulations include a section on the move-in and move-out requirements for assisted living facility conditions, each state has a different interpretation of the regulations. Administrators will need to consult their state regulations to ensure that the rights of residents to facility transfer are maintained.

Residents in assisted living facilities are entitled to rights related to financial affairs. As noted in the Nursing Home Bill of Rights (Code of Federal Regulations, Title 42, Section 483.10), residents have the right to secure possessions including the right to manage their own financial affairs, and to not have to pay for services that are covered by Medicare or Medicaid. Again, an issue facing assisted living administrators involves strategies to ensure that these resident rights are protected. State regulations governing assisted living facilities differ in each state. The regulations do not specifically address rights related to financial affairs, meaning that facilities must develop their own policies regarding financial rights for residents. This results in a wide variation in approaches to these important rights.

The right to file a complaint is also guaranteed for residents in long-term care facilities. This includes the ability to file grievances without reprisals, and to have nursing homes promptly address complaints. For residents of assisted living facilities, these rights are important but are not covered in all state regulations. While many facilities have developed individual policies regarding residents' ability to file complaints, there are no national standards currently available for review. Another example of a best practice to improve elder rights in assisted living facilities includes the work done at The Orchards at Bartley Assisted Living in Jackson, NJ. This organization received the Assisted Living Federation of America Best of the Best award for their monthly town meetings project (Redding, 2009). This best practice involved monthly town hall meetings with assisted living facility residents and the company CEO. Residents participating in this project identified a greater sense of ownership and satisfaction with their living arrangements, and improved resident rights when they could discuss and resolve issues with each other as well as the facility CEO.

Residents in assisted living facilities have the right to receive visits from spouses, family members, and friends. As noted in the Nursing Home Bill of Rights (Code of Federal Regulations, Title 42, Section 483.10), residents in nursing homes are entitled to immediate access to relatives and reasonable visits by organizations, in addition to individuals providing health, social, or legal services. Issues may arise for those residents who do not have private rooms, or who have family members wishing to visit at times that may not be convenient for other residents. Again, administrators need to work flexibly with residents and with spouses, family members, and friends to promote these important visits. Many facilities may have their own policies regarding visits. Without state or national standards, individual regulations have the potential to create confusion for both administrators and consumers.

The right for respectful treatment is a right afforded to residents in long-term care facilities along with the rights for dignity, respect, and freedom. Residents in assisted living facilities have the same need for this important right. While some authors (Polzer, 2009) indicate that the right for respectful treatment is implicit in the services that are provided in assisted living facilities, state regulations do not specifically identify respectful treatment for residents within their documents. Many administrators must abide by facility policies, and create a bill of rights for residents to ensure that residents are afforded care that is both dignified and respectful.

Residents in assisted living facilities have the right to privacy as do residents in long-term care facilities. Residents have the right to privacy concerning the receipt of treatment and in regard to personal care. Again, this right is identified in the Nursing Home Bill of Rights (Code of Federal Regulations, Title 42, Section 483.10) and should be implemented in all assisted living facilities. State assisted living regulations address privacy in terms of physical plant requirements, the square footage requirements for resident rooms, the maximum number of residents allowed per resident room, bathroom requirements which detail whether bathrooms may be shared, as well as specifying the number of bathing units required per resident (Polzer, 2009). Again, issues related to variability in state regulations must be addressed by assisted living facility administrators who may augment state assisted living facility regulations with their own policies regarding privacy.

Residents in assisted living facilities also have their privacy protected through implementation of the Health Insurance Portability and Accountability Act (HIPPA) of 1996 (Public Law 104–191). Designed to recognize that privacy and confidentiality are considered to be basic rights for all Americans, this is the first federal legislation designed to protect the privacy of patient health information through the development of requirements and standards for the electronic transmission of patient health records (Tabloski, 2006). There is specific health care information that is considered to be confidential. This information includes the following: (1) information that identifies residents, including resident name and medical record number, or record identification information; (2) health information that is related to the past, present, or future health status or problem of the resident; (3) all documentation related to the provision of health care services to residents; and (4) any payments for health care that may be in the past, present, or future (Tabloski, 2006). Additionally, residents in assisted living facilities have the right to review their medical records and to ask questions regarding any of the information contained within those documents. Residents in assisted living facilities have the right to dignity, respect, and freedom, including the right to be free from both mental and physical abuse (Code of Federal Regulations, Title 42, Section 483.10). While much attention has been paid to the rights of residents in long-term care facilities to avoid the use of physical and chemical restraints, administrators in assisted living facilities should have an awareness of these practices as well. Researchers have demonstrated that the use of physical and chemical restraints may be related to the increased risk for injury and for falls (Linton & Lach, 2007). Current practice encourages changes in a resident's environment to minimize the need for restraints, and for careful monitoring of residents who otherwise may be candidates for restraints. The autonomy of residents can best be protected by avoiding the use of physical and chemical restraints, and by administrators recognizing that the use of these devices impedes upon the rights of residents.

PROFESSIONAL RESOURCES TO ADDRESS RESIDENT RIGHTS

Administrators in assisted living facilities can ensure that the rights of residents are protected in part through an understanding of professionals who work to protect residents and resident rights. Chief among these professionals is the Ombudsman. Other professionals including nurses, geriatric specialists, and social workers also assume a role in protecting resident rights. The roles of these professionals will be briefly discussed.

The Ombudsman serves as an advocate for the rights of residents and also investigates resident complaints in a number of settings including long-term care facilities, assisted living facilities, board, and care homes. Established under the auspices of the Older American Act, the National Long-Term Care Ombudsman Program has served as a national forum for resident advocacy (Miller, 2009). Developed as a federally mandated response to substandard conditions in American nursing homes, the Ombudsman model is now established in all states with the use of many volunteer workers (Nelson, 1995). In 1992, the Older Americans Act (OAA) was amended (PL-102–375) and merged the Ombudsman, legal services, and elder abuse programs into Title VII, the Vulnerable Elder Rights Protection Activities, a federally legislated addition to the patient and consumer rights movement (Netting, Huber, Patton, & Kautz, 1995).

The role of the Ombudsman consists of a number of advocacy and problem solving functions including the following: (1) identify, investigate, and resolve resident complaints; (2) provide information to residents about long-term care services; (3) protect resident rights through advocacy at governmental agency levels; (4) analyze and recommend changes in laws and regulations that relate to the health, safety, welfare, and rights of residents; (5) educate both consumers and the general public about issues and concerns related to long-term care; (6) promote the development of citizen organizations; (7) provide technical support for the development of family and resident councils to protect the well-being and rights of residents; and (8) advocate for improvements in resident's quality of life and care (Agency on Aging, 2006).

Ombudsmen face issues in their current roles. While Ombudsman programs are mandated through the Older Americans Act, implementation of programs occurs at both the state and local level. Because state implementation of programs differ even within the state, data collection and reporting systems are not standardized, making reporting more arduous, and the quality of data varying from state to state. Additionally, some Ombudsmen have experienced problems is obtaining data from long-term care and assisted living facilities despite federal legislation guaranteed access to resident medical records (Netting, Huber, Patton, & Kautz, 1995). Challenges in the collection and dissemination of data required for role completion, means that Ombudsmen will be less effective in their advocacy efforts on behalf of residents. Volunteers are hired to fill many of the Ombudsman positions and their roles are defined at either the state or the local level. Training, certification, and continuing education for these individuals are all determined at the state level. Additionally, volunteers must be recruited, trained, supervised, and supported by professional staff working to maintain the quality of Ombudsmen programs (Netting, Huber, Patton, & Kautz, 1995). Despite these and other issues that Ombudsmen must deal with, the services that they perform for elders, especially elders in assisted living facilities are critical to ensuring the rights of these vulnerable individuals.

Many health care professionals serve in roles designed to advocate and protect the rights of residents in facilities including assisted living facilities. Some nurses specialize in gerontological nursing work to protect the rights of older adults. Additionally, nurses involved in the care of elders provide ethical nursing care by: (1) focusing on patients, and actively listening and using good communication skills; (2) respecting residents worth, individuality, and the value of individual choices; and (3) providing care services that are necessary and accountable (Miller, 2009). Geriatric specialists can advocate and protect the rights of assisted living facility residents through their comprehensive understanding of the needs and the rights of assisted living facility residents. Social workers provide services that support rights of residents through a number of resident advocacy roles, and frequently work with Ombudsmen to provide educational, advisory, and support roles.

Administrators in assisted living facilities can obtain additional information regarding the rights of residents from a number of web sites and on-line resources. The National Institute on Aging, the American Geriatrics Society, and the American Association for Retired People are examples of resources that may be of benefit to assisted living facility administrators.

CASE STUDY

The staff in an assisted living facility located in an affluent community expressed concerns to the administrator about SG, an 80-year-old resident. SG has been noted to have facial and upper arm bruising over the past several months. When questioned, SG stated that her vision is failing, she has been walking into her bathroom door and that is why she has some bruises that do not hurt or cause her any problems. The administrator decided to follow a best practice in the screening of elders for mistreatment through the implementation of the Elder Assessment Instrument, a 41 item assessment instrument designed to identify signs, symptoms, and complaints of elder abuse, neglect, abandonment, and exploitation (Fulmer, 2008). Elders are referred for assistance if data from administration of the instrument reveals evidence of mistreatment, elder complaints of abuse, or if a high risk of abuse exists.

When assisted living staff administered the Elder Assessment Instrument to SG, they found the presence of new and healing bruises on SG's face, arms, and chest. Evidence of financial exploitation and misuse of SG's money was also noted. Further questioning revealed that the bruises occurred following visits by SG's daughter who had been taking money from SG's checking account and was also trying to access SG's savings accounts. SG stated that her daughter was really a "good girl with a little drug problem" and she was ashamed to admit that her daughter was abusing her and spending money from her checking account. SG finally revealed that her daughter had recently been physically abusive in attempts to get additional money from SG's saving account.

The administrator was able to use the information collected from the Elder Assessment Instrument to contact SG's other family members and local authorities regarding SG's mistreatment and the misuse of SG's funds. The daughter was arrested for both elder abuse and drug abuse and SG's other family members worked on strategies to protect SG's financial assets. SG also spent time with members of the social services staff to address the problems related to the abuse. The staff has reported to the administrator that no new bruising has been noted following these interventions.

CONCLUSIONS

Protecting the rights of elders residing in assisted living facilities is critical, and is the responsibility, in part, of administrators. Comprehension of federal legislation, including the Civil Rights Act, the Nursing Home Reform Act, and the Patient Self-Determination Act, as well as state legislation as described earlier, will augment important care provided to residents. Understanding social and ethical rights, and the issues related to the protection of elder's rights as presented in this chapter, will also serve to enhance the services that are provided by administrators in assisted living facilities.

REFERENCES

Agency on Aging. (2006). Retrieved from http://www.aoa.gov/eldfam/Elder_Rights/LTC/LTC.asp

Burke, M. M., & Walsh, M. B. (1997). *Gerontologic nursing. Holistic care of the older adult.* St. Louis, MO: Mosby.

Fulmer, T. (2008). Screening for mistreatment of older adults. *American Journal of Nursing, 108*(12), 52–59.

Health Insurance Portability and Accountability Act of 1996, Pub.L. No 104–191, 1171, (1996).

Miller, C. A. (2009). *Wellness in older adults* (5th ed.). Philadelphia: Wolters Kluwer Lippincott Williams & Wilkins.

Nelson, H. W. (1995). Long-term care volunteer roles on trial: Ombudsman effectiveness revisited. *Journal of Gerontological Social Work, 23*(3–4), 25–46.

Netting, E. F., Huber, R., Paton, R. N., & Kautz III, J. R. (1995). Elder rights and the long-term care ombudsman program. *Social Work, 40*(3), 351–357.

Nursing Home Residents' Bill of Rights in the Omnibus Budget Reconciliation Act of 1987 42, CFR, 483.10 (1987).

Polzer, K. (2009). *Assisted living state regulatory review.* Washington, DC: National Center for Assisted Living.

Redding, W. (2009). Best of the best. *Assisted Living Executive,* 11–19.

Tabloski, P. A. (2006). *Gerontological nursing.* Upper Saddle River, NJ: Pearson Education, Inc.

U.S. National Archives & Records Administration. (2009). *Teaching with documents: The Civil Rights Act of 1964 and the Equal Employment Opportunity Commission.* Retrieved from http://www.archives.gov/education/lessons/civil-rights-act/index.html?template=print

Glossary of Financial Management Terms

- **Absorption**: the sharing out of the costs of a cost center amongst the products which use the cost center.
- **Accelerating Depreciation**: is a methodology of computing depreciation, such as the "sum of the year's digits" or "double declining balance", where the asset losses value more rapidly than would occur by the "straight line" depreciation method.
- **Account**: a record in a double entry system that is kept for each (or each class) of asset, liability, revenue and expense.
- **Accounting**: the field of study and work that comprises accurate bookkeeping, financial report preparation as well as the proper interpretation of the financial data and reports of the business.
- **Accounting Equation**: an expression of the equivalence, in total, Assets = Liabilities + ALF Stockholder's Equity. It is the basic foundation for the balance sheet and income statement that comprises "double entry accounting.
- **Accounting Period**: that time period, typically 1 year, to which financial statements are related. It can also be a month or quarter (3) months.
- **Accounting Policies**: the specific accounting bases selected and followed by a business enterprise (e.g., straight line or reducing balance depreciation).
- **Accounting Rate of Return**: a ratio sometimes used in investment appraisal but based on profits not cash flows.
- **Accounting Standards**: Prescribed methods of accounting by the accounting standards or financial reporting standards regulation body in your jurisdiction. It is also considered standard collection or rules, laws and conventions which determine how accounting transactions are recorded as well as how they are presented in the financial statements.
- **Accounts Payable**: the amount of monies owed to vendors for either physical goods or services purchased on credit.
- **Accounts Receivable Collection Report**: a table or spreadsheet that depicts the ALF outstanding accounts receivables by the length of time (days, months) that have not been paid and need to be collected.

417

■ **Accounts Receivable Turnover Ratio**: used in ratio analysis to determine the efficiency of how the ALF utilizes its assets. Here, the receivables turnover is an indication of how quickly the facility collects on its resident's rent owed. It can be expressed as "rent charges to resident's accounts during a given period divided by the amount of accounts receivables."

■ **Accruals**: (that which has accrued, accumulated, grown) expenses which have been consumed or enjoyed but which have not been paid for at the accounting date.

■ **Accruals Convention**: the convention that revenues and costs are matched with one another and dealt with in the Profit and Loss (P&L) Account of the period to which they relate irrespective of the period of receipt or payment.

■ **Accumulated Depreciation**: that part of the original cost of a fixed asset which has been regarded as a depreciation expense in successive Profit and Loss (P&L) Accounts: cost less accumulated depreciation = net book value. It is also considered the cumulative depreciation expense to date, or the total portion of the original cost of the ALF depreciable assets that have already been allocated to depreciation expense in the prior and current period.

■ **Acid Test**: The ratio of current assets (excluding stock) to current liabilities. It is also known as the "quick rate or quick current ratio" and measures the immediate solvency or debt-paying ability of a company.

■ **Acquisitions**: operations of a reporting entity that are acquired in a period. Separate disclosure of turnover, profits, etc., must be made.

■ **Adjusting Entry**: a journal entry to the general ledger that is necessary to adjust the book account balances to conform with the actual balances and accrual basis at the end of accounting periods.

■ **Aging Schedule**: table that separates and categorizes resident accounts according to the length of time (days, weeks, months) they are outstanding.

■ **Allocation**: the charging of discrete, identifiable costs to cost centers or cost units. A cost is allocated when it is unique to a particular cost center.

■ **Allowable Charge**: the maximum fee that a third-party payer (state Medicaid and a long-term care insurer) had negotiated with Facility to reimburse for resident care.

■ **Amortization of Debts**: the repayment of a debt (e.g., bank loan, mortgage) by the Facility over a period of time by making regular payments of the principal and interest. It is another word for depreciation: commonly used for depreciation of the capital cost of acquiring leasehold property.

■ **Apportionment**: the division of costs among two or more cost centers in proportion to estimated benefit on some sensible basis. Apportionment is for shared costs.

- **Assets**: resources of value owned by a business entity.
- **Assets Turnover Ratio**: a ratio which purports to measure the intensity of use of business assets. Calculated as sales over net operating assets. Can be expressed as sales as a percentage of net operating assets. Asset turnover ratios also provide information of how efficiently the assisted living facility utilizes its assets. They are sometimes referred to as "efficiency ratios, asset utilization ratios or asset management ratios." Two commonly used asset turnover ratios are the "accounts receivable turnover ratio" and the "inventory turnover."
- **Asset Value**: a term which expresses the money amount of assets less liabilities of a company attributable to one ordinary share.
- **Avoidable Costs**: the specific costs of an activity or sector of a business which would be avoided if that activity or sector did not exist.
- **Auditing**: the independent examination of, and expression of an opinion on, the financial statements of an enterprise by an appointed auditor or accountant in pursuance of that appointment and in compliance with any relevant statutory obligation.
- **Auditors**: outside independent accountants that are either an outside independent accounting firm (e.g., Ernst & Young, LLP) or certified professional accountants (CPAs) hired by the assisted living facility in order to cross-check the accuracy of the facility's bookkeepers to ensure that the ALF's financial statements are accurate.
- **Bad Debts**: debts known to be irrecoverable and therefore treated as losses by inclusion in the Profit and Loss (P&L) Account as an expense.
- **Balance Sheet**: a financial statement showing the financial position of a business entity in terms of assets, liabilities, and capital at a specified date.
- **Bank Statement**: financial statement produced by bank to checking and savings accounts depicting deposits, expenses, balances, interest earned, and any service fees.
- **Bankruptcy**: a legal status imposed by a court. Usually a trustee is appointed to receive and realize the assets of the bankrupt, and to distribute the proceeds to his creditors according to the law.
- **Benefits in Kind**: things or services supplied by a company to its directors and others in addition to cash remuneration. A good example is the provision of and free use of a motor car. The value of benefits in kind are taxable.
- **Bidding**: the facility requesting responses from vendors to their written specifications for goods (e.g., cleaning supplies) or services (e.g., outside auditor).
- **Bill of Lading**: a document issued by a carrier to a shipper upon acceptance of goods for shipment that represents a receipt for the goods and the contract stating the terms of carriage.

■ **Board-Designated Funds**: unrestricted funds set aside by the facility's governing board (e.g., corporation's board of directors) for specific purposes.

■ **Bond**: a formal written document that provides evidence of a loan. It is a written promise by issuing entity (e.g., U.S., state and local governments, corporation like assisted living company, etc.) under legal seal to repay a sum of monies (principal and interest) at some specific time in the future.

■ **Book Value**: the amount at which an asset is carried on the accounting records and balance sheet. The usual book value for fixed assets is cost less accumulated depreciation. Alternative words include written down value, net book value, and carrying value. Book value rarely if ever corresponds to saleable value.

■ **Break-even Chart**: a chart which illustrates costs, revenues, profit, and loss at various levels of activity within a relevant range.

■ **Break-even Point**: the level of activity (e.g., level of sales) at which the business makes neither a profit nor a loss (i.e., where total revenues exactly equal total costs).

■ **Budget**: a formal quantitative expression of management's plans or expectations. Master budgets are the forecast or planned Profit and Loss Account and balance sheet. Subsidiary budgets include those for sales, output, purchases, labor, cash, etc.

■ **Capital**: an imprecise term meaning the whole quantity of assets less liabilities owned by a person or a business. It is thus the funds used in the business.

■ **Capital Allowances**: deductions from profit for fixed asset purchases. In effect, capital allowances is a standard system of depreciation used instead of depreciation for tax purposes only.

■ **Capital Budgeting**: the process of planning or appraising possible fixed asset acquisitions.

■ **Capital Employed**: a term describing the total net assets employed in a business. Various definitions are used, so beware when talking at cross purposes.

■ **Capital Expenditure**: expenditure on fixed assets which is chargable to an asset account where the asset acquired has an estimated life in excess of 1 year and is not intended for sale in the normal running of the business operations.

■ **Capital Structure Ratios**: financial ratios showing the realtionship of long-term debt to total assets or to capital/equity.

■ **Cash**: strictly coins and notes but used also to mean all forms of ready money including bank balances.

- **Cash Disbursement Journal**: records the expenditures of cash.
- **Cash Discount**: a reduction in the amount payable by a debtor to induce prompt payment (equivalent to settlement discount).
- **Cash Flow**: a vague term (compare cash flow difficulties) used for the difference between total cash in and total cash out in a period.
- **Cash Flow Forecast**: a document detailing expected or planned cash receipts and outgoings for a future period.
- **Cash Flow Statement**: a formal financial statement showing a summary of cash inflows and outflows under certain required headings.
- **Chart of Accounts**: the complete listing of names of the accounts in the general ledger.
- **Coinsurance Clause:** an insurance policy clause which limits the liability of the insurance company to a determinable percentage of the medical loss suffered by the resident (insured).
- **Committed Costs**: those fixed costs which cannot be eliminated or even cut back without having a major effect on the enterprise's activities (e.g., rent).
- **Composition ratios**: indicate the relationships between various types of assets and current or total assets.
- **Conservatism**: (also known as **prudence**) the convention whereby revenue and profits are not anticipated, but provision is made for all known liabilities (expenses and losses) whether the amount of these is known with certainty or is a best estimate. Essentially- future profit, wait until it happens- future loss, count it.
- **Consideration**: the amount to be paid for anything sold including businesses. May be cash, shares or other securities.
- **Consistency**: convention that there is consistency of accounting treatment of like items within each year and from year to year.
- **Consolidation**: the aggregation of the financial statements of the separate companies of a group as if they were a single entity.
- **Contingent Liabilities**: possible future debts which may arise due to some future event that is considered possible but not probable.
- **Contra Account:** an auxiliary account which is an offset to a related account (i.e., allowance for uncollectable accounts offset resident accounts receivable).
- **Contractual Discount**: the uncollectable difference between the amount the facility charges for its services and the reduced/lower amount the facility has agreed to accept as reimbursement for either Medicaid/ long-term care insurer.
- **Contributed Capital**: amounts paid intp the assisted living facility by investors.

- **Contribution**: a term used in marginal costing – the difference between sale price and associated variable costs.
- **Contribution Clause**: an issurance policy clause that limits the liablity of the issuer to a pro rata portion of a loss of property insured by more than one company.
- **Control Account**: a general ledger account, the detail of which is contained in a subsidiary ledger (e.g., accounts receivable).
- **Controllable costs** (also known as **managed costs**): costs, chargeable to a budget or cost centre, which can be influenced by the actions of the persons in whom control is vested.
- **Controller**: the title usually given to the financial management executive responsible for the accounting function within the facility. This position usually reports the Chief Financial Officer (CFO) of the assisted living facility.
- **Conversion cost**: the cost of bringing a product or service into its present location or condition. May include a share of production overheads.
- **Convertible loan stock**: loans where, at the option of the lender, the loan can be converted into ordinary shares at specified times and specified rates of conversion.
- **Cost Basis**: the use of historical, objectively determined cost as the basis of accounting for most assets.
- **Cost Behavior**: the change in a cost when the level of output changes.
- **Cost Center**: a location, function, or item of equipment in respect of which costs may be ascertained and related to cost units.
- **Cost Control**: the attempt to maintain actual costs at, or below, budgeted levels.
- **Cost Convention**: the accounting convention whereby Balance Sheet assets are mostly valued at input cost or by reference to input cost.
- **Credit**: commonly used to refer to a benefit or gain also the practice of selling goods and expecting payment at a later date.
- **Credit Control**: those measures and procedures adopted by a firm to ensure that its credit customers pay their accounts.
- **Creditors**: those persons, firms, or organizations to whom the enterprise owes money.
- **Creditors Payment or Settlement Period**: a ratio (usually creditors/inputs on credit in a year x 365) which measures how long it takes the firm to pay its creditors.
- **Current Assets**: cash + those assets (stock, debtors, prepayments, bank accounts) that the management intend to convert into cash or consume in the normal course of business within 1 year or within the operating cycle.

- **Current Cost Accounting (CCA)**: a system of accounting which recognizes the fluctuating value of money by measuring current value by applying specific indices and other devices to historical costs. A valid method which is complex and difficult to understand intuitively.
- **Current Liabilities**: debts or obligations that will be paid within 1 year of the accounting date. Another term used to describe the same is Creditors: amount falling due within 1 year.
- **Current Ratio**: the ratio of current assets to current liabilities.
- **Cut-off**: the difficulties encountered by accountants in ensuring all items of income and expense are correctly ascribed to the right annual profit statement.
- **Day's Revenue in Receivable**: the average number of days of billings in accounts receivable and uncollected at a given point in time.
- **Debenture**: a document which creates or acknowledges a debt. Commonly used for the debt itself.
- **Debt**: a sum due by a debtor to his creditor. Commonly used also as a generic term for borrowings.
- **Debt to Equity Ratio**: is Long-Term Liabilities divided by Total Assets. It should be noted that Debt to Equity ratio of 0.5 or better is considered good.
- **Debit**: amount shown in the left side of a T-account, increasing assets and expense accounts and decreasing owner's equity and liability.
- **Debtors**: those who owe money.
- **Debtors Payment (Settlement) Period**: a calculation of the average time taken by credit customers to pay for their goods. Calculated by debtors/credit sales in a year x 365.
- **Depletion Method**: a method of depreciation applicable to wasting assets such as mines and quarries. The amount of depreciation in a year is a function of the quantity extracted in the year compared to the total resource.
- **Depreciation**: a measure of the wearing out, consumption or other loss of value whether arising from use, passage of time or obsolescence through technology and market changes. Depreciation should be allocated to accounting period so as charge a fair proportion to each accounting period during the expected useful life of the asset.
- **Direct Costs**: those costs comprising direct materials, direct labor, and direct expenses which can be traced directly to specific jobs, products, or services.
- **Discontinued Operations**: operations of the reporting entity that are sold or terminated in a period. Turnover and results must be separately disclosed.

- **Discount**: a monetary deduction or reduction. Settlement discount (also known as cash discount) is given for early settlement of debts. Debentures can be redeemed at a discount. Trade discount is a simple reduction in price given to favored customers for reasons such as status or bulk purchase.
- **Discounted Cash Flow**: an evaluation of the future cash flows generated by a capital investment project, by discounting them to their present value.
- **Discounting of Receivables**: a method of short-term financing where resident receivables are used to secure a loan (which is less than the aface amount of the receivables) from a financial institution. It is also known as "factoring."
- **Discretionary Costs:** expenses such as advertisement, sales promotions, donations, etc.
- **Dividend**: a distribution of earnings to its shareholders by a company.
- **Dividend Cover**: a measure of the extent to which the dividend paid by a company covered by its earnings (profits).
- **Dividend Policy Ratios**: provides insight into the dividend policy of the assisted living facility as well as its prospects for future growth. Two commonly used ratios are the "dividend yield ratio" and the "payout ratio."
- **Dividend Yield**: a measure of the revenue earning capacity of an ordinary share to its holder. It is calculated by dividend per share as a percentage of the quoted share price.
- **Double Entry Accounting**: a system of recording both the debit and credit aspect of each transaction.
- **Earnings**: another word for profits, particularly for company profits.
- **Earnings Per Share**: an investor ratio, calculated as after tax profits from ordinary activities / number of shares.
- **Equity Convention**: the convention that a business can be viewed as a unit that is a separate entity and apart from its owners and from other firms.
- **Equity**: the ordinary shares or risk capital of an enterprise.
- **Equity Financing**: raising funds by issing capital stock, or ownership shares in the assisted living facility.
- **Exceptional Items**: material items which derive from events or transactions that fall within the ordinary activities of the reporting entity and which need to be disclosed by virtue of their size or incidence if the financial statements are to give a true and fair view. Examples are profits or losses on termination of an operation, costs of a fundamental reorganization and profits and losses on disposal of fixed assets.

- **Expense**: a cost which will be in the Profit and Loss (P&L) Account of a year. It is the cost of operating a business, including capital, administrative and other operating expenditures.
- **Exposure Draft**: a document issue on a specific accounting topic for discussion.
- **Extraordinary Items**: material items possessing a high degree of abnormality which arise from events or transactions that fall outside the ordinary activities of the reporting entity and which are not expected to recur. They should be disclosed but are very rare indeed.
- **Factoring**: the sale of debtors to a factoring company to improve cash flow. Factoring is a method of obtaining finance tailored to the amount of business done but factoring companies also offer services such as credit worthiness checks, sales and debtor recording, and debt collection.
- **FICA**: Federal Insurance Contributions Act, commonly known as Social Security.
- **FIFO: first in first out** – a method of recording and valuation of fungible assets, especially stocks, which values items on the assumption that the oldest stock is used first. FIFO stocks are valued at most recent input prices.
- **Finance Lease**: a leasing contract which transfers substantially all the risks and rewards of ownership of an asset to the lessee. In effect the lessee is really buying the assets with the aid of a loan and the lease installments are really payments of interest and repayments of capital. They are accounted for as such in accordance with the accounting convention of substance over form.
- **Financial Leverage Ratio**: provides information of the long-term solvency of the assisted living facility. Dissimilar to liquidity ratios that focus with short-term assets and liabilities, financial leverage ratios measure the extent to which the Facility is utilizing it's long-term debt. Two primary financial leverage ratios are the "debt ratio" and the "times interest earned ratio."
- **Financial Ratio Analysis**: the analysis of quanitative indicators of the financial health of the organization. These ratios depict liquidity or the ability of the ALF to satisfy short-term obligations.
- **Financial Statements**: Balance Sheets, Profit and Loss Account, Income and Expenditure Accounts, Cash Flow Statements, and other documents that formally convey information of a financial nature to interested parties concerning an enterprise. In companies, the financial statements are subject to audit opinion.
- **Fixed Assets**: business assets which have a useful life extending over more than 1 year. Examples are land and buildings, plant and machinery, vehicles.

- **Fixed Cost**: a cost which in the short term, remains the same at different levels of activity. Examples are rent, real estate tax, depreciation.
- **Flexible Budget**: a budget which is flexed to recognize the difference in behavior of fixed and variable costs in relation to levels of output. Total budgeted costs changed to accord with changed levels of activity.
- **Floating Charge**: an arrangement whereby a lender to a company has a floating charge over the assets generally of the company gives the lender priority of repayment from the proceeds of sale of the assets in the event of insolvency. Banks frequently take a floating charge when lending.
- **Format**: a specific layout for a financial statement. Several alternatives are often prescribed by the prevailing governing authority or law of the country in which the enterprise operates or reports its financial performance.
- **Functional Classification**: the grouping of expenses according to the operating purposes (administrative, property, and related, etc.) for which costs are incurred. Revenues are also classified functionally.
- **Fund**: a self-containing accounting entity set up to account for a specific activity.
- **Fund Balance**: the excess of assets over liabilities (i.e., net equity). An excess of liabilities over assets is known as a deficit in fund balance.
- **Funded Debt**: also known as Long-Term Debt.
- **Funded Depreciation**: the setting aside of a portion of retained earnings in a special account to be used for the purpose of new or replacement capital assets.
- **Funds Flow Statement**: a financial statement which links Balance Sheets at the beginning and end of a period with the Profit and Loss (P&L) Account for that period. Now replaced by the cash flow statement.
- **Gearing**: also known as leverage, the relationship between debt and equity in the financing structure of a company.
- **General Ledger**: a book which summarizes all journal entries for an accounting period in order to arrive at a trial balance.
- **Goal Congruence**: the situation in which each individual, in satisfying his or her own interests, is also making the best possible contribution to the objectives of the enterprise.
- **Going Concern**: the accounting convention which assumes that the enterprise will continue in operational existence for the foreseeable future. This means in particular that the Profit and Loss (P&L) Account and Balance Sheet (BS) assume no intention or necessity to liquidate or curtail significantly the scale of operation.

- **Goodwill**: an intangible asset which appears on the Balance Sheet of some businesses. It is valued at (or below) the difference between the price paid for a whole business and the fair value of the net assets acquired.
- **Gross**: usually means before or without deductions. For example, Gross Salary or Gross Profit.
- **Gross Income**: Gross receipts of the assisted living facility before deductions or expenditures.
- **Gross Profit**: sales revenue less cost of sales but before deduction of overhead expenses. In a manufacturing company it is sales revenue less cost of sales but before deduction of nonmanufacturing overheads.
- **Gross Margin**: (or gross profit ratio), gross profit expressed as a percentage of sales.
- **Group**: a set of interrelated companies usually consisting of a holding company and its subsidiary and sub-subsidiary companies.
- **Group Accounts**: the financial statements of a group wherein the separate financial statements of the member companies of a group are combined into consolidated financial statements.
- **Historical Cost**: the accounting convention whereby goods, resources, and services are recorded at cost. Cost is defined as the exchange or transaction price. Under this Convention, realizable values are generally ignored. Inflation is also ignored. The almost universal adoption of this convention makes accounting harder to understand and lessens the credibility of financial statements.
- **Hurdle**: a criteria that a proposed capital investment must pass before it is accepted. It may be a certain interest rate, a positive NPV, or a maximum payback period.
- **Income and Expenditure Account**: the equivalent to Profit and Loss (P&L) Accounts in nonprofit organizations such as clubs, societies, and charities.
- **Indirect Costs**: costs which cannot be traced to particular products. An example is rent or management salaries. They are usually shared by more than one product and are called overheads.
- **Insolvency**: the state of being unable to pay debts as they fall due. Also used to describe the activities of practitioners in the fields of bankruptcy, receivership, and liquidations.
- **Intangible Assets**: assets which have long-term value but no physical identity. Examples are goodwill, patents, trademarks, and brands.
- **Interim Dividend**: a dividend paid during a financial year, generally after the issue of un-audited profit figures half way through the year.

■ **Interim Financial Statements**: financial statements prepared at a date other than the end of the fiscal year (e.g., monthly/quarterly balance sheets and income statements).

■ **Internal Rate of Return**: the rate of discount which will just discount the future cash flows of a proposed capital investment back to the initial outlay.

■ **Inventory**: a detailed list of things. Used by accountants as another word for stock.

■ **Inventory Turnover**: the Cost of Supplies Used divided by the Average Inventory for the Period.

■ **Invested Capital:** equity capital which is supplied by the owner(s) or shareholders of the assisted living facility.

■ **Investment Appraisal**: the use of accounting and mathematical methods to determine the likely returns for a proposed investment or capital project.

■ **Invoice**: a document portraying the details of a sale.

■ **Journal:** the book of original entry.

■ **Labor Hour Rate**: a method of absorption where the costs of a cost centre are shared out amongst products on the basis of the number of hours of direct labor used on each product.

■ **Lease:** a contract in which the lessee (user) pays the lessor (owner) for the use of an asset.

■ **Ledger:** the collection of all accounts used in the assisted living facility.

■ **Leverage**: another word for gearing.

■ **Lien:** a claim on particular property for payment of a debt or obligation.

■ **LIFO: Last in first out** – a valuation method for fungible items where the newest items are assumed to be used first. Means stocks will be valued at old prices.

■ **Line of Credit**: an arrangement whereby a financial institution commits itself to lend the assisted living facility a specified maximum amount for a specified period of time.

■ **Liquidation**: the procedure whereby a company is wound up, its assets realized and the proceeds divided up amongst the creditors and shareholders.

■ **Liquidity**: the ease with which funds can be raised by the sale of assets.

■ **Liquidity Ratios**: ratios which purport to indicate the liquidity of a business. These ratios provide information about the assisted living facility's ability to meet its short-term financial obligations. They are of particular interest to those financial institutions extending short-term credit (i.e., bank loans) to the Facility. Two frequently-used liquidity ratios are the "current ratio (or working capital) ratio" and the "quick ratio."

- **Long-Term Investments**: investments, generally in securities, which the assisted living facility intends to own for longer than 1 year or more from the Balance Sheet.
- **Long-Term Liabilities:** debts and obligations of the assisted living facility not due for more than 1 year or more.
- **Management Accounting**: the provision and interpretation of information which assists management in planning, controlling, decision making, and appraising performance.
- **Management by Exception**: control and management of costs and revenues by concentrating on those instances where significant variances by actual from budgets have occurred.
- **Marginal Costing**: a system of cost analysis which distinguishes fixed costs from variable costs.
- **Marginal Cost**: the additional cost incurred by the production of one extra unit.
- **Marginal Return**: the point at which income equals expenses. It is also referred to as the "break-even point."
- **Margin of Safety**: the excess of budgeted activity over break-even activity. Usually expressed as a percentage of budgeted activity.
- **Matching Convention**: the idea that revenues and costs are accrued, matched with one another as far as possible so far as their relationship can be established or justifiably assumed, and dealt with in the Profit and Loss (P&L) Account of the period in which they relate. An example is the matching of sales of a product with the development costs of that product. The appropriate periods would be when the sales occur.
- **Master Budgets**: the overall budgets of an enterprise comprising cash budget, forecast Profit and Loss (P&L) Account and forecast Balance Sheet (BS). They are made up from subsidiary budgets.
- **Material Management**: the integration of the processes of planning, acquiring, moving, and controlling materials.
- **Materiality**: the accounting convention that recognizes that accounting is a summarizing process. Some items and transactions are large (i.e., material) enough to merit separate disclosure rather than inclusion with others in a lump sum. Examples are an exceptionally large bad debt or an exceptionally large loss on sale of a fixed asset.
- **Minority Interest**: the interests in the assets of a Group relating to shares in group companies not held by the holding company or other members of the group.
- **Modified Accounts**: financial statements which are shortened versions of full accounts. Small and medium sized companies can file these with the Registrar of Companies instead of full accounts.

■ **Money Measurement**: the convention that requires that all assets, liabilities, revenues and expenses shall be expressed in money terms.

■ **Mortgage**: a pledge of designated property as security for a loan (e.g., motgage bonds).

■ **Natural Expenditures Classification**: a method of classifing expenditures according to their natural classification such as salaries, utilities and supplies.

■ **Net**: usually means after deductions.

■ **Net Book Value**: the valuation on the Balance Sheet of an asset. Also known as the carrying value or written down value.

■ **Net Income**: the excess of revenue over related expenses during an accounting period.

■ **Net Present Value**: the value obtained by discounting all cash inflows and outflows attributable to a proposed capital investment project by a selected discount rate.

■ **Net Realizable Value**: the actual or estimated selling price of an asset less all further costs to completion (e.g., Cost of a repair if it needs to be repaired before sale) and all costs to be incurred before and on sale (e.g., commission).

■ **New Worth**: can be calculated by Total Assets minus Total Liabilities.

■ **Nominal Value**: the face value of a share or debenture as stated in the official documents. Will not usually be the same as the issue price which may be at a premium and which will almost never correspond to actual value.

■ **Objectivity**: the convention of using reliable and verifiable facts (e.g., the input cost of an asset) rather than estimates of 'value' even if the latter is more realistic.

■ **Occupancy Rate**: a key utilization measurement of success for assisted living facilities that is the ratio of Actual Number of Resident Days to the Total Possible Resident Days.

■ **Operating Budget**: includes anticipated incomes by source and anticipated expenses by category.

■ **Operating Cycle**: the period of time it takes a firm to buy inputs, make or market a product and sell to and collect the cash from a customer.

■ **Operating Ratio**: Total operating expenses divided by total operating revenues.

■ **Opportunity Cost**: the value of a benefit sacrificed in favor of an alternative course of action.

■ **Outsourcing**: the use of services (such as administration or computing) from separate outside firms instead of using the enterprise's own employees.

- **Overheads**: Indirect cost.
- **Payback**: the number of years which will elapse before the total incoming cash receipts of a proposed project are forecast to exceed the initial outlays.
- **Periodicity**: the convention that financial statements are produced at regular intervals usually at least annually.
- **Petty Cash Fund:** a small fund of cash maintained by the assisted living facility for the purpose of making minor disbursements (e.g., less than $25 or $50) for which the issuance of a bank check would not be practical.
- **Physical Inventory**: the actual inventory as determined by physical count by auditors, usually at the end of a reporting period (usually annually).
- **Planning Variance**: a variance arising because the budgeted cost is now seen as out of date. Examples are wage or price rises.
- **Pledging of Receivables**: the use of resident account receivables as security or collateral for a bank loan.
- **Position Control Plan**: a management tool for controlling the number of employees on the assisted living facility payroll and for assuring the utilization of each employee to the point of maximum effectiveness. It is also known as a "staffing plan."
- **Posting:** transfer from general journal to the ledger.
- **Prepayments**: expenditure already made on goods or services but where the benefit will be felt after the Balance Sheet (BS) date. Examples are rent or rates or insurances paid in advance.
- **Price Earnings Ratio**: an investor ratio calculated as – share/earnings per share.
- **Private Company**: any company that is not a public company.
- **Profitability Index**: in investment appraisal, the net present value of cash inflows/the initial out lays.
- **Profitability Ratios**: provides information on several different measures of success of the assisted living facility at generating profits. Two key profitability ratios are the "return on assets ratio" and the "return on equity ratio."
- **Profit and Loss (P&L) Account**: a financial statement which measures and reports the profit earned over a period of time.
- **Provision**: a charge in the Profit and Loss (P&L) Account of a business for an expense which arose in the past but which will only give rise to a payment in the future. To be a provision the amount payable must be uncertain as to amount or as to payability or both. An example is possible damages awardable by a court in a future action over a past incident (e.g., a libel).

- **Prudence** (or **conservatism**): the convention whereby revenue and profits are not anticipated, but provision is made for all known liabilities (expenses and losses) whether the amount of these is known with certainty or is a best estimate. Essentially future profit, wait until it happens – future loss, count it now.
- **Purchase Order:** document issued by the assisted living facility authorizing a vendor to deliver goods with payment to be made later.
- **Qualified Audit Report:** an audit report including one or more qualifications or exceptions.
- **Quantity Discount:** a reduction in unit purchase cost received by those who acquire supplies in a quantity in excess of a specific amount.
- **Quick Ratio:** also known as acid test ratio, current assets (except stock)/current liabilities.
- **Realizable Value:** the amount that an asset can be sold for.
- **Realization:** to sell an asset and hence turn it into cash.
- **Realization Convention:** the concept that a profit is accounted (or when a good is sold and not when the cash is received).
- **Receiver:** an insolvency practitioner who is appointed by a debenture holder with a fixed or floating charge when a company defaults.
- **Reconciliation:** the procedure of checking bank accounts, deposits and withdrawals against the bank statement.
- **Redemption:** repayment of shares, debentures or loans.
- **Redemption Yield:** the yield given by an investment expressed as a percentage and taking into account both income and capital gain or loss.
- **Reducing Balance:** a method of depreciation whereby the asset is expensed to the Profit and Loss (P&L) Account over its useful life by applying a fixed percentage to the written down value.
- **Relevant Costs:** costs that will only be incurred if a proposed course of action is actually taken. The only ones relevant to an actual decision.
- **Relevant Range:** the range of activity which is likely. Within it variable costs are expected to be linearly variable with output and fixed costs are expected to be unchanged.
- **Reporting:** the process whereby a company or other institution seeks to inform shareholders and other interested parties of the results and position of the entity by means of financial statements.
- **Reserves:** a technical term indicating that a company has total assets which exceed in amount the sum of liabilities and share capital. This excess arises from retained profits or from revaluations of assets.
- **Resource Accounting and Budgeting:** the use of normal accruals accounting and Balance Sheets in federal/government departments and agencies.

- **Responsibility Accounting**: a system of accounting which accumulates financial and statistical information according to the organizational units generating the revenues and responsible for incurring the expenses. The primary purpose is to obtain optimal financial management control.
- **Retained Profits**: also known as retentions, the excess of profits over dividends.
- **Return on Capital Employed**: a profitability ratio being income expressed as a percentage of the capital which produced the income.
- **Return on Sales**: the ratio of profit to sales expressed as a percentage.
- **Returns**: the income flowing from the ownership of assets. May include capital gains.
- **Revenue**: amounts charged to customers for goods or services rendered.
- **Revenue Expenditure**: expenditure that benefits only the current period and which will therefore be charged in the Profit and Loss (P&L) Account.
- **ROP**: known as the Reorder Point. In inventory management, the point in time at which a new order should be placed for supplies and/ or services.
- **Safe Harbor Regulations**: federal regulations describing investment interest and other business transactions which are not violations of the Medicare and Medicaid anti-fraud and abuse laws.
- **Salvage Value**: also known as residual value, the amount estimated to be recoverable from the sale of a fixed asset at the end of its useful life.
- **Secured Liabilities**: liabilities secured by a fixed or floating charge or by other operation of law such as hire purchase commitments.
- **Securities**: financial assets such as shares, debentures, and loan stocks.
- **Sinking Fund**: funds required by external sources to be set aside to meet debt service charges and the retirement of indebtedness on plant assets.
- **State of Changes in Financial Position**: a financial statement summarizing the movement of funds (working capital) within the assisted living facility for a given period of time.
- **Stockholder's Equity**: the excess of assets over liabilities that consists mainly of invested capital and retained earnings.
- **Subchapter S Corporation**: a corporation that is taxed by the Internal Revenue Service as a private individual.
- **Subsidiary Ledger**: a group of accounts which is contained in a separate ledger that supports a single account (a control account) in the general ledger.

- **Tangible Asset**: an asset that has physical characteristics as equipment, land, and buildings.
- **Third-Party Payer**: someone else paying for the ALF bill other than the resident. It could either be a commercial insurance company that offers long-term care insurance or state Medicaid. Medicare general does not pay for assisted living facility's expenses.
- **Trial Balance**: a financial statement indicating name and balance of all ledger accounts arranged according to whether they are debts or credits. Debits must equal credits.
- **Turnover ratios**: financial indicators that measure the efficient management of assets by indicating the number of times assets (inventories, accounts receivables, etc.) are replaced during a period.
- **Useful Life**: an estimate of the number of years an item of plant and equipment will be used by the assisted living facility.
- **Variable Cost**: an operating cost which varies in direct proportion to change in volume. Examples are salary costs, supplies, etc.
- **Variance Analysis**: managerial control technique which identifies deviations from the original budget projections.
- **Voucher System**: a system for the processing and control of cash disbursements.
- **Weighted-Average Costing**: a method that determines the cost of supplies used and the valuation of inventory.
- **Working Capital**: available excess assets left over from subtracting current assets from current liabilities that the assisted living facility can use in operations.
- **Write Off**: the removal of a bad debt from revenues that reduces its value to zero. An example is resident room & board charges that written off because of nonpayment after failure of collection efforts by the facility.
- **Yield**: the actual rate of return on an investment as opposed to the nominal rate of return.

Index

Xend. of the 15